Sonny

MILADY STANDARD COSMETOLOGY

Study Guide:

The Essential Companion

MILADY STANDARD COSMETOLOGY

Study Guide:

The Essential Companion

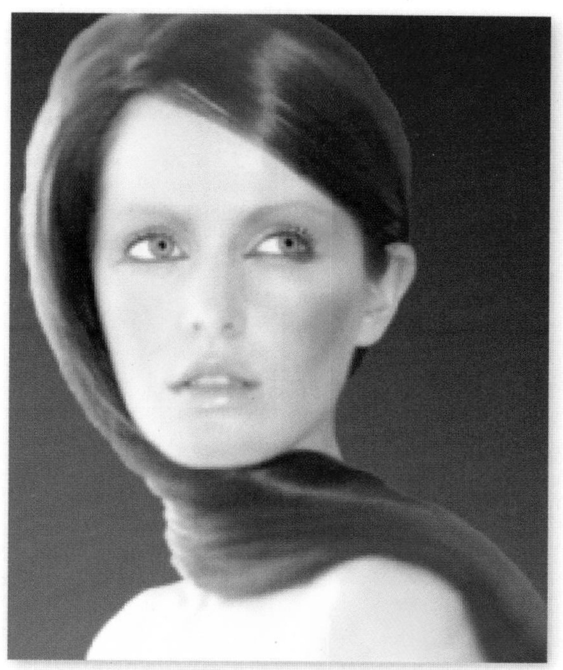

Author for 2012 Edition
Letha Barnes

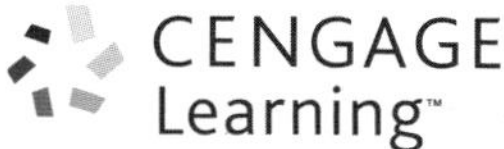

Australia • Brazil • Japan • Korea • Mexico • Singapore • Spain • United Kingdom • United States

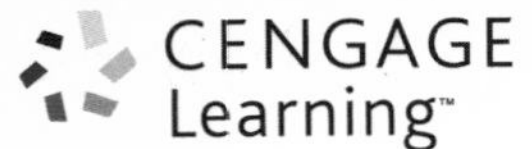

Milady Standard Cosmetology Study Guide: The Essential Companion
Letha Barnes

President, Milady: Dawn Gerrain

Acquisitions Editor: Martine Edwards

Associate Acquisitions Editor: Philip Mandl

Editorial Assistant: Maria K. Hebert

Director of Beauty Industry Relations: Sandra Bruce

Executive Marketing Manager: Gerard McAvey

Production Director: Wendy Troeger

Senior Content Project Manager: Angela Sheehan

Art Director: Benj Gleeksman

Composition and Text Design: Silver Editions

Cover Photo: ©Adrianna Williams/Corbis

Library of Congress Control Number: 2010903896

ISBN-13: 978-1-4390-5924-1

ISBN-10: 1-4390-5924-1

Milady
5 Maxwell Drive
Clifton Park, NY 12065-2919
USA

Cengage Learning products are represented in Canada by Nelson Education, Ltd.

For your lifelong learning solutions, visit **milady.cengage.com**

Visit our corporate website at **cengage.com**

Printed in the United States of America
1 2 3 4 5 15 14 13 12 11

Table of Contents

Preface

Introduction

Congratulations! As a student of cosmetology you now hold in your hands one of the most essential tools available to successfully progress through your course of study. You have chosen to embark upon a career in cosmetology, and that can be a life-transforming event. In this journey, you deserve the best possible education, and that can be accomplished by using the best possible educational tools available. The *Milady Standard Cosmetology Study Guide: The Essential Companion* is just such a tool.

Purpose

The purpose of *The Essential Companion* is to act as a study guide for you to achieve the objectives of each lesson presented by your instructors. Each chapter of the *Essential Companion* is designed to be a critical companion to the chapter you are assigned in the *Milady Standard Cosmetology* textbook. The study guide is designed to emphasize active, conceptual learning and to consolidate your understanding of the textbook. Information presented is provided in an informal tone allowing the study guide to take on the role of a private tutor or companion to aid you in mastering the textbook content.

Design

Each chapter of *The Essential Companion* is divided into sections as follows:

Essential Objectives

The objectives set forth for the textbook chapter are restated to help students focus on the goals for the lesson.

Essential Subject

This section provides a brief overview about why the subject matter contained in the chapter is essential in the life of a successful cosmetologist.

Essential Concepts

This section provides a conversational outline or brief overview of the chapter content.

Essential Experiences

This section contains activities, projects, and puzzles which are designed to reinforce the content contained in the textbook chapter and increase learner retention of the material studied. Each **Essential Experience** is designed to help students retain important information on a given subject through fun and interesting activities. The activities include personal research projects, mind mapping, windowpaning, matching exercises, crossword puzzles, word search puzzles, word scramble puzzles, role playing, and so much more.

To help you understand some of the active learning exercises you will use throughout the study guide, a brief explanation is provided here.

Mind mapping is used for developing an innovative and more creative approach to thinking. It simply creates a free-flowing outline of material or information. It is easy to learn, and when the technique is mastered, students will be able to organize an entire project or chapter in a matter of minutes. Mind mapping will allow students to release their creativity and engage both hemispheres of their brain. This technique has proved more effective than the linear form of note taking for most students. When mind mapping, the central or main idea is more clearly defined. The map lays out the relative importance of each idea or element of the subject matter. For example, the more important ideas or material will be nearer the center, and the less important material will be located in the outer parameters. Proximity and connections are used to establish the links between key concepts or ideas. The result is that review and recall will occur more quickly and be more effective. As you develop the art of mind mapping, you will see that each one takes on a unique appearance, which even adds to your recall ability of different topics or subjects. An example of how all the qualities, skills, and characteristics of an educator could be placed in a mind map is provided below.

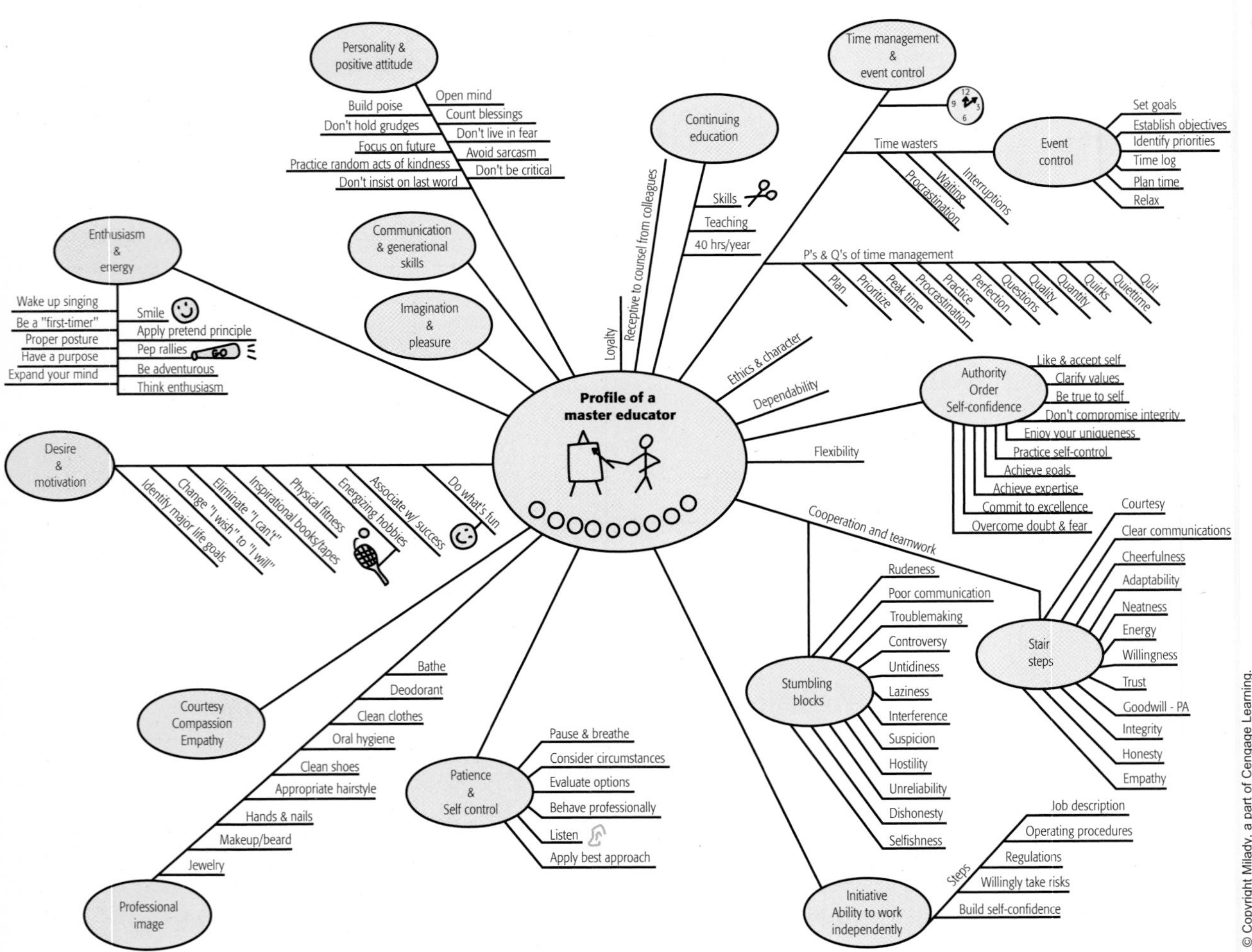

Windowpaning is the process of transferring key elements, points, or steps in a lesson into visual images that are then hand sketched into the squares or *panes* of a matrix. Your mind thinks in pictures or images. Research indicates that people can retain in their short-term memory an average of seven bits of information with a variation of two on the plus or minus side. Therefore, it is recommended that students complete windowpanes with no more than nine panes for a given topic. Refer to the example below of a windowpane on how to perform cardiopulmonary resuscitation (CPR).

Ask, call 911
1
Tilt head, lift chin, open airway
2
Look, listen, feel
3
Two full breaths
4
If airway blocked, use Heimlich maneuver
5
Check carotid pulse
6
Administer rescue breathing
7
No pulse, chest compressions, 15 to 2 breaths
8
Continue until help arrives
AMBULANCE
9

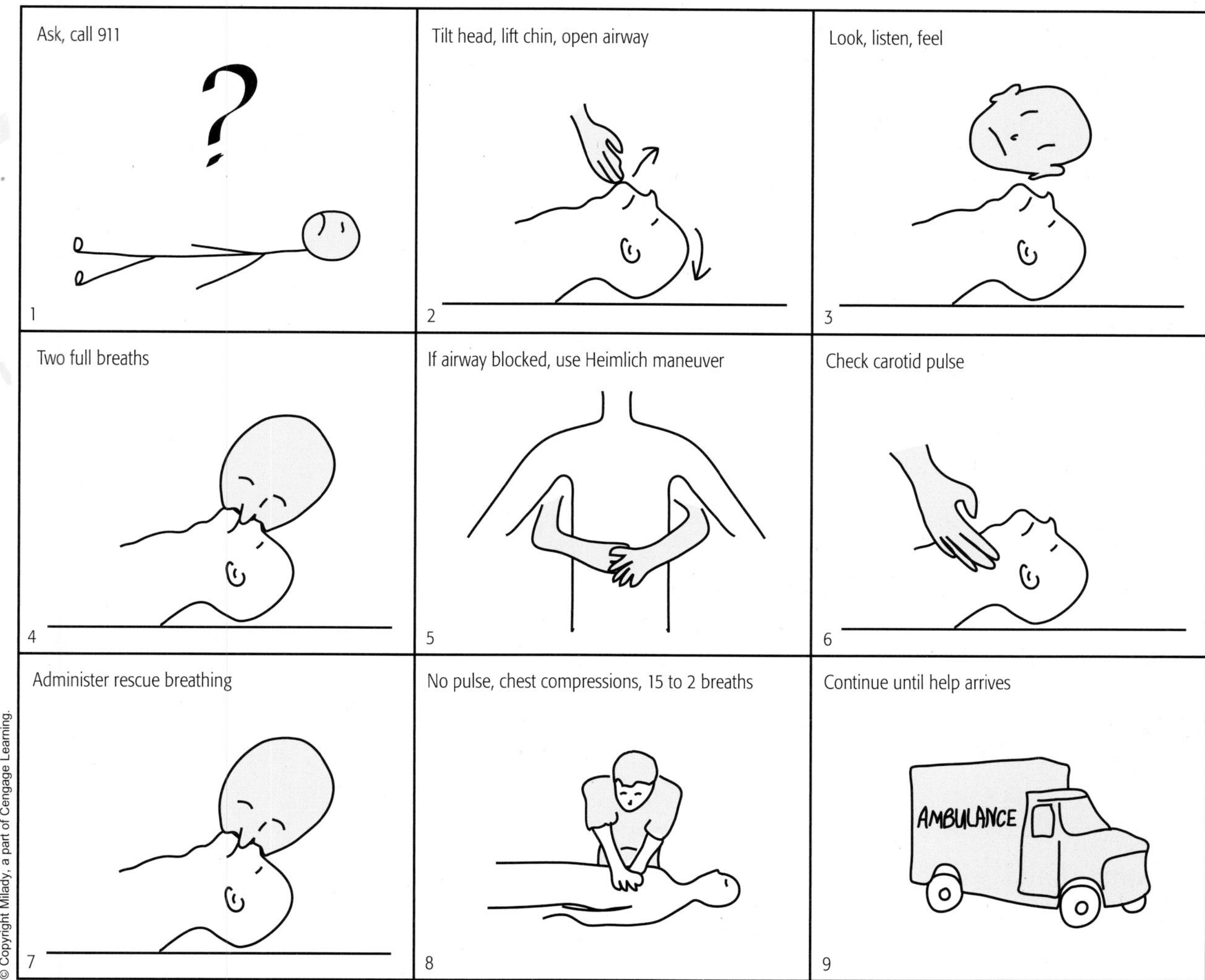

Essential Rubrics

Rubrics are used in education for organizing and interpreting data gathered from observations of student performance. It is a clearly developed scoring document used to differentiate between levels of development in a specific skill performance or behavior. A rubric is provided in the practical skills chapters of this study guide as a self-assessment tool to aid you in your behavior development.

You will be asked to rate your performance according to the following scale:

(1) Development Opportunity: There is little or no evidence of competency; assistance is needed; performance includes multiple errors.

(2) Fundamental: There is beginning evidence of competency; task is completed alone; performance includes few errors.

(3) Competent: There is detailed and consistent evidence of competency; task is completed alone; performance includes rare errors.

(4) Strength: There is detailed evidence of highly creative, inventive, mature presence of competency.

Space is provided for comments to assist you in improving your performance and achieving a higher rating.

Essential Review

This section contains a quiz, which may include multiple choice or completion questions, designed to help you measure your understanding of the key concepts presented in the textbook chapter.

Essential Discoveries and Accomplishments

This section is the learner's personal journal regarding the material studied. We suggest that students jot notes about the concepts in the chapter that were the hardest to understand or remember. Students are asked to consider themselves in the role of the "teacher" and think about what they would tell their "students" to help them ***discover*** and understand these difficult concepts. We suggest that students share their Essential Discoveries with other students in their class and to determine if what they have discovered is also beneficial to them. As a result of feedback from other students, you may want to revise your journal and include some of the good ideas received from your peers. Under accomplishments, students are asked to list at least three things they have accomplished since their last entry that relate to their career goals.

Students may find it helpful to read the **Essential Subject** and **Essential Concepts** sections found in the study guide before reading the actual chapter in the textbook. Upon completion of the chapter, you will then want to complete the Essential Experiences, Review, and Discoveries and Accomplishments.

By choosing an institution that uses educational materials published by Milady, a part of Cengage Learning, the industry leader in cosmetology education and technology, you have taken a significant step toward providing yourself with a rewarding and successful career. You have chosen proven performance and longevity by choosing Milady. You have chosen wisely and well. May success and good fortune accompany you in every step you take with *Milady Standard Cosmetology* and *The Essential Companion*. We believe that with the right tools, your commitment to the best education possible, and your passion for an exciting industry, you will experience all the joys and rewards possible in a great career!

Combined Chapters

Please note that this edition of the Study Guide contains information and activities related to every chapter of *Milady Standard Cosmetology*, 2012 edition. For the sake of efficiency and clarity, Chapter 25, Manicuring, and Chapter 26, Pedicuring, have been combined into one chapter in this Study Guide. In addition, the advanced nail chapters (Chapter 27, Nail Tips and Wraps; Chapter 28, Monomer Liquid and Polymer Powder Nail Enhancements; Chapter 29, UV Gels) have also been combined into one chapter as well.

Best wishes for success!

Letha Barnes, Master Educator and Consultant

ACKNOWLEDGMENTS

My thanks to the many educators and students I have had the privilege of teaching and learning from over my long career. Each time I enter a classroom to facilitate, I end up taking away much more than I bring to the room. Thanks to all of those who have shared their wisdom, experiences, and humor with me. Much of what they have offered is reflected in this Study Guide to help you become the best you can be.

CHAPTER 1

History & Career Opportunities

A Motivating Moment: "The person who gets the farthest is generally the one who is willing to do and dare. The sure-thing boat never gets far from shore."
— Dale Carnegie

Essential Objectives

After studying this chapter and completing the Essential Companion components, you will be able to:

1. **Explain the origins of appearance enhancement.**
2. **Name the advancements made in cosmetology during the nineteenth, twentieth, and early twenty-first centuries.**
3. **List several career opportunities available to a licensed beauty practitioner.**

Essential History and Career Opportunities

Why is knowing about the history and evolution of this industry so important to my success in cosmetology or a related field?

Cosmetologists should study and have a thorough understanding of the history of cosmetology and the career opportunities available because:

- Many old and even ancient techniques have evolved into techniques used today. Understanding their origin and why they were developed can be useful in understanding and using them today.
- Knowing where your profession has been will help you to predict and forecast where it is going.
- You'll appreciate just how much things have changed very recently.
- By understanding different career paths now, you'll see why many areas of study deserve your full attention.

As a professional in this industry, your overall knowledge about the field in general will enhance your credibility with your clients and help you serve them better. A study of the trends throughout history will also establish that many of these trends repeat themselves, either decades or even centuries later. Thus, the more you know about the history of cosmetology, the more prepared you will be for the changing trends throughout your career.

Society as a whole now has access to professional hair, skin, and nail care services. Therefore, it is important for today's professional to know about all the various career paths available to you in order to make the best personal choice.

Essential Concepts

What are the essential concepts about the industry's history and the career opportunities available?

Nearly every society has found it necessary to confine, cut, or manage the hair in order to keep it out of the way. The human species has essentially always had a basic desire to look good. As we look at history, that desire for personal adornment has varied in form from the ornately curled, blond wigs of Roman matrons to the sleek, waved heads of the flappers in the 1920s.

In preindustrial societies, hairstyling was used to indicate a person's social status. For example, primitive men would fasten bones, feathers, and other items into their hair for the purpose of impressing the lowly and frightening the enemy with their rank and prowess. Caesar made the noblemen of ancient Gaul cut off their hair as a sign of submission after he conquered them. In addition, occupational associations have been indicated by hair throughout history as manifested by the gray wigs worn by the barristers of England and the lacquered, black wigs worn by Japanese geisha.

Hair arrangement has also been used to indicate age or marital status. Adolescence was shown by shaved heads for young Hindu men, while boys in ancient Greece simply cut their hair. Until the twentieth century, generally only the upper classes enjoyed fashionable hairstyles. However, in the first half of the twentieth century, nearly all classes of women followed the trend set by film stars like Jean Harlow or Marilyn Monroe.

Because of the general increase in wealth, the improvement of mass communication, greater individualism, and overall attitude of informality, men and women of all classes can choose the style and color of hair that suits their interests, their needs, and their best image. This change in perspective has greatly increased the demand for the services of licensed professionals in the cosmetology industry.

1 Essential Experience

Historical Timeline

Using the material contained in the textbook and any other resources available to you, create a visual timeline of the history of hairdressing from the beginning of its recorded history to the present. The top of the timeline will indicate the year, decade, or century. The bottom of the timeline will contain drawings or pictures (cut and pasted) of hairstyles or tools and implements that represent that era.

Use large poster board, colored markers, and any other items you can think of to re-create the history of hairdressing in a colorful and interesting manner. Additional historical data is provided here. Use Figure 1–9 in the *Milady® Standard Cosmetology* textbook as a guide.

Essential Experience 2

Mind Mapping Career Opportunities

Mind mapping simply creates a free-flowing outline of material or information with the central or key point being located in the center. (Refer to the Preface for more details on how to create a mind map.) The key point of this mind map is you as a licensed beauty professional. Diagram the different career opportunities awaiting you upon your completion of your course of training. Identify the different disciplines and branches of each, including the different positions that may be obtained in that field. Use terms, pictures, and symbols as desired. Using color will increase the mind's retention and memory of the information. Keep your mind open and uncluttered and don't worry about where a line or word should go. The organization of the map will usually take care of itself.

3 Essential Experience

Character Study and Report

Select a twenty-first century industry icon (such as John Paul DeJoria or Nick Arrojo) and conduct research on their life and career in cosmetology. Again, use the library, the Internet, trade magazines, or other resources to obtain your information. Explain the impact this person has had on the industry and why or why not he/she should be respected within the industry. Don't limit yourself to a written report. Get creative and use illustrations, photos, drawings, diagrams, and color to enhance your report and make it more meaningful.

Essential Experience

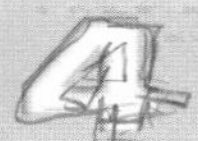

Word Scramble

Using the clues provided, unscramble the terms below.

KEY:

Scramble	**Correct Word**
msiekksoto	_ _ _ _ _ _ _ _ _ _
	Clue: Greek term.
mngipste	_ _ _ _ _ _ _ _
	Clue: Made from berries.
tsreyo lesshl	_ _ _ _ _ _ _ _ _ _ _ _
	Clue: Used to make implements.
mlaain wsine	_ _ _ _ _ _ _ _ _ _ _
	Clue: Used to tie hair back.
feemprsu	_ _ _ _ _ _ _ _
	Clue: Used in Grecian religious rites.
nniarcba	_ _ _ _ _ _ _ _
	Clue: Made into red pigment.
laemtoa	_ _ _ _ _ _ _
	Clue: Used to make masks.
zttdrsiiiaaonniul	_ _ _ _ _ _ _ _ _ _ _ _ _ _ _ _ _
	Clue: Brought new prosperity.
aapetrclo	_ _ _ _ _ _ _ _ _
	Clue: Erected a personal cosmetics factory near the Dead Sea.
selarhc noserv	_ _ _ _ _ _ _ _ _ _ _ _ _
	Clue: Marketed nail lacquer.

Essential Review

Using the following words, fill in the blanks below to form a thorough review of Chapter 1, History & Career Opportunities. Words or terms may be used more than once or not at all.

austere	**esthetician**	**processes**
barber	**fastest-growing**	**pulling teeth**
bare brow	**fourteenth**	**red**
beeswax	**full-service salon**	**restrictive**
berries	**hair color**	**spa**
black	**ice**	**stone**
bloodletting	**irons**	**surgery**
braiding	**kohl**	**texture**
classes	**lacquered**	**towering headdresses**
curl	**leaves**	**tree bark**
dentistry	**lips**	**trends**
desire	**nuts**	
educators	**pancake**	

1. If business is your calling, you will find that management opportunities in the salon and ____________ environment are quite diverse.
2. Archeological studies reveal that haircutting and hairstyling were practiced in some form as early as the ____________ age.
3. Ancient records show that coloring matter was made from minerals, insects, ____________, herbs, and leaves to color the hair, skin, and nails.
4. Roman noblewomen tinted their hair ____________.
5. During the golden age of Greece, women applied white lead on their faces, ____________ on their eyes, and vermillion on their cheeks and lips.
6. The poor class of ancient Rome wore their hair ____________.
7. The modern barber pole was originally the symbol of the ____________ surgeon.
8. Up until the nineteenth century, ____________ was performed by barbers.

9. The barber pole has its roots in the medical procedure known as ____________.

10. The Middle Ages showed women wearing ____________________.

11. During the Renaissance, a ____________ was thought to give women a look of greater intelligence.

12. The Victorian Age was one of the most austere and ____________ periods in history.

13. During the Shang Dynasty, aristocrats rubbed a tinted mixture of gum arabic, gelatin,____________, and egg whites onto their nails to turn them crimson or ebony.

14. In 1935, Max Factor created ____________ makeup to make actors' skin look natural on color film.

15. Beyond defining your area of expertise, you must also decide whether or not you want to work in a specialty salon, ______________, or day spa.

Essential Discoveries and Accomplishments

In the space below, jot some notes about what concepts of this chapter were hardest for you to understand or remember. Imagine finding yourself suddenly in the role of "teacher" and consider what you would tell your "students" about these concepts. Share your Essential Discoveries with some of the other students in your class and ask if they are helpful to them. You may want to revise your discoveries based on any good ideas shared by your peers.

Discoveries:

List at least three things you have accomplished since you decided to enroll in school.

Accomplishments:

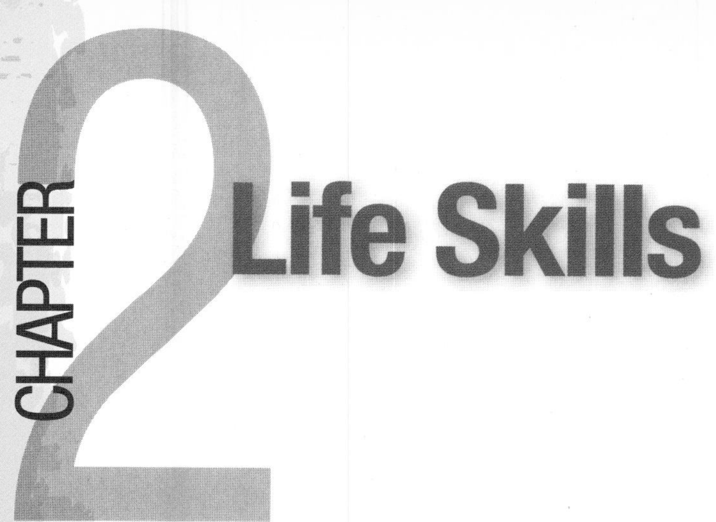

Life Skills

A Motivating Moment: "The greatest discovery of any generation is that a human being can alter his life by altering his attitude."

—William James

Essential Objectives

After studying this chapter and completing the Essential Companion components, you will be able to:

1. List the principles that contribute to personal and professional success.
2. Explain the concept of self-management.
3. Create a mission statement.
4. Explain how to set long-term and short-term goals.
5. Discuss the most effective ways to manage time.
6. Describe good study habits.
7. Define *ethics*.
8. List the characteristics of a healthy, positive attitude.

Essential Life Skills

Why do I need to learn about life skills in order to be successful as a cosmetologist?

Cosmetologists should have a thorough understanding of life skills because:

- Practicing good life skills will lead to a more satisfying and productive career in the beauty industry.
- Hair stylists work with many different types of clients and life skills help you keep those interactions positive, no matter what you are thinking and feeling.
- The ability to deal with difficult clients, coworkers, and even friends comes from well-developed life skills.
- Having good life skills builds high self-esteem, which in turn helps you achieve your goals.

Life skills are essential for increasing your effectiveness, career success, and personal satisfaction in your personal life as well as on the job. You may be able to achieve the highest quality technical skills, but if you are unable to manage the big picture of your life in general, those technical skills will yield little or no results.

For example, research shows that stress has reached epidemic proportions in the United States and is having a negative impact on all of society, especially in the workplace and even in the field of cosmetology. Our goal in this chapter is to provide ideas, tools, and the best practices that you can use to increase your effectiveness, enhance your career, and feel more fulfilled with your life in general.

Essential Concepts

What do I need to know about life-skills management in order to be effective as a licensed professional?

Managing your life skills includes a plethora of qualities, characteristics, and skills. In addition to all the technical skills you will need to master for your new career, you will need to practice general principles that form the foundation for both personal and business success. You will need to understand personal motivation and what is meant by self-management.

You will develop skills useful in expanding your creativity. Yale psychologist Robert Sternberg argues that successful intelligence goes beyond cognitive intelligence to include what he calls "creative and practical intelligence." He says that people with creative intelligence know how to leverage their cognitive intelligence by *applying* what they learn in *new* and *creative* ways. Therefore, this chapter introduces you to some strategies that will help you do just that. Goal setting is an integral part of any successful person's career. Thus, you need to learn how to set goals, monitor them, and expand them throughout your journey.

All of these life skills will be better managed if you also learn how to manage the events in your life. By event control, we really mean what has long been referred to as time management. Tips from the experts on time management will be useful in planning your personal quest for success.

You are now enrolled in a career program of study. Therefore, you will need to ensure that your personal study skills are up-to-speed and adequate to see you successfully through the course. You will even need to identify your own personal learning style in order to maximize the time spent in both study and in the classroom.

You will realize after completion of this chapter that other key ingredients to success are affected by your personality, your attitude, your approach to professional ethics, and, possibly more than anything else, your ability to interact effectively with others, which is also known as human relations. Your future will be much richer if you look at your training as the opportunity to learn to manage your life in the same manner as those successful professionals who have attained many of the goals you aspire to achieve.

1 Essential Experience

Goal Setting

If you have not already done so, make a chart of your short-term and long-term goals as well as your action plan for achievement of those goals in the space provided. Your action plan should include the education you need to attain, as well as target dates for completion. Remember a goal is anything you can *have, be,* or *do*. For most people, goals are divided into several categories, including: Career/Job, Salary/Earnings, Personal/Family Relationship, Health/Weight, Education/Skills, Knowledge, Personal Free-Time, Travel, Financial/Material Assets, Home, Transportation, and Spirituality. (Make you own chart if more space is needed.)

Short-Term Goals: Less Than 1 Year	Long-Term Goals: 1 to 10 Years	Action Plan: Education Required

Essential Experience 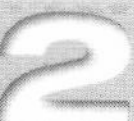

Collage of Goals

It is a well-known belief that in order to obtain goals, we need to visualize ourselves as having already attained them. Therefore, we should picture ourselves at that desired weight, or driving that fancy sports car that appeals to us, or living in that special home we want. With that in mind, and referring back to the goals you set for yourself in Essential Experience 1, create a collage that depicts having attained that success. For example, if you have visualized a special home in your future, cut out a picture that represents that dream and paste it on a poster board. If you have a goal of driving a Porsche, find a picture of a Porsche in a magazine and cut it out and park it in front of the house. Cut out a picture of yourself as well and place it in the sports car!

If you dream of having a wonderful spouse and two children, cut out a picture of that significant other and two children and yourself and place them in front of the house as well. Perhaps you will have a picture of a successful platform artist performing on stage with your head overlaid on the body! Get the idea? Once you have completed the collage that holds all your dreams and goals, place it in a prominent place in your life where you will see it each and every day. By seeing the visualization of achieved goals, your subconscious works even harder to help you accomplish the activities set out in your action plan and finally reach your goals.

3 Essential Experience

Mind Map of Yourself Today

Mind mapping simply creates a free-flowing outline of material or information with the central or key point being located in the center. (Refer to the Preface for more details on how to create a mind map.) The key point of this mind map is you at this point in your life. Diagram the different aspects of your life as they exist today. Use terms, pictures, and symbols as desired. Using color will increase your mind's retention and memory of the information. Keep your mind open and uncluttered and don't worry about where a line or word should go. The organization of the map will usually take care of itself.

To begin, draw a stick figure that represents you in the middle of the page and encircle it. Draw a line out from the center and insert another circle where you write *student*. Off the student circle, you will draw lines that might say things like *attend class, study, work with clients*, etc. Another line from the center circle might say *Mom* or *Dad* (if you are a parent), and the lines off that circle might reflect your role as a parent with tasks such as *drive car pool*, *coach little league*, etc. Consider all the aspects of your life and put them into the mind map in the space provided.

4 Essential Experience

Mind Map Your Future

Using the collage you created in Essential Experience 2, create another mind map using the guidelines presented in the previous experience. This time, however, draw the map as you see yourself in ten years. Upon completion of these drawings, place them in a safe place for reflection later. Take another look at the end of your course of study and then on New Year's Day each year until the time that you had scheduled for reaching the goals you defined in Essential Experience 1 has elapsed.

Essential Experience 5

Track Your Attendance

Managing your life skills also includes something called *impulse management.* In this context, impulses are defined as anything that isn't an integral part of your goals and may actually interfere with the accomplishment of your goals. According to *Merriam-Webster,* a goal is defined as "the end toward which effort is directed." An impulse is defined as a "sudden spontaneous inclination or incitement to some usually unpremeditated action." History indicates that students often act on impulse when they decide to not attend school as scheduled. With that in mind, consider tracking your attendance one month at a time using the following form. This will give you clear, first-hand documentation if you are committed to achieving your goals or if you are letting *impulse management* rule your life.

Date	Hours Missed	Reason for Absence	If action was *impulse management*, what actions will prevent the absence in the future?

6 Essential Experience

Self-Assessment of Personal Characteristics

Consider the qualities and characteristics you now possess and list them either as strengths or weaknesses in the space provided. If the characteristic is a strength, state the benefits received from it. If the characteristic is a weakness, identify steps you can take to improve. Refer to the example to get started.

Strength	Benefit	Weakness	Action Plan
Promptness	Maximum use of my time; respect from others.	Tardiness	Get up earlier; implement better time-management strategies; be more conscientious and respectful of those who are expecting me on time.

Essential Experience 7

Time Management

For one week, track your time in thirty-minute increments. While this may seem like drudgery and cause you to groan, you will find the results totally enlightening. Take a look at how much time you spent in class, how much time you spent (or didn't spend) studying, how much time you spent eating and sleeping, how much quality time you spent with your family, and how much time you wasted on busy work or unimportant activities.

Time Utilization Log

Time	Sun	Mon	Tue	Wed	Thu	Fri	Sat
7:00 am							
7:30 am							
8:00 am							
8:30 am							
9:00 am							
9:30 am							
10:00 am							
10:30 am							
11:00 am							
11:30 am							
12:00 pm							
12:30 pm							
1:00 pm							
1:30 pm							
2:00 pm							
2:30 pm							
3:00 pm							
3:30 pm							
4:00 pm							
4:30 pm							
5:00 pm							

7 Essential Experience continued

Time Utilization Log							
5:30 pm							
6:00 pm							
6:30 pm							
7:00 pm							
7:30 pm							
8:00 pm							
8:30 pm							
9:00 pm							
9:30 pm							
10:00 pm							
10:30 pm							
11:00 pm							

Essential Experience 8

Action Plan for Time Management

After you have analyzed the time utilization log thoroughly, develop a personal action plan (using the chart below) for better managing your time this week. To help you do that, you need to identify the activities you wish to complete in the next seven days. Then you need to prioritize those activities as: A) greatest importance; B) average importance; C) least importance. As you progress through the week, indicate when each of the tasks has been completed.

Priorities for the Current Week		
Activities to Complete	Priority Rank	Date Completed

9 Essential Experience

Is Your Bad Attitude an Addiction?

Experts tell us that the first step in addressing any addiction is recognizing, defining, and admitting the problem. Note the following definitions.

Addict: to devote or surrender (oneself) to something habitually or obsessively.

Addiction: the compulsive need for (or dependence on) and use of a habit-forming substance (or behavior) characterized by tolerance and by well-defined physiological symptoms upon withdrawal.

Dependence: the quality or state of being subordinate to something else.

Please answer the following questions as honestly as you can.

- Do you lose productive time due to your bad attitude? ___ **Yes** ___ **No**
- Is your bad attitude making your home life unhappy? ___ **Yes** ___ **No**
- Have you ever felt remorse because of your bad attitude? ___ **Yes** ___ **No**
- Have you gotten into financial difficulties because of your bad attitude? ___ **Yes** ___ **No**
- Do you turn to lower companions and an inferior environment because of your bad attitude? ___ **Yes** ___ **No**
- Does your bad attitude make you careless with your family's welfare? ___ **Yes** ___ **No**
- Has your ambition decreased because of your bad attitude? ___ **Yes** ___ **No**
- Does your bad attitude cause you difficulty in sleeping? ___ **Yes** ___ **No**
- Has your efficiency ever decreased because of your bad attitude? ___ **Yes** ___ **No**
- Is your bad attitude jeopardizing your job or business? ___ **Yes** ___ **No**
- Do you use your bad attitude to escape from worries or troubles? ___ **Yes** ___ **No**
- Have you ever experienced memory loss due to your bad attitude? ___ **Yes** ___ **No**

Essential Experience continued

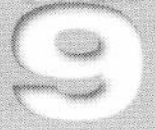

- Has your supervisor ever counseled you because of your bad attitude? ___ **Yes** ___ **No**
- Is your bad attitude an absolute must in your daily life? ___ **Yes** ___ **No**
- Have you ever been to a hospital or institution because of your bad attitude? ___ **Yes** ___ **No**

If you have answered yes to any ONE of these questions, this is a definite *warning* that you may be dependent upon your bad attitude.

If you answered yes to any TWO of these questions, the chance that you are dependent on your bad attitude is high.

If you answered yes to THREE or more of these questions, you are definitely dependent upon your bad attitude.

To begin immediate recovery from this dependency, *smile*, think positive thoughts, speak positive self-affirmations, and visualize personal health, happiness, and success!

**Questions adapted from Johns Hopkins University Hospital.*

Essential Review

Using the following words, fill in the blanks below to form a thorough review of Chapter 2, Life Skills. Words or terms may be used more than once or not at all.

accomplishment	**friends**	**self-esteem**
attitude	**game plan**	**short-term**
caring	**integrity**	**small tasks**
communication	**long-term**	**social**
competent	**moral**	**strengths**
creative	**motivation**	**technical**
decisions	**passion**	**test**
desire	**perfectionism**	**time-out**
diplomacy	**personality**	**uninterrupted**
discipline	**prioritized**	**values**
discretion	**problem-solving**	**visualize**
down time	**procrastination**	**vocabulary**
education	**professional**	
energetic	**respect**	

1. By nature, the salon is a ____________ workplace where you are expected to exercise your artistic talent.
2. One important life skill is that of being genuinely____________ and helpful to other people.
3. Another necessary life skill is that of making good ____________.
4. You can have all the talent in the world and still not be successful if your talent is not fueled by the ____________ for your work that will sustain you over the course of your career.
5. ____________ helps you achieve your goals.
6. The more you ____________ yourself as a success, the easier it is to turn your goals into realities.
7. Principles or guidelines for helping you achieve success include building on your ____________, being kind to yourself, defining success as you see it, practicing new behaviors, and separating your personal life from your work.

8. Successful people make a point of relating to everyone they know with a conscious feeling of ____________.
9. ____________ keeps you from maintaining peak performance.
10. An unhealthy compulsion to do things perfectly is called ____________.
11. Having a ____________ is the conscious act of planning your life.
12. To enhance skill creativity, you should stop criticizing yourself, stop asking others what to do, change your ____________, and not try to go it totally alone.
13. A personal mission statement sets forth the ____________ you plan to live by and establishes future goals.
14. Goals which take several years to accomplish are called ____________ goals.
15. To manage time more effectively, tasks should be ____________, which means making a list of tasks that need to be done in the order of most to least important.
16. Give yourself some ____________ whenever you are frustrated, overwhelmed, irritated, worried, or feeling guilty about something.
17. Learn ____________ techniques that will save you time and needless frustration.
18. If you find studying overwhelming, focus on ____________.
19. Studying should take place in a quiet spot where you can work ____________.
20. Studying is best done when you feel ____________ and motivated.
21. Retention of important material is best accomplished when you ____________ yourself on each section of a chapter.
22. Ethics are the ____________ principles of good character, proper conduct, and judgment we live by.
23. Self-care, integrity, ____________, and communication are key qualities of ethics.
24. Maintain your ____________ by making sure your behavior and actions match your values.
25. Ingredients for a healthy, well-developed attitude include ____________, a pleasing tone of voice, emotional stability, sensitivity, high values and goals, receptivity, and communication skills.

Essential Discoveries and Accomplishments

In the space below, jot some notes about what concepts of this chapter were hardest for you to understand or remember. Imagine finding yourself suddenly in the role of "teacher" and consider what you would tell your "students" about these concepts. Share your Essential Discoveries with some of the other students in your class and ask if they are helpful to them. You may want to revise your discoveries based on good ideas shared by your peers.

Discoveries:

___

___

___

___

___

___

___

___

___

___

List at least three things you have accomplished since your last entry that relate to your career goals.

Accomplishments:

___

___

___

___

___

CHAPTER 3 Your Professional Image

A Motivating Moment: "To simplify, you have to clarify. Simplification is the new competitive advantage."
— Jack Trout

Essential Objectives

After studying this chapter and completing the Essential Companion components, you will be able to:

1. **Understand the importance of professional hygiene.**
2. **Explain the concept of dressing for success.**
3. **Demonstrate an understanding of ergonomic principles and ergonomically correct postures and movements.**

Essential Professionalism

Why are professionalism and my image so important to my success in cosmetology or a related field?

Professionalism has been defined as the conduct, aims, or qualities that characterize or mark a professional person. The cosmetology industry and all related fields such as nail technology, barbering, esthetics, and massage therapy represent the *image* industry. There is no other profession in which image and communication skills (which we will learn more about in Chapter 4, Communicating for Success) are more essential. As a student in training and as a professional, you will come in contact with numerous clients on a daily basis.

Cosmetologists should study and have a thorough understanding of the importance of a professional image because:

- Clients rely on beauty professionals to look good, well-cared for, and contemporary.
- Clients will feel confident that a professional who has a pleasant, professional image can be trusted to perform their beauty services.
- Finding a salon and salon environment with a compatible idea of professional image and behavior is vitally important to working and flourishing in your career.
- Behaving professionally includes having a genuine interest in your own day-to-day activities, being concerned about and for others, and knowing how to interact with managers, coworkers, and clients appropriately.
- Understanding ergonomics will help keep you healthy and gainfully employed.

Psychologists tell us that people form an opinion of us in the first few seconds of meeting us. It is up to us to make that first impression a positive one. It is also up to us to make that positive impression a lasting one. We can accomplish that by understanding how to enjoy both personal and professional health. This chapter will help you do just that.

Essential Concepts

What are the essential concepts about image and professional development?

As a professional in the beauty industry, it will be essential for you to concentrate on your personal and professional health. You will need to be aware of your physical presence, your nutrition, and your ability to manage personal stress. In the process, you will realize the importance of developing a positive winning attitude and practicing professionalism at all times. Chapter 3, Your Professional Image, in the *Milady® Standard Cosmetology* textbook and this Essential Companion will provide the road map for helping you achieve all these important personal and professional goals.

1 Essential Experience

What Does Your Professional Image Say About You?

Professional image is the impression you project and consists of your outward appearance as well as the conduct you exhibit in the workplace. It is essentially the code of behavior by which you conduct yourself. It relates to proper conduct and business dealings with employers, clients and coworkers, and others with whom you come in contact. Professionalism will help you establish a well-respected reputation. Ask yourself the following questions to help you evaluate your professionalism and your professional image.

- Do you treat others honestly and fairly at all times?
- Are you courteous and do you show respect for the feelings, beliefs, and rights of others?
- Do you keep your word when you make a promise?
- Do you set an example of good conduct and behavior at all times?
- Are you loyal to your family, your friends, your school, and your fellow students?
- Do you obey all the rules and standards of conduct set forth by your institution?

If you answered no to any of the above questions, you may want to re-evaluate your commitment to a professional career. If you answered yes to all, give yourself a pat on the back. You practice many qualities required for projecting a professional image.

Essential Experience

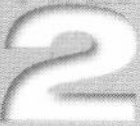

Policy Development

Imagine yourself the owner of a professional establishment and write a detailed dress code that you would require all employees to follow.

Dress Code: ____

____

____

____

____

____

____

____

____

____

____

____

____

____

3 Essential Experience

Word Scramble

Using the clues provided, unscramble the terms below.

KEY:

Scramble	**Correct Word**
csexeeirs	_ _ _ _ _ _ _ _ _ *Clue:* Help relieve stress from repetitive movements.
ggnmoior	_ _ _ _ _ _ _ _ *Clue:* An extension of personal hygiene.
oeptrus	_ _ _ _ _ _ _ *Clue:* Position or bearing of the body.
csimongreo	_ _ _ _ _ _ _ _ _ _ *Clue:* The study of human characteristics for the specific work environment.
niosfesorpliams	_ _ _ _ _ _ _ _ _ _ _ _ _ _ _ *Clue:* Business conduct.
ehhtal	_ _ _ _ _ _ *Clue:* Well-being.
neegyih	_ _ _ _ _ _ _ *Clue:* Practicing cleanliness.
ressst	_ _ _ _ _ _ *Clue:* Caused by repetitive movements.
zssaceeoric	_ _ _ _ _ _ _ _ _ _ _ *Clue:* Secondary to dressing.

Essential Experience 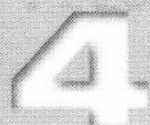

Rate Your Image

On a scale of 1 to 5, with 5 being considered the best, rate your appearance in the following categories:

_____ Clothing is clean, pressed, and free of stains or damage.

_____ Dress is in compliance with the dress code established by the institution.

_____ Shoes are clean, polished, and in good repair.

_____ Makeup (if applicable) is tasteful and neatly applied.

_____ Hair is properly groomed and styled appropriately for current trends.

_____ Facial hair (beard or mustache, if applicable) is properly trimmed and neat.

_____ Hands and nails are properly manicured; nails are clean and trimmed appropriately.

_____ Fragrance is appropriate, not overpowering.

_____ Hygiene is maintained (daily bath, proper use of deodorant, teeth are brushed, etc.).

_____ Jewelry is kept to a minimum and not overdone or too trendy.

Add your scores and evaluate your image according to the following guidelines.

45 to 50	Your image is excellent.
40 to 44	Your image is above average.
30 to 39	Your image is average.
Below 30	Improvement is needed. Evaluate the chart and pay particular attention to any category rated less than 3. Make a personal commitment to improvement in those areas.

5 Essential Experience

Analyze Your Personal Lifestyle

Answer the following questions thoughtfully and honestly.

- How many hours of sleep do you get on average nightly?
- What kind of exercise you get daily/weekly, if any?
- What methods do you use for relaxation, and how often?
- What is your daily personal hygiene and grooming regimen, including the care of your hands and feet?
- Think back over the past three days and report on your nutrition habits. What did you eat for breakfast, lunch, and dinner over that period of time?
- Evaluate and list other lifestyle components such as the use of alcohol, tobacco, or drugs. Do they have a negative impact on your life?

As a result of this analysis, write a Plan of Action for improving your routines and habits to make the most of a healthy and balanced physical, mental, and emotional lifestyle.

PLAN OF ACTION

____

____

____

____

Essential Experience 6

Your Attitude—What Does It Say About You?

One way to determine whether or not you possess and convey a positive attitude is to ask yourself the following questions daily. They have been adapted from a well-known poem "I Promise Myself" by an unknown author.

- Do you promise yourself to be so strong that nothing can disturb your peace of mind?
- Do you promise yourself to talk health, happiness, and prosperity to every person you meet?
- Do you promise yourself to make all your friends feel that there is something special in them?
- Do you promise yourself to look at the sunny side of everything and make your optimism come true?
- Do you promise yourself to think only of the *best,* to work only for the *best,* and to expect only the *best?*
- Do you promise yourself to be just as enthusiastic about the success of others as you are about your own success?
- Do you promise yourself to forget the mistakes of the past and press on to the greater achievements of the future?
- Do you promise yourself to wear a cheerful countenance at all times and greet every living creature you meet with a smile?
- Do you promise yourself to give so much time to the improvement of yourself that you have no time to criticize others?
- Do you promise yourself to be too large for worry, too noble for anger, too strong for fear, and too happy to permit the presence of trouble in your life?

If you make these ten promises daily, you will live a life full of prosperity and rewards too great to count!

Essential Review

Using the following words, fill in the blanks below to form a thorough review of Chapter 3, Your Professional Image.

balance	**image**	**repetitive**
blend	**impression**	**sleep**
disconnect	**jingle**	**stress**
energy	**mask**	**tension**
ergonomics	**personal**	**thirty**
health	**pressure**	**work habits**
hygiene pack	**professional**	

1. Your professional image is the ____________ you project and consists of your outward appearance and the conduct you exhibit in the workplace.
2. A good way to ensure that you always smell fresh and clean is to create a ____________.
3. The daily maintenance of cleanliness and healthfulness is known as ____________ hygiene.
4. Stressful ____________ motions have a cumulative effect on muscles and joints.
5. Physical presentation, which includes your posture, your walk, and your movements, is part of your ____________ image.
6. When you obtain employment, strive to ensure your hair, makeup, and clothing style are consistent with the ____________ of the salon.
7. Accessories are best kept simple and attractive, and jewelry should not ____________ while working.
8. Makeup should accentuate your best features and ____________ your less flattering ones.
9. ____________ is the study of how a workplace can best be designed for comfort, safety, efficiency, and productivity.
10. An awareness of your body posture and movements, coupled with better work habits and proper tools and equipment, will enhance your ____________ and comfort.

Essential Discoveries and Accomplishments

In the space below, jot some notes about what concepts of this chapter were hardest for you to understand or remember. Imagine finding yourself suddenly in the role of "teacher" and consider what you would tell your "students" about these concepts. Share your Essential Discoveries with some of the other students in your class and ask if they are helpful to them. You may want to revise your discoveries based on good ideas shared by your peers.

Discoveries:

List at least three things you have accomplished since your last entry that relate to your career goals.

Accomplishments:

CHAPTER 4 Communicating for Success

A Motivating Moment: "To live our lives fully, to work whole heartedly, to refuse directly what we can't swallow, to accept the mystery in all matters of meaning . . . this is the ultimate adventure."

— Peter Block

Essential Objectives

After studying this chapter and completing the Essential Companion components, you will be able to:

1. **List the golden rules of human relations.**
2. **Explain the definition of effective communication.**
3. **Conduct a successful client consultation/needs assessment.**
4. **Handle an unhappy client.**
5. **Build open lines of communication with coworkers.**

Essential Communication Skills

Why do I need to learn about communicating when I just want to cut hair?

Today's professionals, regardless of their chosen field, thrive on the exchange of information. In fact, it is information that acts as the fuel that keeps businesses going, moving, and growing. You must think of managing your career as a professional in the beauty industry as that of managing your own business. Indeed, when you build and retain a loyal clientele, you are building a successful business. Therefore, you need to receive information in order to make decisions, develop strategies, and effectively interact with your clients. You need to send information if you want your decisions and strategies to be followed and accepted.

This exchange of information is called communication. Your technical skills, however outstanding they may be, will not bring back a client who does not feel comfortable, appreciated, and important as a result of a visit to your salon. Thus, you must be able to address these important social and emotional needs through effective communications.

In addition, you cannot provide exceptional technical services if you do not truly understand the client's desires. Therefore, communication skills play a huge role in your quest for success.

Cosmetologists should study and have a thorough understanding of effective communication because:

- Communicating effectively—with a purpose—is the basis of all long-lasting relationships with clients and coworkers.
- Professionals need to build strong relationships based on trust, clarity, and loyalty in order to have a successful career, and they must be able to verbalize their thoughts and ideas to clients, colleagues, and supervisors.
- The close-knit salon environment will present complex and sometimes difficult interpersonal issues, and you will need effective ways to communicate in order to navigate them successfully.
- Practicing and perfecting professional communication ensures that clients will enjoy their experience with you and will encourage their continued patronage.
- The ability to control communication and effectively express ideas in a professional manner is a necessary skill for success in any career, but particularly so in one as personal as cosmetology.

Essential Concepts

What do I need to know about communicating for success in order to provide quality service to my clients and enjoy career success?

We communicate not only by speaking, but also through listening, reading, and writing as well. In order to exchange information with our clients about their hair, skin, and nail care needs, we must be able to exchange information effectively. We send information by speaking and writing. We receive information by listening and reading. In addition to these methods, we also communicate without using words. We can send and receive messages by using gestures, facial expressions, voice intonations, eye contact, personal mannerisms, dress, and posture. Throughout this whole communicating process, we are involved in relationship building. We build relationships with our clients, our coworkers, our supervisors, and salon managers or owners.

Therefore, we must develop exceptional skills in conducting consultations with our clients that will result in their desired outcomes. We must learn to interact effectively on a day-to-day basis with our peers and coworkers in order to participate in a highly productive, team-oriented environment. And, finally, we must know how to respond to and interact favorably with our supervisors in order to ensure our continued career development, growth, and success.

Essential Experience 1

Matching Exercise

Every part of our body has something to add to the message we are trying to send. Hand movements are the most common companions to spoken messages, more so for some than others. Many hand movements are so common they have come to mean the same thing for all of us. From the list below, match the listed hand movements with the nonverbal message they send.

1. Pointing a finger at someone	____ Boredom, nervousness
2. Twiddling thumbs	____ A warning, an accusation
3. Clasping two hands overhead	____ Hopefulness
4. Drumming or tapping fingers	____ Calmness, self-confidence
5. Crossing two fingers	____ A threat
6. Crossing arms across chest	____ Impatience, annoyance
7. Folding hands together on desk	____ "Okay" or "right on"
8. Making a circle with thumb and forefinger	____ Authority, anger
9. Making a fist	____ Victory

2 Essential Experience

Eye Movement

As with our hands, we can use our eyes to send nonverbal messages which might include close attention, anger, admiration, disbelief, or surprise. Study the list of various eye movements below and write in the space provided the nonverbal message you believe the eye movement sends.

- Staring and having a tightened jaw ______________________
- Rolling the eyes ______________________
- Looking directly at someone ______________________
- Opening the eyes wide ______________________
- Staring/glaring at someone for too long ______________________
- Blinking eyes rapidly ______________________
- Looking directly at strangers in close quarters ______________________
- Shifting eyes away to avoid direct contact ______________________

Essential Experience 3

Mind Map Consultation Interference

Mind mapping simply creates a free-flowing outline of material or information with the central or key point being located in the center. The key point of this mind map is a client consultation. Diagram all the things that could interfere with the communication process during a client consultation. Use terms, pictures, and symbols as desired. Use color to increase the mind's retention and memory of the material. Keep your mind open and uncluttered and don't worry about where a line or word should go as the organization of the map will usually take care of itself.

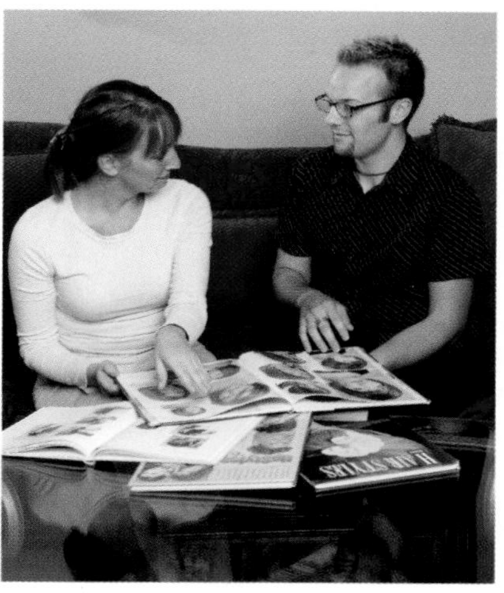

4 Essential Experience

Partner Messaging

Choose another student as your partner and conduct this communication exercise: Spend five minutes talking to each other about any subject you choose. Interact openly and respond to each other naturally. At the conclusion of the five minutes, each of you should make a list of the messages you received. Then review the lists together and compare the messages received to the messages you each intended to send. List the results in the space provided.

Message Received	Message Intended
______________________________	______________________________
______________________________	______________________________
______________________________	______________________________
______________________________	______________________________
______________________________	______________________________
______________________________	______________________________
______________________________	______________________________
______________________________	______________________________
______________________________	______________________________
______________________________	______________________________

Essential Experience 5

Role Playing a Dissatisfied Client

The purpose of role playing is to help you understand the views and feelings of other people with respect to a wide range of personal and social issues. By acting out situations in which people are in conflict, you can begin to understand the other person's point of view. In this activity, there will be three main characters and several other students will be needed to observe. Three of you will perform the role-playing exercise while the other students observe and make notes. Upon completion of the role play, ask the observers what they saw, what worked in the communication exchange, what did not work, and why.

Role-playing scenario: One student will role play the salon stylist, and another student will play a client who has come into the salon for a haircolor service and is clearly dissatisfied with the results. The third character will be the salon supervisor who ultimately has to become involved in the quest for a solution. Upon completion of the role play and discussion with the observers, record your findings from the activity in the space provided. Consider answering the following questions: What did you learn from this experience? Are there certain ways to handle conflict that are more effective than others? If so, what are they and why do they work better?

____

____

____

____

____

____

____

____

____

6 Essential Experience

Windowpane Client Consultation Tools

Windowpaning is the process of transferring key elements, points, or steps in a lesson into visual images that are hand sketched into the squares or *panes* of a matrix. Let your mind think in pictures and sketch the essential concepts printed in each of the following windowpanes. Don't be concerned with your artistic ability. Use lines and stick figures to depict the concepts requested.

Consultation Card	**Styling Books**	**Personal Portfolio**
Photos	**Digital Camera**	**Color Charts**
Color Swatches	**Mirror**	**Mannequin**

Essential Experience 7

Topics to Avoid

In the space provided make a list of at least six topics that you should avoid discussing with clients. Then write a brief explanation as to why these topics would be inappropriate and list alternative topics that you might suggest if the client should bring up any of these.

Essential Review

True or False

Circle the T for true or the F for false as applicable to the following statements to form a thorough review of Chapter 4, Communicating for Success.

T **F** **1.** A fundamental factor in human relations has to do with how secure we are feeling.

T **F** **2.** Communicate from your head; problem solve from your heart.

T **F** **3.** Show people you care by listening to them and trying to understand their point of view.

T **F** **4.** Effective human relations and communication skills build lasting client relationships, aid in your growth, and help prevent misunderstandings.

T **F** **5.** Communication is the act of effectively sharing information between two people, or groups of people, so that it is effectively understood.

T **F** **6.** To earn a client's trust and loyalty, you need to always approach a new client in a formal and reserved manner.

T **F** **7.** The client consultation is the written communication that determines the desired results.

T **F** **8.** The work and consultation area needs to be freshly cleaned and uncluttered.

T **F** **9.** Reflective listening is the process of repeating back to the client, in your own words, what you think she is telling you.

T **F** **10.** If a client doesn't fully realize that her choice in a service will not benefit her, it is your obligation to find a way to bluntly let her know.

T **F** **11.** The verbal communication with a client that is used to determine the client's desired results is called a client consultation.

T **F** **12.** A consultation with a first-time client should be scheduled at least fifteen minutes prior to the actual appointment.

T **F** **13.** Record any formulations or products used, including the strength and any specific techniques followed, on the Rolodex.

Essential Review continued

T F **14.** When meeting a client for the first time, always introduce yourself.

T F **15.** The first step in the client consultation process is to ask the client what he/she likes least and most about his/her current look.

T F **16.** Encouraging a client to flip through photo collections and point out finished looks that he/she likes and why is called the show-and-tell step of the consultation.

T F **17.** If a client arrives late, you should establish a precedent by refusing to complete the service under any circumstances.

T F **18.** If a client shows up at an incorrect time or day, politely explain his/her mistake and offer to reschedule them.

T F **19.** Never argue with a client or try to force your opinion on him/her.

T F **20.** Your job and your relationship with your clients are very specific: the goal is to advise and service clients with their beauty needs, and nothing more.

Essential Discoveries and Accomplishments

In the space below, jot some notes about what concepts of this chapter were hardest for you to understand or remember. Imagine finding yourself suddenly in the role of "teacher" and consider what you would tell your "students" about these concepts. Share your Essential Discoveries with some of the other students in your class and ask if they are helpful to them. You may want to revise your discoveries based on good ideas shared by your peers.

Discoveries:

____

____

____

____

____

____

____

____

____

____

____

List at least three things you have accomplished since your last entry that relate to your career goals.

Accomplishments:

____

____

____

____

____

CHAPTER 5

Infection Control: Principles & Practices

A Motivating Moment: "It is amazing what ordinary people can do if they set out without preconceived notions."
— Charles Kettering

Essential Objectives

After studying this chapter and completing the Essential Companion components, you will be able to:

1. Understand state laws and rules and the differences between them.
2. List the types and classifications of bacteria.
3. Define hepatitis and Human Immunodeficiency Virus (HIV) and explain how they are transmitted.
4. Explain the differences between cleaning, disinfecting, and sterilizing.
5. List the types of disinfectants and how they are used.
6. Discuss Universal Precautions.
7. List your responsibilities as a salon professional.
8. Describe how to safely clean and disinfect salon tools and implements.

Essential Principles and Practices of Infection Control

Why do I need to know about the principles of infection control?

If you work in cosmetology or a related career field, you will come in contact with the public on a regular basis in a variety of ways. Understanding bacteriology, methods of decontamination, and your professional responsibilities will make a big difference in how you protect yourself and your clients from the spread of infection or disease. There has never been a time in our history when the public has been more aware of how easily disease can be spread. Your clients' perceptions of you will be greatly improved if you convey both knowledge and concern about bacteria and the spread of disease.

There is an old saying that you never get a second chance to make a positive first impression. Nothing could be more appropriate for the first impressions you and your establishment make on the public. They will judge you by the cleanliness of the establishment where you work, by the cleanliness of your work station and implements, and by the neat, well-groomed image you present. Today's public demands that their doctors, dentists, optometrists, and beauty service professionals practice the highest levels of infection control and decontamination. So, if you want to build a solid, repeat clientele for the services in which you specialize, you will want to practice obvious cleaning and disinfection measures to build client confidence and trust in you as a knowledgable and skilled cosmetologist. In addition, you must be able to take the necessary steps to protect yourself, your coworkers, and your clients from infection by a person who may have an infectious disease that can't be identified by you.

Cosmetologists should study and have a thorough understanding of infection control principles and practices because:

- To be a knowledgeable, successful, and responsible professional in the field of cosmetology, you are required to understand the types of infections you may encounter in the salon.
- Understanding the basics of cleaning and disinfecting and following federal and state rules will safeguard you and your clients and ensure that you have a long and successful career as a cosmetologist.
- Understanding the chemistry of the cleaning and disinfecting products that you use and how to use them will help keep you, your clients, and your salon environment safe.

Essential Concepts

What are the essential concepts of providing the safest possible environment using effective decontamination and infection control procedures?

As a professional in the cosmetology industry, you will need to understand the difference between nonpathogenic (helpful or harmless) and pathogenic (harmful) bacteria. You will need to know the various classifications of bacteria and how to identify each. It is essential that you develop an understanding of bacterial growth and reproduction, bacterial infections, other infectious agents, immunity, and acquired immune deficiency syndrome (AIDS).

As a successful licensee in the field of cosmetology or related discipline, you will need to know about both prevention and infection control. You need to understand that surfaces may be contaminated even if they appear clean; you will also need to know the steps necessary to make those surfaces germ free. You will learn procedures and products for cleaning and disinfecting as well as sterilizing and will gain knowledge about the tools and implements to accomplish all three. The Occupational Safety and Health Administration (OSHA) plays an important role in the responsibilities each licensed establishment has to ensure a safe work environment both for workers and the public. By taking the approach known as Universal Precautions and following the same infection control practices with all clients, regardless of their health status, you are ensuring the best possible protection for you and the public.

1 Essential Experience

Mind Map Staphylococci

Mind mapping creates a free-flowing outline of material or information. Using the central or key point of *Staphylococci*, diagram the types of illnesses staph is responsible for, sources of staph or how staph can be picked up, and symptoms of staph. Use terms, pictures, and symbols as desired. Using color will increase memory of the material.

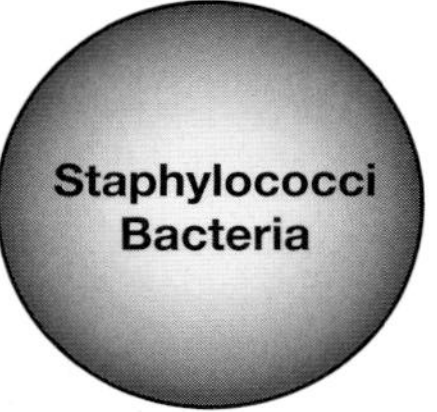

Essential Experience 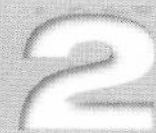

Term Matching

Match the following essential terms with their identifying terms or phrases.

______	**Bacteria**	**1.** Lives and reproduces by penetrating cells
______	**Pathogenic**	**2.** Powerful tuberculocidal disinfectants
______	**Infectious**	**3.** Kills most, but not all, microorganisms on nonliving surfaces
______	**Toxin**	**4.** One-celled microorganisms
______	**Virus**	**5.** An organism that lives on another organism
______	**Efficacy**	**6.** Removing visible dirt and debris, and many disease-causing germs with soap and water
______	**Local infection**	**7.** Elimination of all microbial life including spores
______	**Mildew**	**8.** Contagious disease caused by the itch mite
______	**Parasites**	**9.** Harmful bacteria
______	**Scabies**	**10.** Can be spread from one person to another
______	**Cleaning**	**11.** Poisonous substance
______	**Disinfection**	**12.** The ability to produce an effect
______	**Sterilization**	**13.** Confined to a specific part of the body
______	**Phenolics**	**14.** A type of fungus

3 Essential Experience

Establishment Inspection

Imagine that you own a professional establishment. You are committed to maintaining the highest levels of infection control and client protection possible. Take a tour through your establishment and identify and list the areas in the salon that are most susceptible to pathogenic bacteria.

Essential Experience 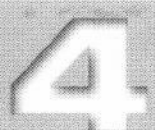

Word Scramble

Using the clues provided, unscramble the terms below.

KEY:

Scramble	**Correct Word**
aasseptir	_ _ _ _ _ _ _ _ _ *Clue:* Require living matter for growth.
fsuoniceti	_ _ _ _ _ _ _ _ _ _ *Clue:* Contagious.
aiarcetb	_ _ _ _ _ _ _ _ *Clue:* Minute, one-celled microorganisms.
alcicyoocshpt	_ _ _ _ _ _ _ _ _ _ _ _ _ *Clue:* Grow in bunches or clusters.
asseibc	_ _ _ _ _ _ _ Clue: Caused by the itch mite.
cpnaiegoht	_ _ _ _ _ _ _ _ _ _ *Clue:* Disease producing.
mrseg	_ _ _ _ _ *Clue:* Microorganism that cause disease.
napnocnghieot	_ _ _ _ _ _ _ _ _ _ _ _ _ *Clue:* Helpful or harmless.
calol fctnoiine	_ _ _ _ _ _ _ _ _ _ _ _ _ _ *Clue:* Contains pus.
seborcim	_ _ _ _ _ _ _ _ *Clue:* Organisms of microscopic or submicroscopic size.
ssriminagoorcm	_ _ _ _ _ _ _ _ _ _ _ _ _ _ *Clue:* Bacteria are one example of this.
ucosaignto	_ _ _ _ _ _ _ _ _ _ *Clue:* Spreads by contact.
uicedsslpoi	_ _ _ _ _ _ _ _ _ _ _ *Clue:* Lice.

4 Essential Experience continued

ieaitnpsct — — — — — — — — — —

Clue: Chemical germicides for skin.

dcgnflaiiu — — — — — — — — — —

Clue: Capable of destroying fungus.

aaiiommnnftl — — — — — — — — — — — —

Clue: Body's response to injury or infection.

ttiisphea — — — — — — — — —

Clue: Bloodborne virus.

oosurp — — — — — —

Clue: Absorbent.

belrtcalduucoi — — — — — — — — — — — — — —

Clue: Type of disinfectant.

Essential Experience 5

Jeopardy

As in the game Jeopardy, write questions which would be correctly answered.

Infection Control for $100.

1. Three types of potentially infectious microorganisms.

   ____

2. Also known as germs and can exist almost anywhere on the skin of the body, in water, air, decayed matter, secretions of body openings, on clothing, and beneath the nails.

   ____

3. Disease producing when they invade plant or animal tissue.

   ____

Infection Control for $200.

1. The life cycle of bacteria.

   ____

2. The stage in which microorganisms grow and reproduce.

   ____

3. Cells that are formed through binary fission.

   ____

Infection Control for $300.

1. Occurs when body tissues are invaded by disease-causing or pathogenic bacteria.

   ____

2. Bacteria normally carried by about a third of the population.

   ____

3. They are responsible for contagious diseases and conditions, such as head lice.

   ____

Infection Control for $400.

1. The ability of the body to destroy bacteria that have gained entrance, and thus resist infection.

   ____

2. Something the body develops after it has overcome a disease, or through inoculation.

   ____

3. A disease that is transmittable by contact.

   ____

Infection Control for $500.

1. A person can be infected with this for many years without having symptoms.

   ____

2. It is transmitted through unprotected sexual contact, IV drug users sharing needles, and accidents with needles in health care settings.

   ____

3. It causes AIDS.

   ____

Essential Experience 6

Safety and Health Inspection Report

Complete the following partial Safety and Health Inspection Report for your institution which is adapted from *Safety and Health in the Salon* by Dennis G. Nelson, published by Milady, a part of Cengage Learning. Write a brief explanation if an area is out of compliance.

Location: ___________ Inspected by: ___________ Date: ___________

All Areas—Housekeeping and Cleaning

- There is evidence the facility has been used for cooking or living quarters. ___ **Yes** ___ **No**
- All areas are orderly, dusted, clean, well-lighted, and rodent free. ___ **Yes** ___ **No**
- Floors are swept clean and hair is swept up after each client service. ___ **Yes** ___ **No**
- Windows, screens, and curtains are cleaned regularly. ___ **Yes** ___ **No**
- Waste materials are deposited in a metal waste receptacle with a self-closing lid. ___ **Yes** ___ **No**
- Waste receptacles are emptied regularly throughout the day. ___ **Yes** ___ **No**
- All sinks and drinking fountains are cleaned regularly. ___ **Yes** ___ **No**
- Separate or disposable drinking cups are provided for clients, employees, and students. ___ **Yes** ___ **No**
- Hot and cold water faucets are clean and leakfree. ___ **Yes** ___ **No**
- Toilets and washing facilities are clean and regularly disinfected. ___ **Yes** ___ **No**
- Toilet tissue, paper towels, and pump-like antiseptic liquid soap are provided. ___ **Yes** ___ **No**
- Door handles are cleaned and disinfected regularly. ___ **Yes** ___ **No**
- Food is stored separately from clinic products. ___ **Yes** ___ **No**
- Eating and drinking are done on clean surfaces separate from chemical handling or where services are being performed. ___ **Yes** ___ **No**

6 Essential Experience continued

- Work area is appropriately ventilated for services provided; fans, humidifiers, and exhaust and ventilation systems are cleaned regularly. ___ **Yes** ___ **No**
- Floors are free of water or other substances that could cause a slip, trip, or fall. ___ **Yes** ___ **No**
- MSDSs are available for all products used in the clinic. ___ **Yes** ___ **No**
- All products are properly stored and all containers are properly labeled. ___ **Yes** ___ **No**
- Appropriate personal protective equipment (eye protection, gloves, dust and organic vapor masks, etc.) is available and used according to manufacturer's directions and salon policy. ___ **Yes** ___ **No**
- Washing machine provides water temperature of at least 160 degrees Fahrenheit. ___ **Yes** ___ **No**
- Hospital-grade tuberculocidal disinfecting solution and instructions are available for disinfecting combs, brushes, plastic capes, and other materials as required. ___ **Yes** ___ **No**

Emergency Precautions and First Aid

- Emergency phone numbers are posted where they can be readily found in an emergency. ___ **Yes** ___ **No**
- Fire evacuation procedures are posted. ___ **Yes** ___ **No**
- First aid kits are readily accessible with necessary supplies. ___ **Yes** ___ **No**
- First aid kit is periodically inspected and replenished as needed. ___ **Yes** ___ **No**
- Emergency eye wash bottles are provided where chemical handling is done and where chemical services are provided. ___ **Yes** ___ **No**
- There is ready access to a sink with tempered water to completely flush the eyes from hazardous materials. ___ **Yes** ___ **No**
- Exit and warning signs (biohazard, fire door, flammable or toxic chemicals) are posted where appropriate. ___ **Yes** ___ **No**

Essential Experience 7

Word Search

After determining the correct word from the clues provided, locate the words in the word search puzzle.

Word	Clue
________________	There are three widely used forms
________________	These can kill bacteria but are not disinfectants
________________	Showing no symptoms or signs of infection
________________	Causes contamination
________________	Surfaces which look clean, may still be this
________________	There are two methods of this
________________	Kills microbes on nonporous surfaces
________________	Destroys harmful organisms (except spores)on nonporous surfaces
________________	Sodium hypochlorite
________________	Provides pertinent information about products
________________	This is part of the United States Department of Labor
________________	Safe and fast-acting disinfectant
________________	Lowest level of decontamination
________________	Most effective decontamination

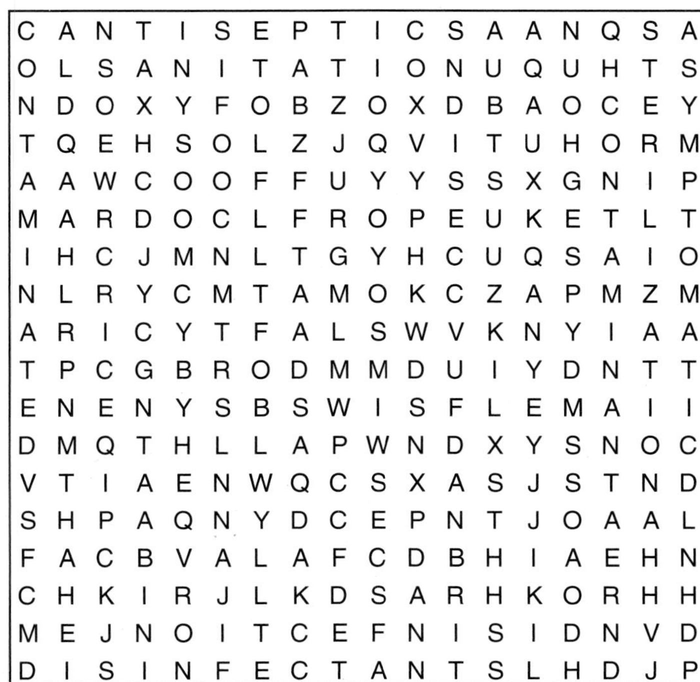

Essential Review

Using the following words, fill in the blanks below to form a thorough review of Chapter 5, Infection Control: Principles & Practices. Words or terms may be used more than once or not at all.

acquired immunity	**local**	**round-shaped**
binary fission	**natural**	**scabies**
boils	**nonpathogenic**	**spherical spores**
contagious	**one-celled**	**streptococci**
daughter cells	**outer covering**	**syphilis**
diphtheria	**parasites**	**systemic**
disinfectant	**pathogenic**	**twelve**
eleven	**pimples**	**virus**
hepatitis B	**pneumonia**	**viruses**
HIV	**protoplasm**	
immunity	**pus**	

1. Staphylococci are pus-forming organisms that grow in clusters and cause ____________ and ____________.
2. A ____________ infection is indicated by a boil or pimple and contains pus.
3. Organisms that live on other living organisms and do not give anything in return are known as ____________.
4. The body's ability to destroy bacteria that have gained entrance is called ____________.
5. Bacteria are ____________ microorganisms found nearly everywhere.
6. ____________ is a fluid created by tissue inflammation.
7. Infectious diseases and conditions such as ____________ should never be treated in a school or salon, but referred to a physician.
8. ____________ are infectious microorganisms smaller than bacteria and capable of infesting almost all plants and animals.
9. The body develops ________________ after it has overcome a disease or through inoculation.
10. A person can be infected with ____________ for many years without having symptoms.

11. ____________ organisms are harmful and produce disease.

12. A ____________ disease affects the body as a whole.

13. When bacteria grow and reach their largest size, they divide and split into two new cells. The division is called ____________ and the new cells formed are called ____________.

14. Immunity against disease can be ____________ or acquired.

15. When a disease becomes ____________ it spreads from one person to another.

For the remainder of the review, circle the correct answer to each question.

16. Any surface that is not free of dirt, hair, or microbes is ____________.

a) sterilized
b) contaminated
c) sterile
d) disinfected

17. The two methods of decontamination are ____________ then sterilizing, or ____________ then disinfecting.

a) washing
b) dusting
c) sweeping
d) cleaning

18. The methods of sterilization include high-pressure steam or ____________.

a) dry heat autoclave
b) gaseous formaldehyde
c) liquid antiseptic
d) dry sanitation

19. Products that kill microbes on contaminated tools and other nonporous surfaces are ____________.

a) antiseptics
b) tablets
c) disinfectants
d) liquids

20. Disinfectants must be registered with the ____________.

a) DOE
b) EPA
c) CDC
d) DOL

21. Federal law requires manufacturers to provide product information on the ____________.

a) MSDS
b) MDSD
c) SMDS
d) MSSD

Essential Review continued

22. The Occupational Safety and Health Administration was created as part of the ____________.

a) DOJ
b) DOE
c) DOL
d) DOA

23. Most QUATS disinfect implements within ____________ minutes.

a) 1 to 3
b) 4 to 5
c) 6 to 8
d) 10

24. If salon implements come into contact with blood, they should be cleaned and then immersed in ____________.

a) quaternary ammonium compounds
b) phenolic disinfectants
c) sodium hypochlorite
d) EPA-registered disinfectant

25. The lowest level of decontamination is known as ____________.

a) disinfection
b) sterilization
c) cleaning
d) immunization

Essential Discoveries and Accomplishments

In the space below, jot some notes about what concepts of this chapter were hardest for you to understand or remember. Imagine finding yourself suddenly in the role of "teacher" and consider what you would tell your "students" about these concepts. Share your Essential Discoveries with some of the other students in your class and ask if they are helpful to them. You may want to revise your discoveries based on good ideas shared by your peers.

Discoveries:

List at least three things you have accomplished since your last entry that relate to your career goals.

Accomplishments:

CHAPTER 6 General Anatomy & Physiology

A Motivating Moment: "Don't go where the path may lead, go instead where there is no path and leave a trail."

— Ralph Waldo Emerson

Essential Objectives

After studying this chapter and completing the Essential Companion components, you will be able to:

1. **Define and explain the importance of anatomy, physiology, and histology to the cosmetology profession.**
2. **Describe cells, their structure, and their reproduction.**
3. **Define tissue and identify the types of tissues found in the body.**
4. **Name the 11 main body systems and explain their basic functions.**

Essential Anatomy and Physiology

Why do I need to know about cells and the anatomy and physiology of the body when I just want to do hair?

As you do hair and perform all the other services you are qualified and trained to perform, almost without exception, you will be affecting the bones, muscles, and nerves of the body. Therefore, it is essential that you understand the basic anatomy and physiology of the body to perform all those services safely and effectively. If you think about it, you will realize that when you cut hair, you must understand the contours of the head and its bone structure. When you apply makeup, you must perform contouring based on the bone and muscle structure of the face. When giving a scalp treatment, you need to know about the circulatory system in order to achieve maximum stimulation of the scalp, and so forth.

Even though you may not consider studying about anatomy and physiology as the most exciting or glamorous part of your training, it is clearly an integral part of your training and will contribute significantly to your effectiveness and success. Certainly your knowledge in this key area will gain your clients' trust and confidence in your credibility.

Cosmetologists should study and have a thorough understanding of anatomy and physiology because:

- Understanding how the human body functions as an integrated whole is a key component in understanding how a client's hair, skin, and nails may react to various treatments and services.
- You will need to be able to recognize the difference between what is considered normal and what is considered abnormal for the body in order to determine whether specific treatments and services are appropriate.
- Understanding the bone and muscle structure of the human body will help you to realize and use the proper application of services and products for scalp manipulations and facials.

Essential Concepts

What do I need to learn about cells and anatomy and physiology to be more effective as a cosmetologist?

The cell is the basic structure from which all other body structures are made. You will want to develop a comfortable knowledge about cell growth and metabolism. You will want a basic knowledge of each of the main systems of the body and of tissue. Once you've gained information about how each organ or system functions and its purpose, you can be more effective in the services you provide.

Essential Experience 1

Mind Map Cell Development

Mind mapping creates a free-flowing outline of material or information. The central or key point is located in the center. The key point of this mind map is process of development from a basic cell to various types of tissue to forming organs to developing systems. Using color will increase the mind's retention of the material. Keep your mind open and uncluttered, and don't worry about where a line or word should go as the organization of the map will generally take care of itself.

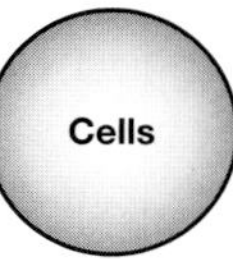

2 Essential Experience

Organs

Label each of the organs indicated in the diagram of a human body. State the purpose of each part of the body in the space provided. You may need to refer to your school's reference library for assistance.

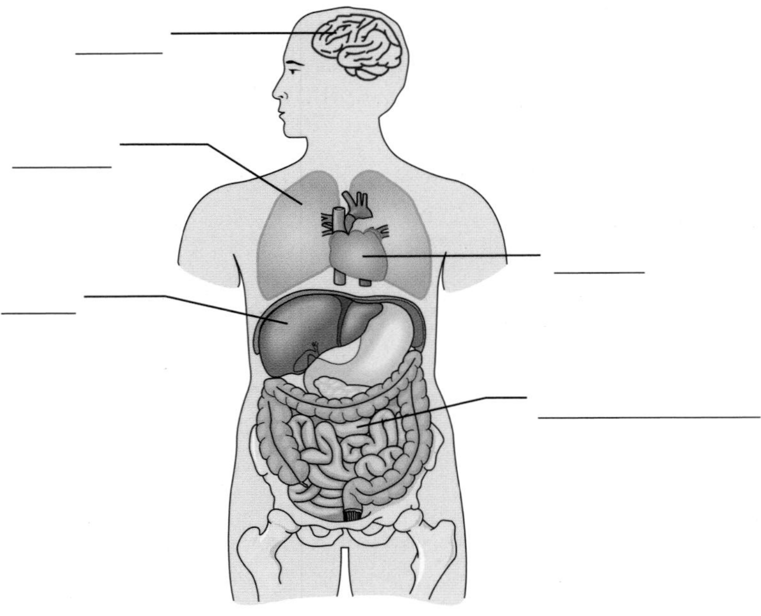

Brain: ________________________________

____

____

Heart: ________________________________

____

Lungs: ________________________________

____

Liver: ________________________________

____

Digestive tract: __________________________

____

Essential Experience 3

Matching Exercise A

Match each of the following essential terms with its definition.

______ Circulatory	**1.** Duct glands and ductless glands
______ Digestive	**2.** Process of converting food into a form that can be assimilated by the body
______ Endocrine	**3.** Physical foundation or framework of the body
______ Excretory	**4.** Situated in the chest cavity, protected by the ribs
______ Integumentary	**5.** Covers, shapes, and supports the skeleton; produces all body movements
______ Muscular	**6.** Made up of the skin and its various accessory organs
______ Nervous	**7.** Organs for reproducing
______ Reproductive	**8.** Carries waste and impurities away from the cells; protects the body from disease by developing immunities and destroying disease-causing microorganisms
______ Lymphatic	**9.** Controls and coordinates the functions of all the other systems and makes them work harmoniously and efficiently
______ Respiratory	**10.** Kidneys, liver, skin, intestines, and lungs; purifies the body by eliminating waste matter
______ Skeletal	**11.** Controls the steady circulation of the blood

4 Essential Experience

Matching Exercise B

Match each of the following essential terms with its function.

	Word	Clue
______	Frontalis	**1.** Enables closing of eye
______	Orbicularis oculi	**2.** Muscle covering lower back
______	Pectoralis	**3.** Assists in swinging of arms
______	Serratus anterior	**4.** Rotates arms
______	Biceps	**5.** Assists in breathing and raising arms
______	Trapezius	**6.** Raises the eyebrows; wrinkles forehead
______	Triceps	**7.** Lifts forearm and flexes elbow
______	Extensors	**8.** Extends arm outward and to side of body
______	Flexors	**9.** Extends forearm
______	Latissimus dorsi	**10.** Allow the wrist to bend and flex
______	Deltoid	**11.** Straighten wrist, hand, and fingers

Essential Experience 5

Matching Exercise C

Match each of the following essential terms with its function.

	Word	Clue
_______	Pronators	**1.** Draw fingers together
_______	Supinator	**2.** Draws the scalp backward
_______	Abductors	**3.** Covers, shapes, and supports skeleton
_______	Muscular system	**4.** Coordinates opening and closing of mouth
_______	Occipitalis	**5.** Rotates palm upward
_______	Epicranial aponeurosis	**6.** Separate the fingers
_______	Masseter	**7.** Lowers jaw and lip
_______	Adductors	**8.** Lowers and rotates the head
_______	Platysma	**9.** Turn hands inward
_______	Sternocleidomastoideus	**10.** Draws eyebrow down and wrinkles forehead vertically
_______	Corrugator	**11.** Connects occipitalis and frontalis

6 Essential Experience

Bones and Muscles of the Cranium

Using a shaved mannequin or a Styrofoam head block, draw a line from the center front hairline to the center nape. On side one, draw in and label the bones of the head. On side two, draw in and label the muscles of the head. (Refer to your text for assistance.) In the absence of a mannequin or head block, use the diagrams below.

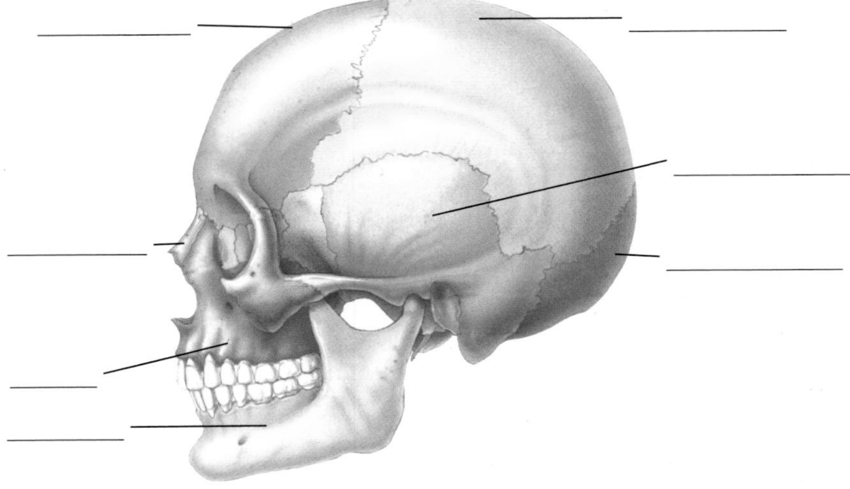

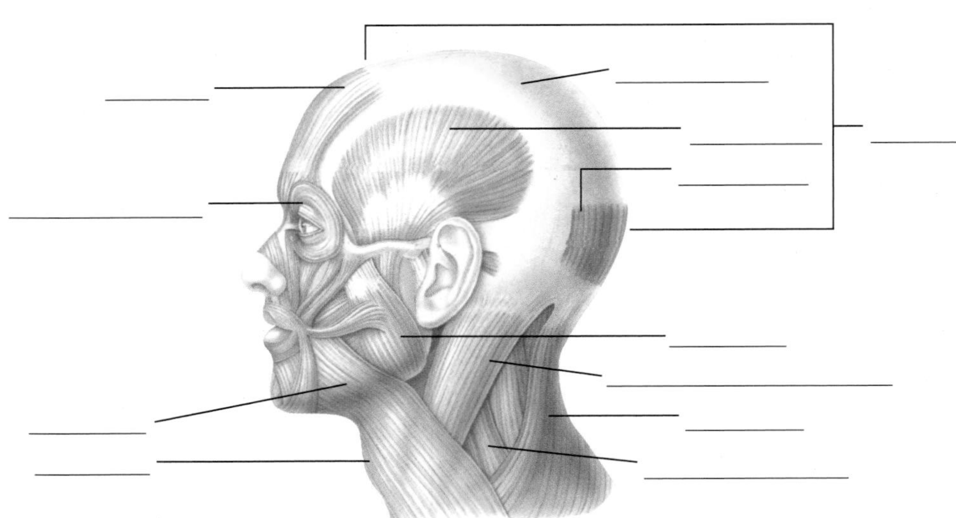

Essential Experience 7

Word Search A

After determining the correct word from the clues provided, locate the words in the word search puzzle.

Word	Clue
______________	Thick-walled muscular and elastic tubes that carry pure blood from the heart to the capillaries
______________	Right or left upper thin-walled chambers of the heart
______________	The nutritive fluid circulating through the circulatory system
______________	Minute, thin-walled blood vessels that connect smaller arteries to veins
______________	The main source of blood supply to the head, face, and neck

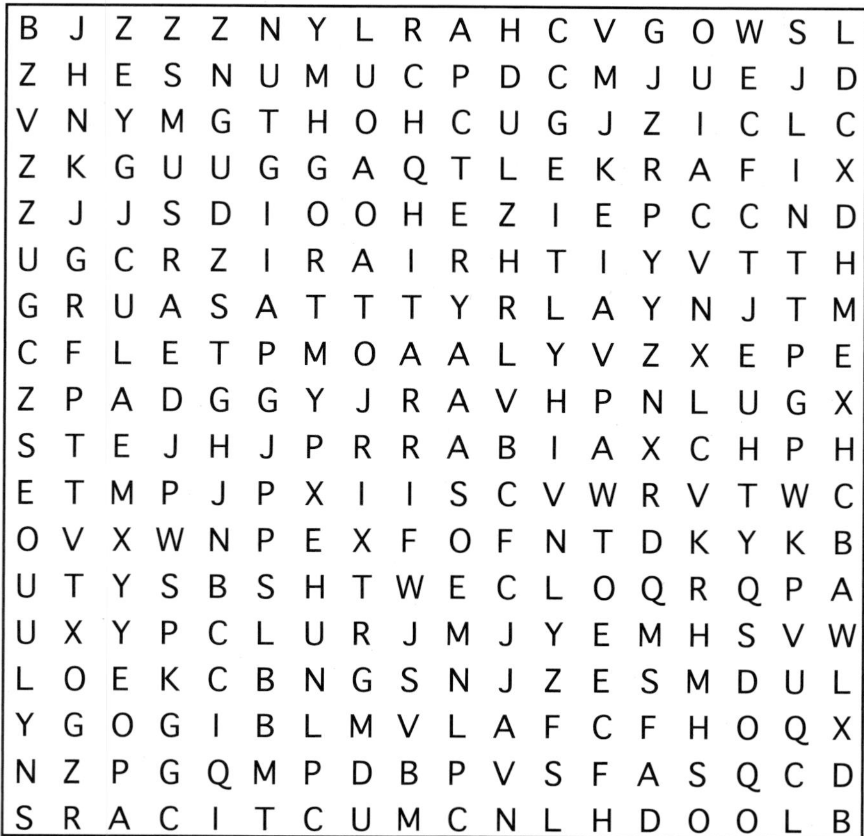

8 Essential Experience

Word Search B

After determining the correct word from the clues provided, locate the words in the word search puzzle.

Word	Clue
________________	A clear, yellowish fluid that carries waste and impurities away from the cells
________________	The fluid part of the blood in which the red and white blood cells and blood platelets flow
________________	Blood circulation that goes from the heart to the lungs to be purified
________________	Artery that supplies the thumb side of the arm and the back of the hand
________________	Artery that supplies the little finger side of the arm and the palm of the hand
________________	Allow blood to flow in only one direction
________________	The circulatory system
________________	Thin-walled blood vessels that are less elastic than arteries
________________	Right or left lower thick-walled chambers of the heart

G	T	G	O	D	V	D	M	N	R	A	X	Z	M	H	V	Z	V
F	Z	I	E	X	E	A	N	G	K	B	M	N	P	A	U	Q	V
J	R	I	K	O	M	B	L	S	I	C	O	M	C	U	H	M	J
L	P	U	S	S	V	H	X	V	A	I	Y	A	H	A	Y	R	E
Q	N	D	E	B	T	C	O	Y	E	L	H	W	O	H	N	C	V
D	T	F	Q	F	I	B	I	V	R	S	E	S	R	B	X	T	U
D	R	I	S	Z	H	S	E	V	S	A	A	W	U	A	F	L	G
Y	Q	B	Y	X	D	N	A	Z	G	D	N	M	A	C	T	H	V
D	J	M	F	O	T	S	S	J	Z	Q	Z	O	S	C	B	Y	P
C	U	G	H	R	C	L	B	F	H	Z	X	R	M	A	K	Q	F
D	R	M	I	U	A	C	U	E	O	S	H	K	A	L	L	B	D
N	B	C	L	I	S	X	B	V	U	W	J	S	O	Z	U	P	N
V	L	A	D	C	W	F	H	Q	N	P	U	J	S	L	C	P	J
E	R	A	L	S	A	B	A	U	H	K	Y	P	F	P	Y	O	X
B	R	G	F	V	L	U	D	J	P	B	E	F	X	F	L	F	R
Y	A	A	D	P	W	X	P	W	P	M	T	A	R	A	N	L	U
O	A	R	C	G	G	R	Q	Q	T	P	Z	I	S	N	I	E	V
J	Q	R	K	C	G	J	R	U	X	D	J	X	Z	D	N	M	P

Essential Review

Complete the following review of Chapter 6, General Anatomy & Physiology, by circling the correct answer to each statement.

1. The uppermost and largest bone of the arm is the ____________.

a) humerus
b) radius
c) ulna
d) metacarpus

2. The structure of the cell found in the center, which plays an important part in cell reproduction, is the ____________.

a) nucleus
b) centrosome
c) cell membrane
d) nucleolus

3. The involuntary muscles that function automatically are called ____________.

a) striated
b) striped
c) nonstriated
d) cardiac

4. To grow and thrive, the cell must receive an adequate supply of food, oxygen, and ____________.

a) toxins
b) poisons
c) pressure
d) water

5. A group of cells of the same kind are ____________.

a) organs
b) tissues
c) systems
d) groups

6. The artery that supplies the back of the head up to the crown is the ____________.

a) supraorbital
b) occipital
c) facial artery
d) posterior auricular

7. The process of building up larger molecules from smaller ones is called ____________.

a) anabolism
b) homeostasis
c) catabolism
d) secretion

8. The small bone on the thumb side of the forearm is the ____________.

a) humerus
b) radius
c) ulna
d) metacarpus

9. The muscle that produces the contour of the front and inner side of the upper arm is called the

a) cardiac b) tricep
c) bicep d) epicranius

10. The epicranius consists of two parts, the frontalis and the ____________.

a) aponeurosis b) dorsalis
c) corrugator d) occipitalis

11. Structures designed to accomplish a specific function are ____________.

a) organs b) tissues
c) systems d) groups

12. Cells are made up of a colorless, jellylike substance called ____________.

a) nucleolus b) nucleus
c) protoplasm d) centrosome

13. The study of the structure of the body and what it is made of is ____________.

a) physiology b) histology
c) anatomy d) osteology

14. The ____________ system changes food into soluble form, suitable for use by the cells of the body.

a) endocrine b) respiratory
c) excretory d) digestive

15. The wrist, or ____________, is a flexible joint composed of eight small, irregular bones.

a) metacarpus b) ulna
c) carpus d) digits

16. The ____________ vascular system consists of the heart and blood vessels for the circulation of the blood.

a) lymph b) circulatory
c) lymphatic d) blood

17. The process of breaking down larger substances or molecules into smaller ones is ____________.

a) anabolism
b) homeostasis
c) catabolism
d) secretion

18. The study of the minute structural parts of the body, such as tissues, hair, nails, sweat glands, and oil glands is ____________.

a) physiology
b) histology
c) anatomy
d) osteology

19. The fingers, or ____________, consist of three phalanges in each finger, and two in the thumb, totaling 14 bones.

a) metacarpus
b) ulna
c) carpus
d) digits

20. The scientific study of bones, their structure, and functions is ____________.

a) physiology
b) histology
c) anatomy
d) osteology

21. The elastic, bony cage that serves as a protective framework for the heart, lungs, and other internal organs is the ____________.

a) sternum
b) clavicle
c) scapula
d) thorax

22. The part of the cell that contains food materials necessary for growth, reproduction, and self-repair is the ____________.

a) cytoplasm
b) centrosome
c) nucleolus
d) cell membrane

23. The ____________ system's function is to produce all movements of the body.

a) circulatory
b) skeletal
c) muscular
d) nervous

24. The physical foundation of the body is the ____________ system.

a) circulatory
b) skeletal
c) muscular
d) nervous

25. Voluntary muscles that are controlled by will are called ____________.

a) striated b) smooth
c) nonstriated d) cardiac

26. The ____________ bone forms the lower back part of the cranium.

a) parietal b) temporal
c) frontal d) occipital

27. The part of the muscle that moves is the ____________.

a) origin b) belly
c) insertion d) middle

28. The ____________ system is made up of the skin and its various accessory organs.

a) endocrine b) excretory
c) integumentary d) reproductive

29. The muscle that completely surrounds the margin of the eye socket is the ____________.

a) corrugator b) orbicularis oculi
c) procerus d) orbicularis oris

30. The ____________ vertebrae form the top part of the spinal column located in the neck region.

a) cervical b) thorax
c) hyoid d) thoracic

31. The ____________ bone forms the forehead.

a) parietal b) temporal
c) frontal d) occipital

32. The muscle that forms a flat band around the upper and lower lip is the ____________.

a) caninus b) mentalis
c) orbicularis oris d) buccinator

33. A broad muscle that extends from the chest and shoulder to the side of the chin is the ____________.

a) pectoralis
b) serratus anterior
c) platysma
d) supinator

34. The ____________ turn the hand outward and palm upward.

a) pectoralis
b) serratus anterior
c) platysma
d) supinator

35. The muscle that straightens the wrist, hand, and fingers to form a straight line is the ____________.

a) opponent
b) adductor
c) extensor
d) abductor

36. The ____________ muscles draw the fingers together.

a) opponent
b) adductor
c) extensor
d) abductor

37. The ____________ system controls and coordinates the functions of all the other systems and makes them work harmoniously.

a) circulatory
b) skeletal
c) muscular
d) nervous

38. The ____________ and the temporalis coordinate in opening and closing the mouth and are referred to as chewing muscles.

a) triangularis
b) risorius
c) zygomaticus
d) masseter

39. There are three main divisions of the nervous system: the central, the ____________, and the autonomic nervous systems.

a) peripheral
b) sympathetic
c) parasympathetic
d) brain

40. The ____________ assists the swinging movements of the arm.

a) pectoralis nubir
b) serratus anterior
c) platysma
d) supinator

Essential Review continued

41. The ____________ nerve supplies the thumb side of the arm and back of hand.

a) ulnar
b) radial
c) median
d) digital

42. The lower thick-walled chambers of the heart are the left and right ____________.

a) atrium
b) ventricle
c) auricle
d) valves

43. Minute, thin-walled blood vessels that connect the smaller arteries to the veins are the ____________.

a) arteries
b) veins
c) capillaries
d) blood

44. The ____________ system is situated within the chest cavity, which is protected on both sides by the ribs.

a) endocrine
b) respiratory
c) excretory
d) digestive

45. ____________ circulation is the blood circulation from the heart throughout the body and back again to the heart.

a) Systemic
b) Plasma
c) Pulmonary
d) Platelet

46. The fluid part of the blood in which the red and white blood cells and blood platelets flow is ____________.

a) lymph
b) corpuscles
c) leukocytes
d) plasma

47. Gland-like structures that help fight infection are known as ____________.

a) lymph nodes
b) corpuscles
c) leukocytes
d) plasma

48. The artery that supplies the crown and side of the head is the ____________.

a) parietal
b) transverse
c) temporal
d) frontal

Essential Review continued

49. The system that purifies the body by eliminating waste material is the ____________ system.

a) endocrine
b) respiratory
c) excretory
d) digestive

50. The collar bone that joins the sternum and scapula is called the ____________.

a) humerus
b) ulna
c) radius
d) clavicle

Essential Discoveries and Accomplishments

In the space below, jot some notes about what concepts of this chapter were hardest for you to understand or remember. Imagine finding yourself suddenly in the role of "teacher" and consider what you would tell your "students" about these concepts. Share your Essential Discoveries with some of the other students in your class and ask if they are helpful to them. You may want to revise your discoveries based on good ideas shared by your peers.

Discoveries:

List at least three things you have accomplished since your last entry that relate to your career goals.

Accomplishments:

CHAPTER 7

Skin Structure, Growth, & Nutrition

A Motivating Moment: "Work as though you would live forever, and live as though you would die today."

— Og Mandino

Essential Objectives

After studying this chapter and completing the Essential Companion components, you will be able to:

1. **Describe the structure and composition of the skin.**
2. **List the functions of the skin.**
3. **List the classes of nutrients essential for good health.**
4. **List the food groups and dietary guidelines recommended by the U.S. Department of Agriculture (USDA).**
5. **List and describe the vitamins that can help the skin.**

Essential Histology of The Skin

Why do I need to learn about the skin structure and growth when I really want to specialize as a hair designer?

You actually do not need the level of knowledge that a scientist would have on this subject matter. However, a thorough knowledge of the underlying structures of the skin, nails, and hair will benefit you in your role as a professional cosmetologist. The skin is the largest and one of the most important organs of the body. Therefore, it becomes one of the most important subjects about which you need to know because so many cosmetology services deal directly with the skin—whether you are providing hair and/or scalp service, facial or skin care service, or nail care service. All these services require you to come in direct contact with clients' skin. Knowledge of the skin will help you achieve the best possible results when performing these treatments, while also providing the safest care for your clients. Remember, happy clients come back and often bring their friends with them. That means greater financial success for you.

Cosmetologists should study and have a thorough understanding of skin structure, growth, and nutrition because:

- Knowing the skin's underlying structure and basic needs is crucial in order to provide excellent skin care for clients.
- You will need to recognize adverse conditions, including skin diseases, inflamed skin, and infectious skin disorders so that you can refer clients to medical professionals for treatment when necessary.
- Twenty-first century skin care has entered the realm of high technology, so you must learn about and understand the latest developments in ingredients and state-of-the-art delivery systems in order to help protect, nourish, and preserve the health and beauty of your clients' skin.

Essential Concepts

What do I need to know about the structure and growth of the skin in order to perform professionally as a cosmetologist?

Skin care is one of the fasting growing areas of the cosmetology industry. By thoroughly analyzing the functions, structure, and components of the skin, you will better understand how the skin actually works. You will learn that with proper care, your skin and the skin of your clients can remain young and look radiant for many years. You will need to understand how the skin is nourished and how the various glands affect the functions of the skin.

1

Essential Experience

Analysis of the Epidermis

Using the chart below, analyze the structure of the epidermis. The first column lists each layer; in the second column, explain what quality this structure adds to the skin; and in the third column, list the purpose of the layer.

Layer	Composition	Purpose
Stratum corneum		
Stratum lucidum		
Stratum granulosum		
Stratum spinosum		
Stratum germinativum		

Essential Experience 2

Skin Layer Reconstruction

Using various household items or food products, create a model cross-section of the following layers of the skin.

- Basal cell layer (stratum germinativum)
- Stratum spinosm
- Stratum granulosum
- Stratum lucidum
- Stratum corneum
- Papillary layer
- Reticular layer
- Subcutaneous tissue

Either paste your items in the space provided or use poster board to make a larger model. (Hint: Items you might use include Rice Krispies, corn flakes, Fruit Loops, honey, a slice of bread, and/or a soft flour tortilla.) Once you've built your model, compare it to Figure 7–2 in your textbook.

3 Essential Experience

Matching Exercise

Match each of the following essential functions of the skin with its description.

_______ Protection	**1.** Sebum or oil that lubricates the skin keeping it soft and pliable; oil keeps hair soft; emotional stress can increase the flow of sebum
_______ Sensation	**2.** Perspiration from the sweat glands is eliminated through the skin; water lost through perspiration takes salt and other chemicals with it
_______ Heat regulation	**3.** The skin shields the body from injury and bacterial invasion; outermost layer of the epidermis is covered with a thin layer of sebum, thus rendering it waterproof; resistant to wide variations in temperature, minor injuries, chemically active substances, and many forms of bacteria
_______ Excretion	**4.** Through the nerve endings, skin responds to heat, cold, touch, pressure, and pain; when nerve endings are stimulated, a message is sent to the brain that directs you to respond accordingly
_______ Secretion	**5.** An ingredient or chemical can enter the body through the skin and influence it to a minor degree; fatty materials, such as lanolin creams, are taken in largely through hair follicles and sebaceous gland openings
_______ Absorption	**6.** The skin protects the body from the environment by maintaining a constant internal body temperature of about 98.6 degrees Fahrenheit; as changes occur in the outside temperature, the blood and sweat glands make necessary adjustments and the body is cooled by the evaporation of sweat

Essential Experience 4

Crossword Puzzle

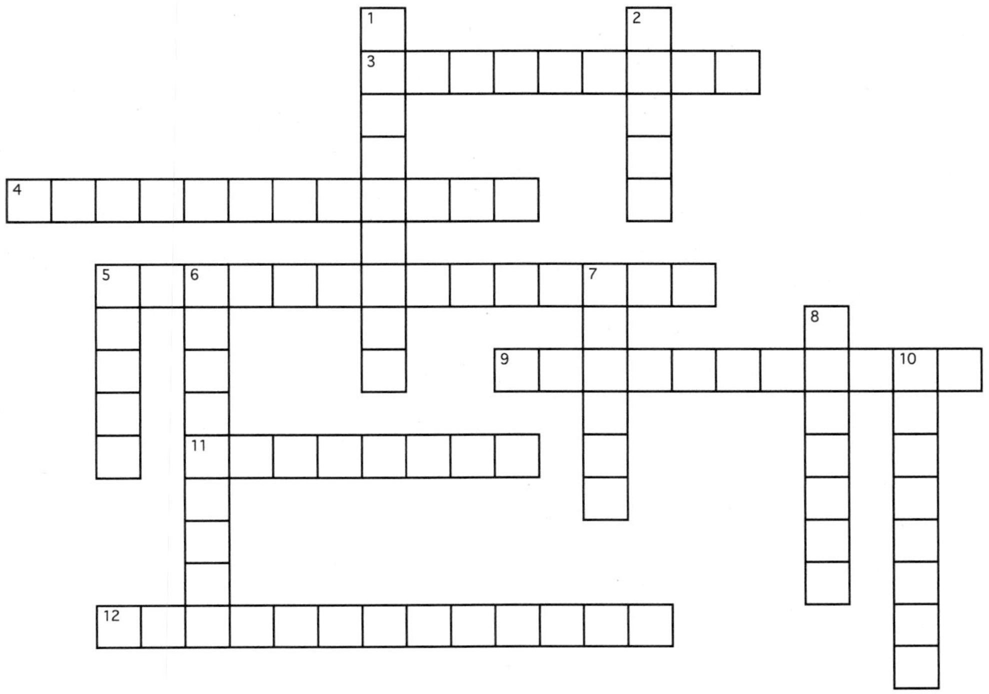

Across

Word	Clue
____________	**3.** Cuticle layer of the dermis
____________	**4.** Fatty layer found below the dermis
____________	**5.** Clear, transparent layer of skin
____________	**9.** Medical branch of science that deals with the study of skin
____________	**11.** Fibrous protein that gives the skin form and strength
____________	**12.** Physician engaged in the science of treating the skin, its structures, functions, and diseases

Down

Word	Clue
____________	**1.** Outermost layer of the skin
____________	**2.** Layer of skin referred to as the stratum germinativum
____________	**5.** Layer of skin referred to as the stratum spinosum
____________	**6.** The deeper layer of the dermis
____________	**7.** Underlying or inner layer of the skin
____________	**8.** Protein base similar to collagen; forms elastic tissue
____________	**10.** Layer of skin referred to as the stratum granulosum

Essential Review

Complete the following review of Chapter 7, Skin Structure, Growth, & Nutrition, by circling the correct answer to each statement.

1. The clear layer of the epidermis, consisting of small transparent cells, is the ____________.

a) stratus lucidum b) stratum granulosum
c) stratum corneum d) stratum germinativum

2. The basal cell layer, composed of several layers of different shaped cells, is the ____________.

a) stratum lucidum b) stratum granulosum
c) stratum corneum d) stratum germinativum

3. The outermost layer of the skin is the ____________.

a) dermis b) subcutaneous
c) epidermis d) adipose

4. The dermis is about ____________ times thicker than the epidermis.

a) 10 b) 25
c) 35 d) 40

5. The ____________ layer of the dermis houses the nerve endings that provide the body with the sense of touch.

a) papillary b) reticular
c) corium d) cutis

6. The ____________ layer of the skin contains numerous blood vessels, lymph vessels, nerves, sweat glands, oil glands, and hair follicles as well as arrector pili muscles.

a) subcutaneous b) dermis
c) adipose d) epidermis

7. The underlying or inner layer of the skin is the ____________.

a) dermis b) subcutaneous
c) epidermis d) adipose

8. ____________ is secreted by the sudoriferous glands.

a) Perspiration b) Blood
c) Odor d) Sebum

9. The ____________ controls the excretion of sweat.
   a) circulatory system b) nervous system
   c) excretory system d) respiratory system

10. A fatty layer found below the dermis is the ____________.
   a) dermis b) subcutaneous tissue
   c) epidermis d) true skin

11. The skin responds to heat, cold, touch, pressure, and pain through stimulation of the ____________.
   a) internal body temperature b) sudoriferous glands
   c) sensory nerve endings d) body fluid absorption

12. No oil glands are found in the ____________.
   a) palms b) face
   c) forehead d) scalp

13. Vitamin ____________ has been shown to improve the skin's elasticity and thickness.
   a) A b) B
   c) C d) D

14. Vitamin ____________ enables the body to properly absorb and use calcium.
   a) A b) B
   c) C d) D

15. Drinking pure water sustains the health of the cells, aids in the elimination of toxins and waste, helps regulate body temperature, and aids in proper ____________.
   a) osmosis b) metabolism
   c) digestion d) congestion

16. The secretory nerves, which are distributed to the sweat and oil glands of the skin, are part of the ____________.
   a) circulatory system b) autonomic nervous system
   c) excretory system d) respiratory system

Essential Review continued

17. ____________ supplies nutrients and oxygen to the skin.

a) Lymph | b) Nerves
c) Blood | d) Sweat

18. Vitamin ____________ helps fight against and protect the skin from the harmful effects of the sun's rays.

a) A | b) C
c) D | d) E

19. Vitamin ____________ is vitally important in fighting the aging process and promotes the production of collagen.

a) A | b) C
c) D | d) E

20. Small epidermal structures with nerve endings that are sensitive to touch and pressure are ____________.

a) tactile corpuscles | b) sudoriferous glands
c) subcutaneous tissue | d) sebaceous glands

Essential Discoveries and Accomplishments

In the space below, jot some notes about what concepts of this chapter were hardest for you to understand or remember. Imagine finding yourself suddenly in the role of "teacher" and consider what you would tell your "students" about these concepts. Share your Essential Discoveries with some of the other students in your class and ask if they are helpful to them. You may want to revise your discoveries based on good ideas shared by your peers.

Discoveries:

____

____

____

____

____

____

____

____

____

____

____

List at least three things you have accomplished since your last entry that relate to your career goals.

Accomplishments:

____

____

____

____

____

CHAPTER 8 Skin Disorders & Diseases

A Motivating Moment: "The big lesson of life is never be scared of anyone or anything. Fear is the enemy of logic."
— Frank Sinatra

Essential Objectives

After studying this chapter and completing the Essential Companion components, you will be able to:

1. Recognize common skin lesions.
2. Describe the disorders of the sebaceous glands.
3. Name and describe changes in skin pigmentation.
4. Identify the forms of skin cancer.
5. Understand the two major causes of acne and how to treat them.
6. List the factors that contribute to the aging of the skin.
7. Explain the effects of overexposure to the sun on the skin.
8. Understand what contact dermatitis is and know how it can be prevented.

Essential Disorders of the Skin

Why do I need to learn about skin diseases and disorders when I really want to specialize as a hair designer?

As a practitioner in the field of cosmetology one of your primary responsibilities will be to help clients acquire and maintain healthy attractive skin, but not to actually diagnose skin disorders or diseases. However, becoming aware of basic clinical symptoms of various skin disorders will allow you to better serve your clients. If a condition is not serious, as a professional, you will be trained to make appropriate recommendations for controlling the condition. It is critical for you to be able to recognize those conditions that require a physician's care or might be infectious and spread disease from one person to another. So, yes, while you are not studying to become a dermatologist, you need a thorough knowledge of the skin and its disorders to help you protect both your client and yourself from harm.

Cosmetologists should study and have a thorough understanding of skin disorders and diseases for the following reasons:

- In order to provide even the most basic of skin care services, you must understand the underlying structure of the skin and common skin problems.
- You must be able to recognize adverse conditions, including inflamed skin conditions, skin diseases, and infectious skin disorders, and you must know which of these conditions are treatable by the cosmetologist and which need to be referred to a medical doctor.
- Knowing about and being able to offer skin care treatments adds another dimension of service for your clients.

Essential Concepts

What do I need to know about the histology of the skin in order to perform professionally as a cosmetologist?

You need to become familiar with common disorders and diseases of the skin and recognize those conditions that cannot be treated or serviced by a cosmetologist. You will need to recognize the many disorders the skin can experience and know how to treat them. The chapter also contains a significant number of new terms and definitions that will be meaningful to you in your career as a cosmetologist.

Essential Experience 

Primary and Secondary Lesions

Write the definition of each of the primary and secondary lesions listed.

Macule ______________________________

____

Papule ______________________________

____

____

Wheal ______________________________

____

Tubercle ______________________________

____

Tumor ______________________________

Vesicle ______________________________

____

____

Bulla ______________________________

____

Pustule ______________________________

____

Cyst ______________________________

____

____

Scale ______________________________

Crust ______________________________

____

____

1 Essential Experience continued

Excoriation ______________________________

____

Fissure ______________________________

____

Ulcer ______________________________

____

Nodule ______________________________

____

Scar ______________________________

____

Keloid ______________________________

____

Essential Experience

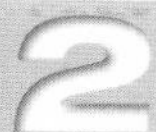

Crossword Puzzle A

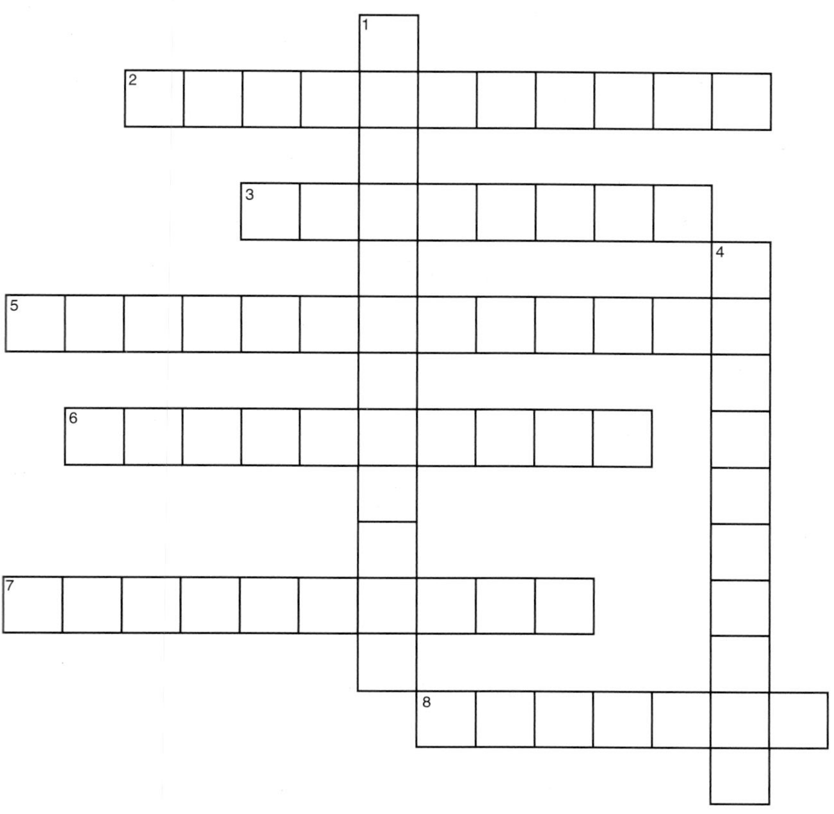

Across

Word	Clue
________________	**2.** Skin sore or abrasion from scratching or scraping
________________	**3.** Blackhead
________________	**5.** Excessive sweating
________________	**6.** Deficiency in perspiration
________________	**7.** Inflammatory skin condition
________________	**8.** Protein that forms elastic tissue

Down

Word	Clue
________________	**1.** Foul-smelling perspiration
________________	**4.** Dry, scaly skin caused by old age and exposure to cold

3 Essential Experience

Crossword Puzzle B

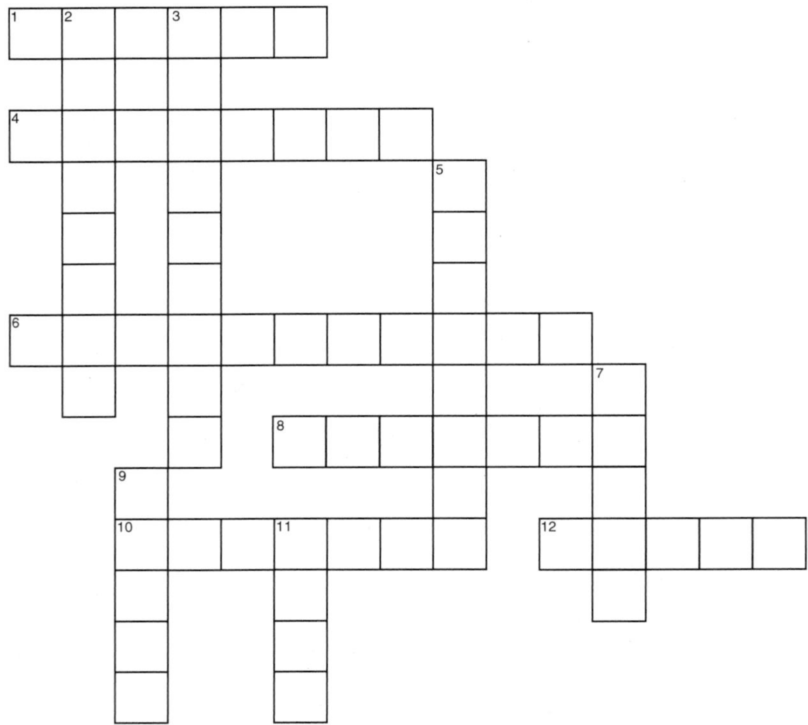

Across

Word	Clue
________________	**1.** Inflammatory, painful itchy disease
________________	**4.** Absence of melanin pigment
________________	**6.** Study of skin
________________	**8.** Crack in the skin
________________	**10.** Chronic congestion on cheeks and nose
________________	**12.** Large blister

Down

Word	Clue
________________	**2.** Protein giving skin form and strength
________________	**3.** Outermost layer of skin
________________	**5.** Increased skin pigmentation in spots
________________	**7.** Malformation of skin due to abnormal pigmentation
________________	**9.** Dead cells that form over a wound
________________	**11.** Characterized by chronic inflammation of the sebaceous glands

Essential Experience

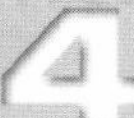

Word Search

After identifying the correct word from the clues provided, locate the words in the word search puzzle.

Word	Clue
________________	Closed, abnormally developed sac, containing fluid, semifluid, or morbid matter, above or below the skin
________________	Abnormal growth of the skin
________________	Skin disorder characterized by light abnormal patches
________________	Small, brownish spot or blemish on the skin
________________	Inflamed pimple containing pus
________________	Skin condition caused by abnormal increase of secretion from the sebaceous glands
________________	Abnormal brown or wine-colored skin discoloration with a circular and irregular shape
________________	Sebaceous cyst or fatty tumor.
________________	Abnormal rounded, solid lump above, within, or under the skin; larger than a papule
________________	An abnormal cell mass resulting from excessive multiplication of cells, varying in size, shape, and color
________________	Open lesion on the skin or mucous membrane of the body, accompanied by pus and loss of skin depth
________________	Technical term for wart; hypertrophy of the papillae and epidermis
________________	Milky-white spots (leukoderma) of the skin; acquired condition
________________	Itchy, swollen lesion that lasts only a few hours; caused by a blow, an insect bite, urticaria, or the sting of nettle

4 Essential Experience continued

K	T	S	V	F	R	E	K	G	K	B	V	Q	A	Y	B	C	W
E	N	L	K	B	C	L	D	I	A	E	L	M	L	M	I	Y	H
U	P	I	U	C	K	I	X	M	R	E	O	F	V	M	D	S	E
Y	L	D	A	Q	L	H	W	R	U	T	E	Y	A	N	T	T	A
M	H	C	B	T	E	Z	U	K	A	V	C	H	X	Y	W	V	L
U	Y	Y	E	O	S	C	O	E	I	K	Y	Z	O	Q	B	I	F
L	R	F	P	R	A	D	T	T	B	C	E	Q	G	O	Z	Y	N
I	U	U	M	E	E	S	I	W	C	J	J	F	I	V	I	K	U
R	P	E	C	R	R	L	F	V	I	Y	I	W	Y	S	T	F	U
C	O	Z	M	R	I	T	A	G	Y	Z	H	R	F	E	T	J	X
L	Z	A	O	G	J	A	R	E	E	W	H	C	G	V	R	W	F
F	U	M	O	C	G	B	G	O	H	L	E	H	X	L	O	P	L
B	U	N	M	V	L	N	X	Y	P	R	C	L	P	R	R	U	K
T	J	K	H	O	T	G	R	Z	E	H	R	R	U	D	W	V	Y
Z	S	E	U	D	V	I	T	A	C	F	Y	O	E	T	U	H	K
E	W	O	Q	Q	Y	R	U	Q	M	B	N	M	B	B	S	T	Z
H	O	Z	P	P	R	I	Z	W	A	Z	Z	R	V	E	U	U	F
M	O	L	E	A	G	O	B	X	T	P	H	X	D	F	S	T	P

Essential Experience 5

Work with a partner and create a word jingle or mnemonic to help you remember the names and descriptions of the primary and secondary lesions. Consider using a familiar tune and inserting the new terminology into it to help you and others remember important key terms.

Essential Review

Complete the following review of Chapter 8, Skin Disorders & Diseases, by circling the correct answer to each statement.

1. A chronic condition that appears primarily on the cheeks and nose and is characterized by flushing is called ____________.

a) rosacea
b) asteatosis
c) seborrhea
d) steatoma

2. An itchy, swollen lesion that lasts only a few hours is a ____________.

a) wheal
b) tubercle
c) bulla
d) macule

3. When checking existing moles for signs of cancer, look for asymmetry, differences in size and shape, and changes in diameter and ______________.

a) feel
b) smell
c) color
d) symmetry

4. Smoking, drinking, taking drugs, and making poor dietary choices greatly influence the ____________ process.

a) developmental
b) stimulation
c) sunscreen
d) aging

5. An abnormal rounded, solid lump above, within, or under the skin that is larger than a papule is known as a ____________.

a) bulla
b) cyst
c) pustule
d) tubercle

6. A thick scar resulting from excessive growth of fibrous tissue is a/an ____________.

a) excoriation
b) fissure
c) ulcer
d) keloid

7. Another name for a scar is ____________.

a) crust
b) excoriation
c) ulcer
d) cicatrix

8. A skin condition caused by an inflammation of the sebaceous glands is ____________.

a) chronic rosacea
b) retention hyperkeratosis
c) seborrheic dermatitis
d) herpes simplex

9. A blister containing a watery fluid, similar to a vesicle, but larger, is a __________.

a) wheal
b) tubercle
c) bulla
d) macula

10. __________ is a skin disease characterized by red patches, covered with silver-white scales.

a) Eczema
b) Psoriasis
c) Dermatitis
d) Herpes simplex

11. An acquired, superficial, round, thickened patch of epidermis commonly know as callus, created by pressure or friction on the hands and feet, is a __________.

a) mole
b) freckle
c) keratoma
d) verruca

12. Benign, keratin-filled cysts that can appear just under the epidermis are called __________.

a) milia
b) blackheads
c) pimples
d) ulcers

13. An acute inflammatory disorder of the sweat glands, characterized by the eruption of small red vesicles and accompanied by burning, itching skin is known as/a __________.

a) closed comedone
b) miliaria rubra
c) contact dermatitis
d) excessive anhidrosis

14. A term used to indicate an inflammatory condition of the skin is __________.

a) eczema
b) psoriasis
c) dermatitis
d) rosacea

15. An abnormal growth of the skin is called __________.

a) hypertrophy
b) hypertrichosis
c) keratoma
d) callus

16. Foul-smelling perspiration is called __________.

a) anhidrosis
b) chloasma
c) bromhidrosis
d) hypertrichosis

17. Deficiency in perspiration is called __________.

a) anhidrosis
b) chloasma
c) bromhidrosis
d) hypertrichosis

Essential Review continued

18. A small brown or flesh-colored outgrowth of the skin is called a ____________.

    a) mole
    b) macule
    c) stain
    d) skin tag

19. An abnormal brown or wine-colored skin discoloration with a circular and irregular shape is called a ____________.

    a) mole
    b) macule
    c) stain
    d) skin tag

20. A spot or discoloration on the skin, such as a freckle, is called a ____________.

    a) mole
    b) macule
    c) stain
    d) skin tag

Essential Discoveries and Accomplishments

In the space below, jot some notes about what concepts of this chapter were hardest for you to understand or remember. Imagine finding yourself suddenly in the role of "teacher" and consider what you would tell your "students" about these concepts. Share your Essential Discoveries with some of the other students in your class and ask if they are helpful to them. You may want to revise your discoveries based on good ideas shared by your peers.

Discoveries:

____

____

____

____

____

____

____

____

____

____

____

List at least three things you have accomplished since your last entry that relate to your career goals.

Accomplishments:

____

____

____

CHAPTER 9

Nail Structure & Growth

A Motivating Moment: "My great concern is not whether you have failed, but whether you are content with your failure."
— Abraham Lincoln

Essential Objectives

After studying this chapter and completing the Essential Companion components, you will be able to:

1. **Describe the structure and composition of nails.**
2. **Discuss how nails grow.**

Essential Nail Structure and Growth

I am going to be a cosmetologist; why do I need to learn about the structure of the nail?

That's a very good question. The fact is that the structure and growth of the nail is certainly not the most glamorous portion of your training in cosmetology, but it could be one of the most essential. More infections are spread through the nails and hands than any other area of the body. To give clients professional and responsible service, you must learn about the structure and function of the nail. You must know when it is safe to work on a client and when they must be referred to a doctor. You should learn about the structure and growth of the nail since it is extremely relevant to your future success and well-being as a professional cosmetologist.

Cosmetologists should study and have a thorough understanding of nail structure and growth because:

- Understanding the structure and growth of natural nails allows you to expertly groom, strengthen, and beautify nails.
- It is important to know the difference between the cuticle and the eponychium before performing nail services.
- Understanding the structure and growth cycles of the natural nail will prepare you for more advanced nail services.

Essential Concepts

What do I need to know about the nail, its structure, and growth in order to provide quality manicuring and pedicuring services?

You will need to recognize that the condition of the nail may actually reflect the general health of the whole body. You need to understand the structure of the nail and also the structures surrounding the nail. Once you understand how the nail grows, you will be better equipped to recognize the malformations, disorders, and irregularities that your clients may bring to the salon. When you've gained that knowledge, you can proceed confidently with appropriate nail services knowing that you and your client are not at risk.

Essential Experience 1

Label Cross-section of the Nail

Label the parts of the nail on the front view and cross-section diagrams using the terms listed below. Note that some essential terms may be used more than once and some not at all.

Nail bed	Eponychium
Free edge	Hyponychium
Matrix	Ligament
Lunula	Nail fold
Nail plate	Nail grooves
Cuticle	Bone

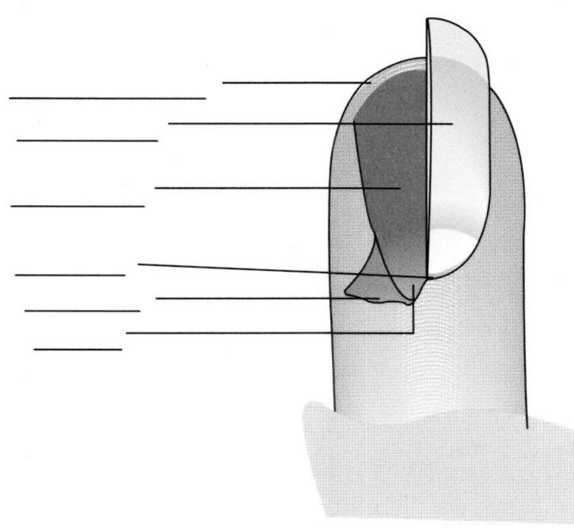

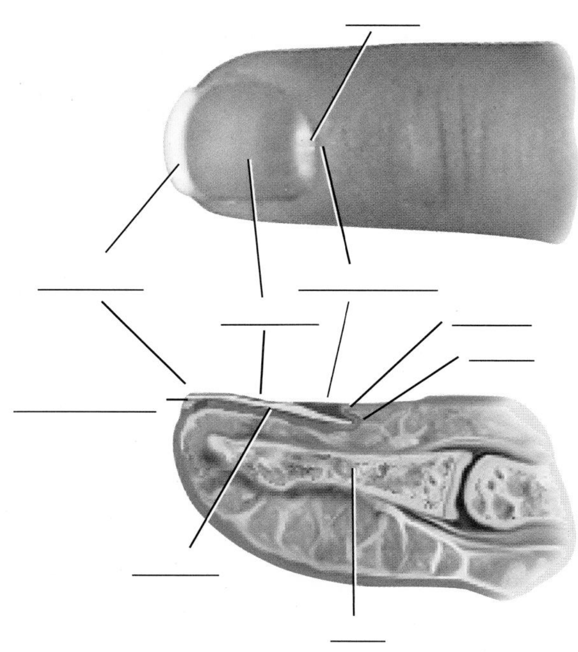

2 Essential Experience

Matching Exercise

Match the following essential terms with their identifying phrases or definition.

______	**Cuticle**	**1.**	Slits or furrows at either side of the nail, upon which the nail moves as it grows
______	**Eponychium**	**2.**	The dead colorless tissue attached to the nail plate
______	**Hyponychium**	**3.**	The slightly thickened layer of skin that lies underneath the free edge of the nail plate
______	**Matrix**	**4.**	Normal skin that surrounds the nail plate
______	**Nail grooves**	**5.**	The portion of the living skin on which the nail plate sits
______	**Nail bed**	**6.**	The living skin at the base of the nail plate covering the matrix area
______	**Nail folds**	**7.**	Where the natural nail is formed
______	**Lunula**	**8.**	The most visible and functional part of the nail
______	**Ligament**	**9.**	The part of the nail plate that extends over the tip of the finger
______	**Free edge**	**10.**	A tough band of fibrous tissue that connects bones or holds an organ in place
______	**Nail plate**	**11.**	The lighter color shows the true color of the matrix

Essential Experience 3

Word Search

After determining the correct word from the clues provided, locate the words in the word search puzzle.

Word	Clue
________________	Composed mainly of keratin
________________	Visible part of the matrix that extends from underneath the living skin
________________	Where the natural nail is formed
________________	Attaches the nail bed and matrix bed to the underlying bone
________________	Dead colorless tissue attached to the nail plate
________________	Helps guide the nail plate along the nail bed as it grows

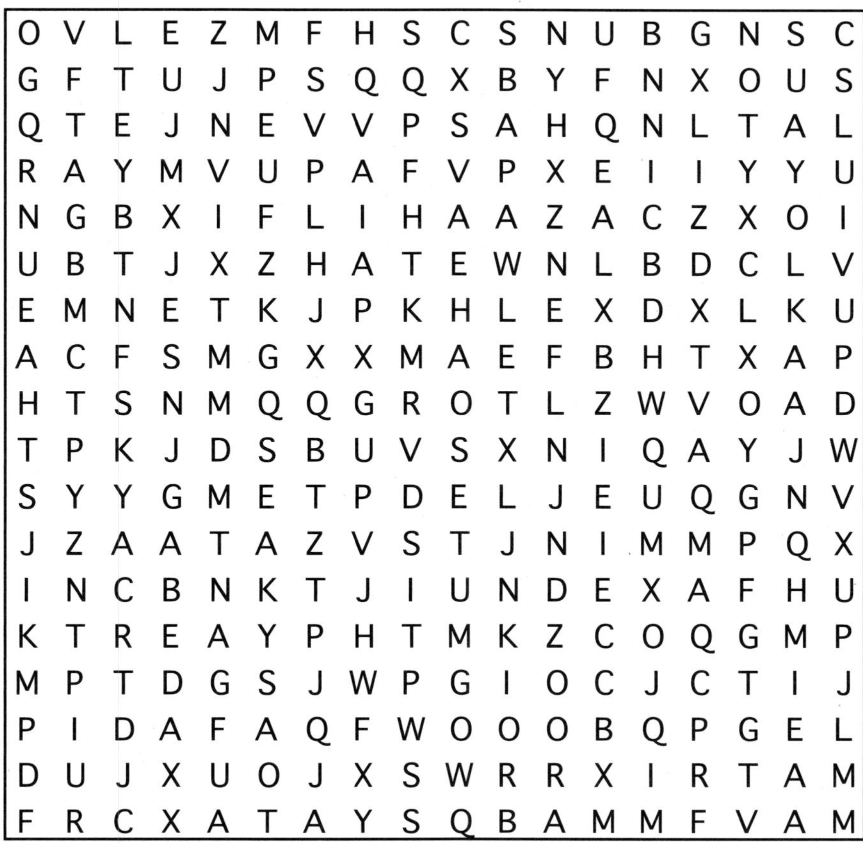

Essential Review

Complete the following review of Chapter 9, Nail Structure & Growth, by circling the correct answer to each statement.

1. The nail is an appendage of the skin and is part of the ____________.

a) circulatory system
b) skeletal system
c) integumentary system
d) muscular system

2. A healthy nail may look dry and hard, but it actually has a water content of between ____________.

a) 10 and 20 percent
b) 15 and 25 percent
c) 20 and 30 percent
d) 25 and 35 percent

3. The matrix is composed of matrix cells that produce the nail ____________.

a) lunula
b) plate
c) grooves
d) mantle

4. The nail bed is supplied with many nerves and is attached to the nail plate by a thin layer of tissue called the ____________.

a) bed epithelium
b) hyponychium
c) nail grooves
d) eponychium

5. The visible part of the matrix that extends from underneath the living skin is the ____________.

a) lunula
b) hyponychium
c) matrix
d) eponychium

6. The slits or furrows on the sides of the nail on which it moves as it grows are called the ____________.

a) nail folds
b) ligaments
c) nail plate
d) nail grooves

7. In an adult, the nail grows at an average of ____________ inch per month.

a) 1/10
b) 1/16
c) 1/4
d) 3/8

8. Ordinary replacement of a natural nail takes about ____________.

a) 2 to 4 months
b) 3 to 5 months
c) 4 to 6 months
d) 5 to 7 months

Essential Review continued

9. Toenails take ____________ months to a year to be fully replaced.

a) 4
b) 6
c) 7
d) 9

10. The sidewall of the nail is also known as the ______________.

a) whitewall fold
b) side fold
c) lateral nail fold
d) overlap fold

Essential Discoveries and Accomplishments

In the space below, jot some notes about what concepts of this chapter were hardest for you to understand or remember. Imagine finding yourself suddenly in the role of "teacher" and consider what you would tell your "students" about these concepts. Share your Essential Discoveries with some of the other students in your class and ask if they are helpful to them. You may want to revise your discoveries based on good ideas shared by your peers.

Discoveries:

List at least three things you have accomplished since your last entry that relate to your career goals.

Accomplishments:

CHAPTER 10

Nail Disorders & Diseases

A Motivating Moment: "The way I see it, if you want the rainbow, you gotta put up with the rain."
— Dolly Parton

Essential Objectives

After studying this chapter and completing the Essential Companion components, you will be able to:

1. **List and describe the various disorders and irregularities of nails.**
2. **Recognize diseases of the nails that should not be treated in the salon.**

Essential Nail Disorders and Diseases

I want to be a hairstylist, not a scientist or doctor; why do I need to learn about nail disorders and diseases?

Nail disorders and diseases are not the most glamorous portion of your training in cosmetology, but it could be one of the most essential. More infections are spread through the nails and hands than any other area of the body. You actually have a greater chance of contracting a nail disease from a client than a skin disease or head lice. Therefore, careful analysis of the client's hands and nails is essential both to your safety and that of your clients. Think about it. If you contract an infection, it may prevent you from working for an extended period of time and that will cost you money, both in lost income and medical expenses. So, learning about the diseases and disorders associated with nails is extremely relevant to your future success and well-being.

Cosmetologists should study and have a thorough understanding of nail disorders and diseases because:

- You must be able to identify any condition on a client's nails that should not be treated in the salon and those which may be treated in the salon.
- You must be able to identify infectious conditions that may be present so that you can take the appropriate steps to protect yourself and your clients from the spread of disease.
- You may be in a position to recognize conditions that may signal mild to serious health problems that warrant the attention of a doctor.

Essential Concepts

What do I need to know about nail disorders and diseases in order to provide quality manicuring and pedicuring services?

You will need to be able to discern between a disorder and an infectious disease, which must be referred to a physician for treatment. When you've gained that knowledge, you can proceed confidently with appropriate nail services knowing that you and your client are not at risk.

1 Essential Experience

Windowpane Nail Conditions

Windowpaning is the process of transferring key elements, points, or steps in a lesson into visual images that are hand sketched into the squares or *panes* of a matrix. Let your mind think in pictures and sketch the essential concepts printed in each of the following windowpanes. Don't be concerned with your artistic ability. Use lines and stick figures to depict the concepts requested for the various conditions of the nail.

Bruised Nails
Ridges
Eggshell Nails
Beau's Line
Hangnail
Leukonychia
Melanonychia
Onychophagy
Plicatured Nail

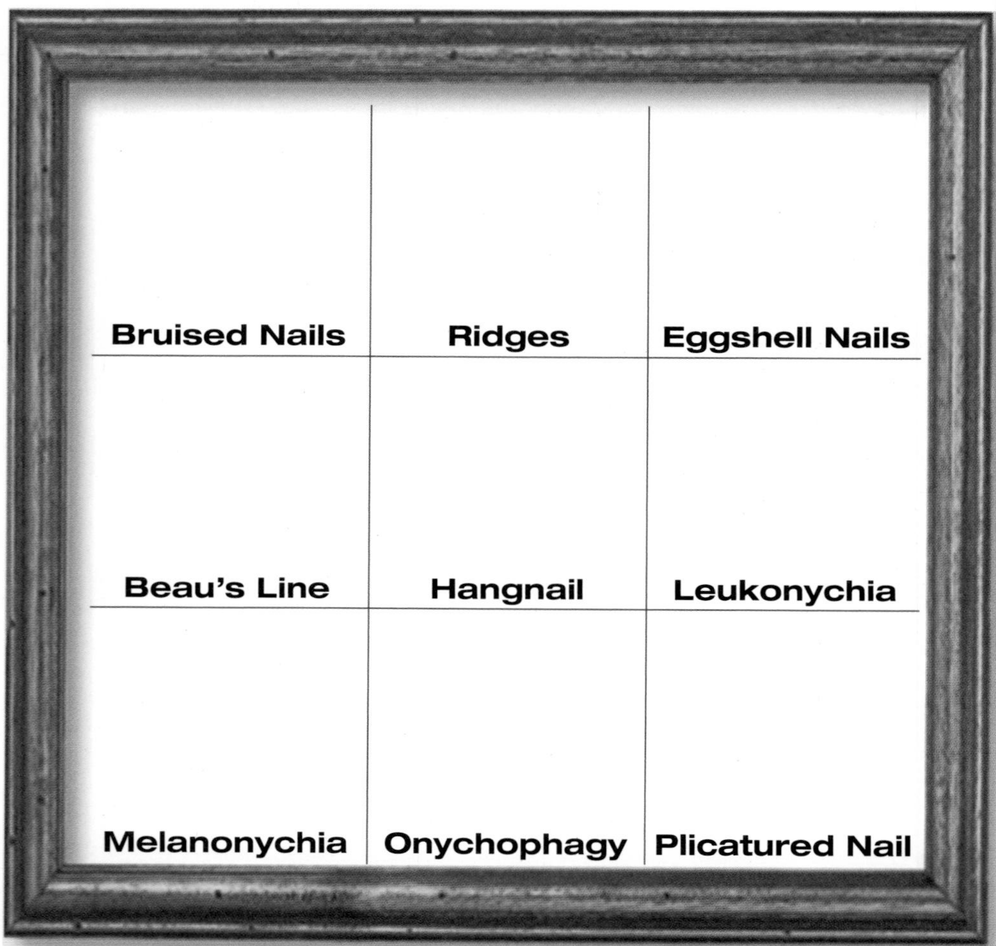

Essential Experience 2

Nail Disorders, Irregularities, and Diseases

Label each of the following pictures or illustrations using the terms below. Use your standard textbook and other references in the school's library to assist you.

Eggshell nail front view	Hangnail	Onychophagy
Eggshell nail end view	Leukonychia spots	Onychorrhexis
Beau's lines	Melanonychia	Plicatured nail

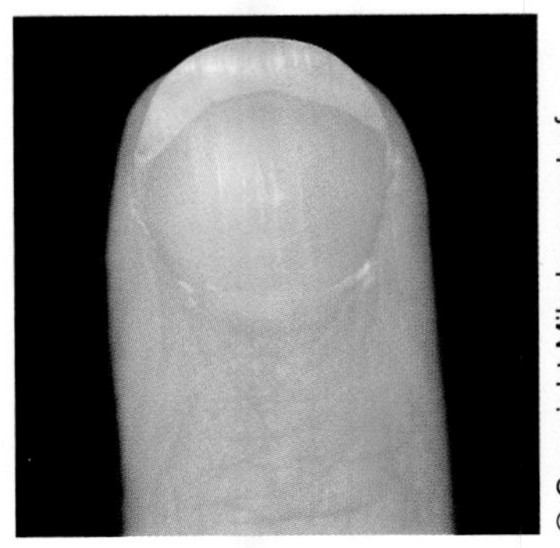

____

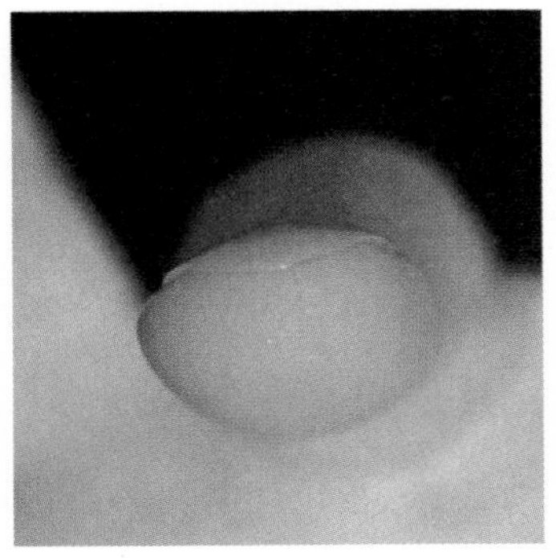

____

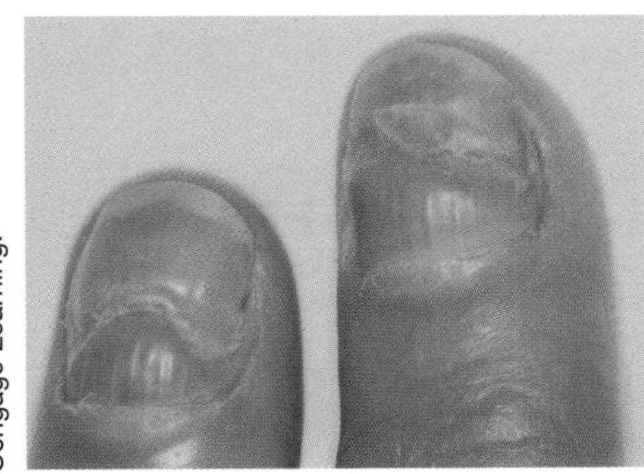

____

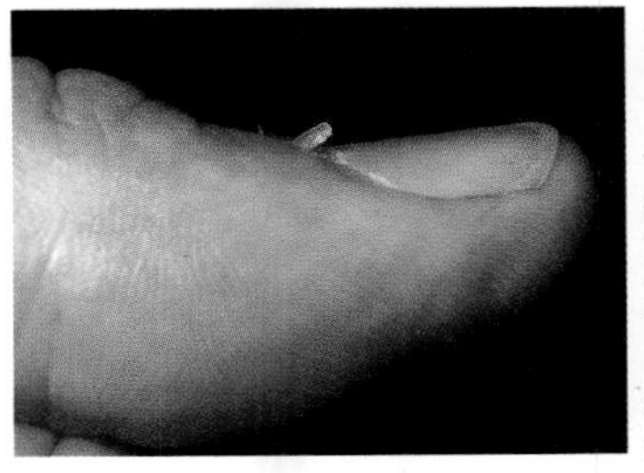

____

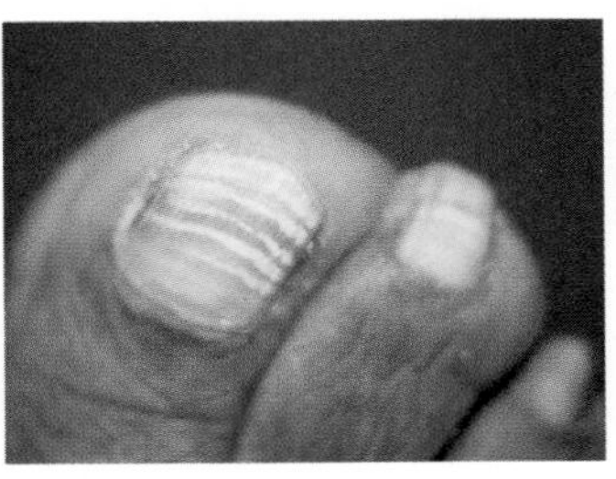

____

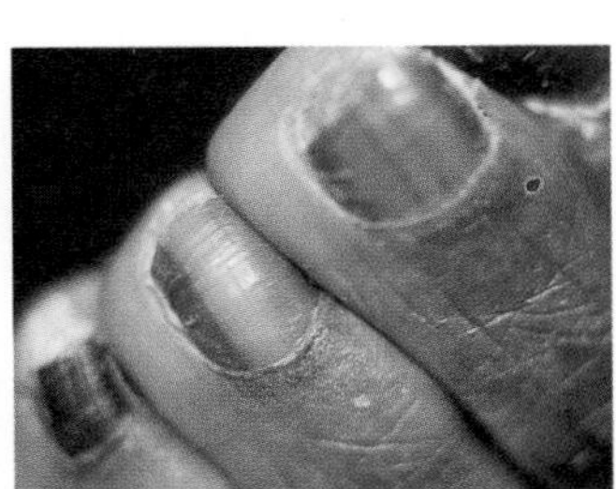

____

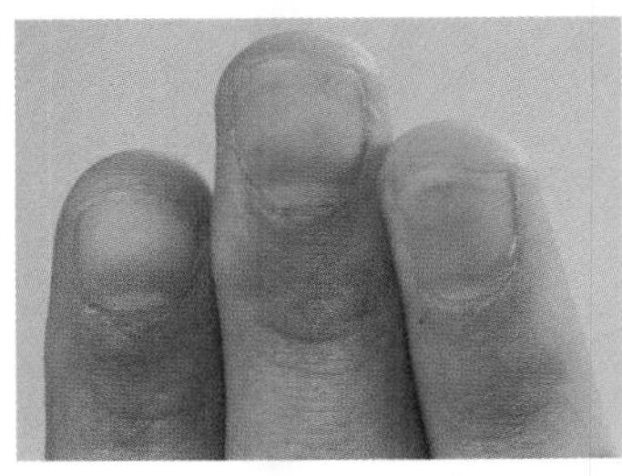

____

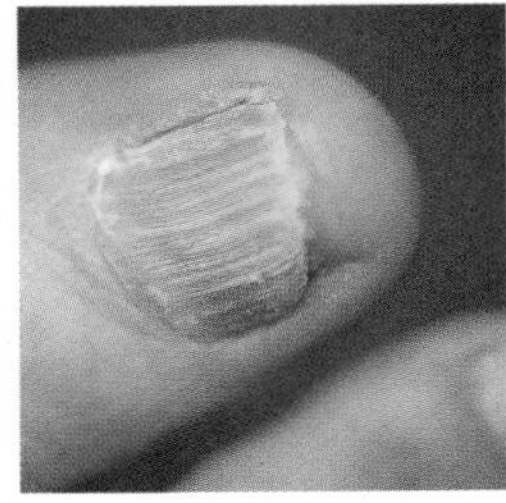

____

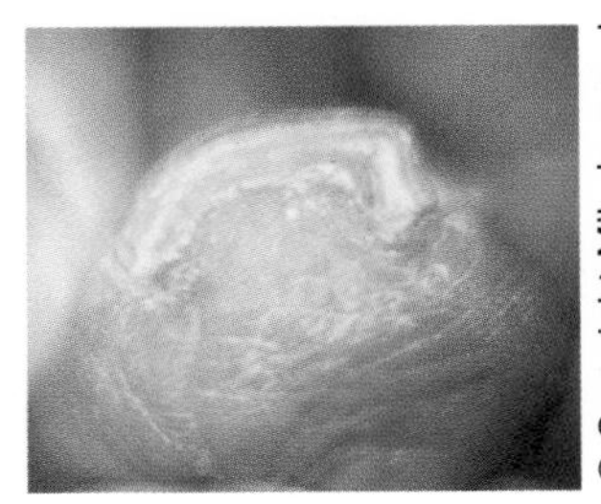

____

2 Essential Experience continued

Onychocryptosis
Onycholysis
Onychomadesis
Nail psoriasis
Paronychia
Pyogenic granuloma
Tinea pedis
Onychomycosis

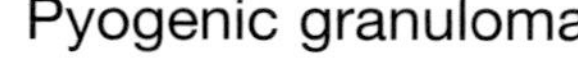

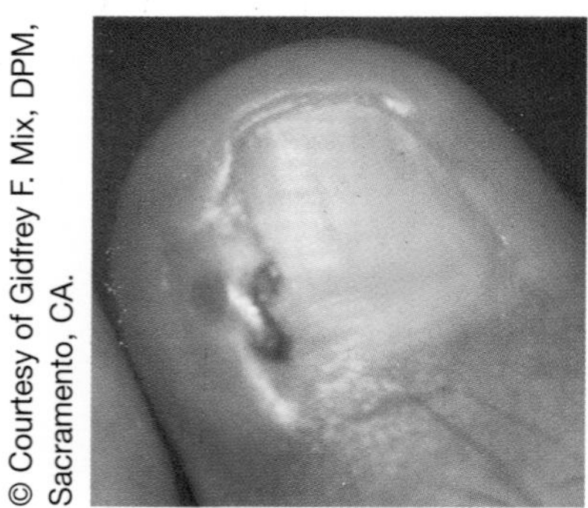

© Courtesy of Gidfrey F. Mix, DPM, Sacramento, CA.

____

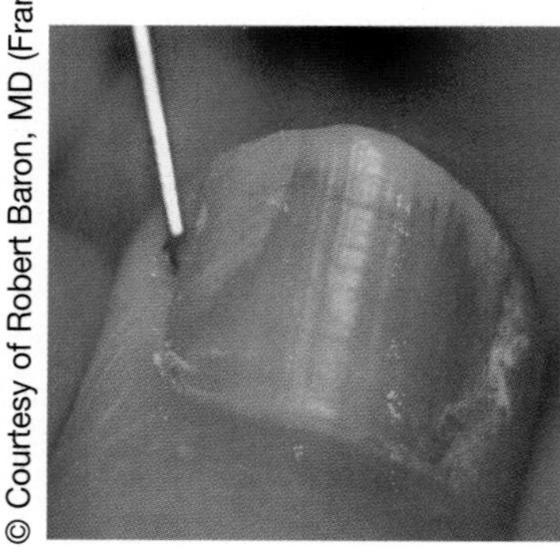

© Courtesy of Robert Baron, MD (France).

____

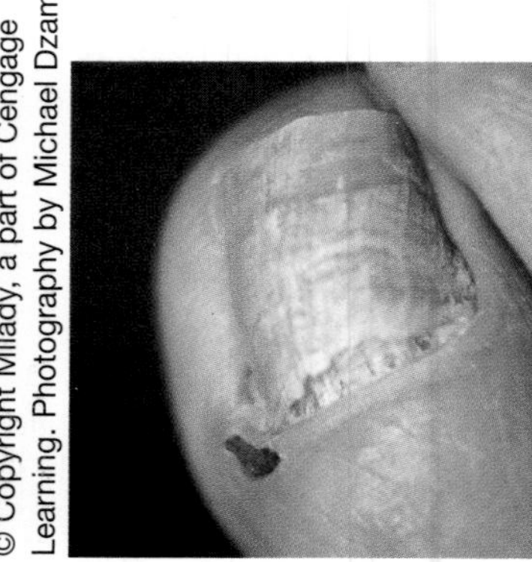

© Copyright Milady, a part of Cengage Learning. Photography by Michael Dzaman.

____

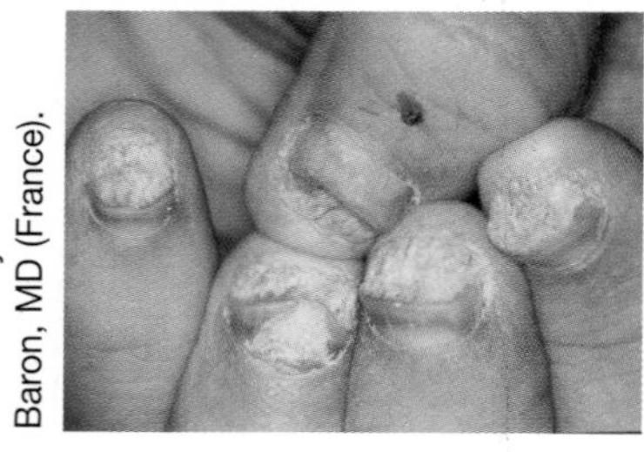

© Courtesy of Robert Baron, MD (France).

____

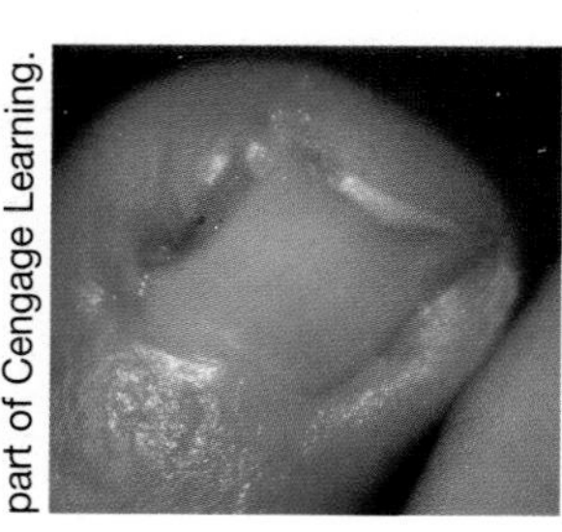

© Copyright Milady, a part of Cengage Learning.

____

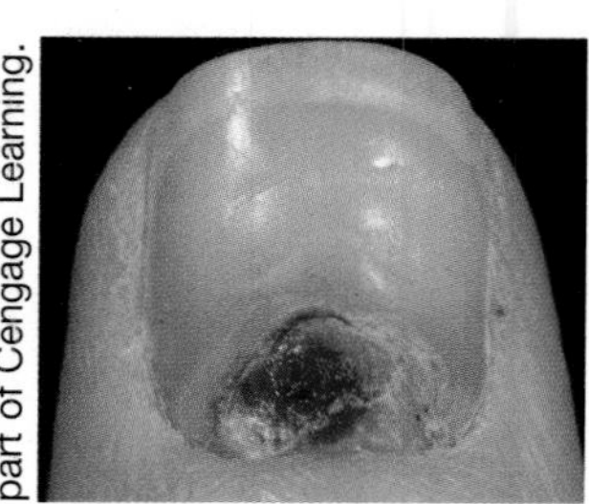

© Copyright Milady, a part of Cengage Learning.

____

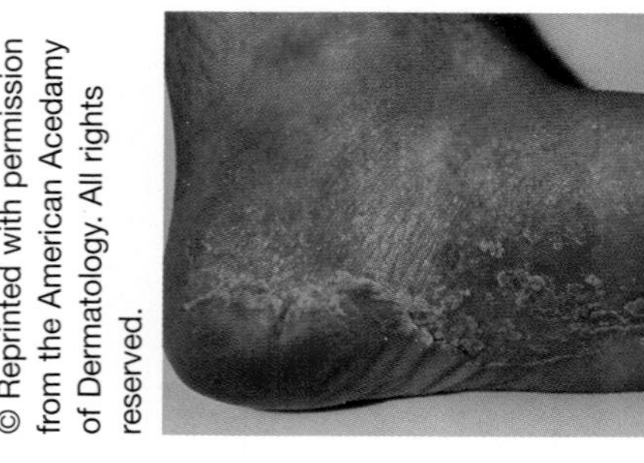

© Reprinted with permission from the American Acedamy of Dermatology. All rights reserved.

____

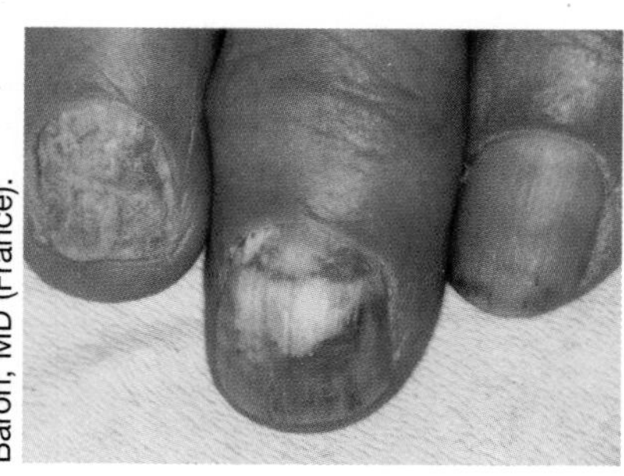

© Courtesy of Robert Baron, MD (France).

____

Essential Experience 3

Matching Exercise

Match the following essential terms with their respective common term or identifying phrase.

______	**Bruised nail**	**1.**	Bitten nails
______	**Melanonychia**	**2.**	Living skin splits around nail
______	**Leukonychia**	**3.**	Surface of nail plate appears rough and pitted
______	**Nail psoriasis**	**4.**	Blood clot under nail plate
______	**Onychomycosis**	**5.**	White spots
______	**Pterygium**	**6.**	Fungal infection
______	**Onychophagy**	**7.**	Darkening of fingernails or toenails
______	**Onychorrhexis**	**8.**	Noticeably thin, white nail plates; more flexible than normal nails
______	**Eggshell**	**9.**	Any deformity or disease of the nails
______	**Hangnail**	**10.**	Inflammation of surrounding tissues
______	**Onychosis**	**11.**	Fungal infections of the feet
______	**Tinea pedis**	**12.**	Ingrown nails
______	**Paronychia**	**13.**	Severe inflammation of the nail in which a lump of red tissue grows up from nail bed to nail plate
______	**Pyogenic granuloma**	**14.**	Skin is stretched by the nail plate
______	**Onychia**	**15.**	Split or brittle nails
______	**Onychocryptosis**	**16.**	Inflammation of matrix with formation of pus and shedding of the nail
______	**Splinter hemorrhages**	**17.**	Associated with hard impact or physical trauma

4 Essential Experience

Word Search A

After determining the correct word from the clues provided, locate the words in the word search puzzle.

Word	Clue
______________	Fungal infection of the feet
______________	Dark purplish spots due to injury
______________	Folded nail
______________	Run vertically down the length of natural nail
______________	Thin, white nail plate and more flexible than normal nails
______________	May cause infections of the feet and hands
______________	White spots in the nail
______________	Split or brittle nails
______________	Darkening of the fingernails or toenails
______________	Visible depressions across the width of the nail plate
______________	Bitten nails

A	G	E	T	I	N	E	A	P	E	D	I	S	J	P	C	F	U
L	R	L	N	P	H	I	Y	Z	H	V	V	H	K	Z	E	N	I
G	X	E	F	I	L	Y	D	M	N	I	K	N	S	B	G	J	S
C	Y	U	O	X	L	I	G	J	Z	I	B	C	L	B	Z	E	N
T	D	K	I	F	L	S	C	Y	K	R	H	Q	E	H	G	E	X
P	Z	O	Z	R	A	T	U	A	N	B	T	A	C	D	G	M	Z
A	J	N	C	X	F	Q	S	A	T	U	M	D	I	G	K	P	X
I	L	Y	Y	O	A	C	H	Y	E	U	Z	R	S	Z	Q	H	K
H	I	C	G	C	T	J	X	Y	W	B	R	H	V	U	H	X	W
C	A	H	A	F	Y	A	B	G	H	E	E	E	S	U	U	A	U
Y	N	I	H	A	V	J	M	R	D	L	C	F	D	R	H	I	U
N	D	A	P	N	V	T	H	D	L	Q	W	K	U	N	R	J	R
O	E	T	O	J	D	H	S	N	U	Z	F	B	J	N	A	Y	R
N	S	N	H	B	C	P	A	D	B	E	F	P	O	Z	G	I	P
A	I	C	C	K	K	I	O	P	Z	G	B	W	O	B	H	I	L
L	U	Z	Y	K	L	P	R	X	N	U	U	D	T	U	A	D	V
E	R	T	N	S	X	J	U	J	E	J	V	S	Y	K	K	K	Z
M	B	V	O	C	S	I	X	E	H	R	R	O	H	C	Y	N	O

Essential Experience 5

Word Search B

After determining the correct word from the clues provided, locate the words in the word search puzzle.

Word	Clue
____________________	Separation or falling off of a nail plate
____________________	Deformity or disease of the nail
____________________	Lifting of the nail plate
____________________	Severe inflammation of the nail
____________________	Inflammation of the nail matrix
____________________	Ingrown nails
____________________	Bacterial inflammation of surrounding tissue of the nail
____________________	Tiny pits or severe roughness
____________________	A fungal infection of the nail plate

O O O L D V Y A I H C Y N O R A P A
I N N O M L C G C M D Y Z B P W M H
E W Y Y K S X B L M W L D U J O A V
P F T C C Y B G X H O W D U L J P J
S S Y O H H I R S L U Y M U C A J F
I B K H Q O I G T G Z Y N R V S Q S
S O N H H I C A Q R Q A M S C U V I
O M D K U E R R L K R H P G Q T S S
C R X Q H P P V Y G P L S D Q O I E
Y N E Q D D Z N C P K M K J J S S D
M Z W W V L U I Q G T V B X T I Y A
O E J I K H N K D P O O J J I S L M
H I L C G E X V I A C F S C D O O O
C W S K G W M B W J A F X I K H H H
Y L J O O H K Z S B Z C Y R S C C C
N W Y C A U W A L F W Z D U W Y Y Y
O P R L F L Z D B C I U N Z M N N N
N A I L P S O R I A S I S X O O O O

6 Essential Experience

Technical Term Mnemonics

Mnemonics are aids that can be used to assist your memory. They can be words or phrase associations, songs, or any other method that will trigger in your memory key terms or information contained in a lesson. For example, if you were trying to remember the three primary areas of haircutting, **b**lunt, **g**raduated, and **l**ayered, you might make up a sentence using the first letter of each type of haircutting. In this case, the mnemonic might be **B**renda **G**ot **L**ost. Using this learning tool, try to develop a mnemonic for each of the following technical terms in the study of the nail. For example: Ony**chop**tosis is the periodic shedding or falling off of the nail. Within the technical term is the word *chop*. You might relate the word *chop* to the chopping off or falling of the nail and remember the meaning of onychoptosis. Give it a try with the other terms. Don't limit yourself to words. You can draw pictures or visualize circumstances that will cause you to remember the technical term.

1. Beau's line

____

____

2. Leukonychia spots

____

____

3. Melanonychia

____

____

4. Onychophagy

____

____

5. Onychorrhexis

____

____

6. Plicatured nail

____

____

7. Pterygium

____

____

8. Onychosis

____

____

9. Onychia

____

____

10. Onychocryptosis

____

____

11. Onycholysis

____

____

12. Onychomadesis

____

____

13. Psoriasis

____

____

14. Paronychia

____

____

15. Onychomycosis

____

____

Essential Review

Complete the following review of Chapter 10, Nail Disorders & Diseases, by circling the correct answer to each statement.

1. A healthy nail appears slightly in __________ color.

a) yellow
b) pink
c) blue
d) purple

2. __________ are caused by uneven growth of the nails.

a) Furrows
b) Depressions
c) Ridges
d) Pterygium

3. __________ on the nails are known as leukonychia.

a) White spots
b) Blue spots
c) White stripes
d) Vertical ridges

4. Bitten nails, a result of an acquired nervous habit, are known as __________.

a) onychauxis
b) onychatrophia
c) onychophagy
d) pterygium

5. __________ is an abnormal condition that occurs when skin is stretched by the nail plate.

a) Onychauxis
b) Onychatrophia
c) Onychophagy
d) Pterygium

6. Hangnails are treated by __________.

a) hot oil manicures
b) filing straight across
c) avoiding polish use
d) firm use of metal pusher

7. Parasites, which under some circumstances may cause infections of the feet and hands, are __________.

a) flagella
b) fungi
c) mold
d) fungus

8. Darkening of the fingernails or toenails is technically known as __________.

a) melanonychia
b) leukonychia
c) onychatrophia
d) onychauxis

9. Onychocryptosis is the technical term for __________.

a) split nails
b) bitten nails
c) bruised nails
d) ingrown nails

Essential Review continued

10. A fungal infection of the nail plate is ____________.

a) onychauxis
b) onychatrophia
c) onychophagy
d) onychomycosis

11. An infectious and inflammatory condition of the tissues surrounding the nails is known as ____________.

a) onychia
b) onychomycosis
c) paronychia
d) onychocryptosis

12. The technical term for loosening of the nail without shedding or falling off is ____________.

a) onycholysis
b) onychogryposis
c) onychomycosis
d) onychophosis

13. A growth of horny epithelium in the nail bed is known as ____________.

a) onycholysis
b) onychogryposis
c) onychophyma
d) onychophosis

14. A condition in which a blood clot forms under the nail plate is known as ____________.

a) hangnail
b) bruised nail
c) eggshell nail
d) plicatured nail

15. A condition which affects the surface of the natural nail plate, causing it to appear rough and pitted, is known as ____________.

a) nail pterygium
b) plicatured nail
c) nail psoriasis
d) pincer nails

Essential Discoveries and Accomplishments

In the space below, jot some notes about what concepts of this chapter were hardest for you to understand or remember. Imagine finding yourself suddenly in the role of "teacher" and consider what you would tell your "students" about these concepts. Share your Essential Discoveries with some of the other students in your class and ask if they are helpful to them. You may want to revise your discoveries based on good ideas shared by your peers.

Discoveries:

____

____

____

____

____

____

____

____

____

____

____

List at least three things you have accomplished since your last entry that relate to your career goals.

Accomplishments:

____

____

____

____

____

Essential Concepts

What are the key concepts a professional cosmetologist must understand in order to properly analyze a client's hair and prescribe appropriate corrective treatments?

Trichology is the technical term for the study of hair. As you proceed through your study of trichology, you will gain important insights into how the hair is distributed over the body and the scalp. You will learn that hair is composed chiefly of the protein called keratin and there are two principal parts of hair, the hair root and the hair shaft. As well as understanding the structure of hair, you will learn how it grows. Most importantly, you will learn to use the senses of sight, touch, hearing, and smell to analyze the condition of a client's hair. Key elements in hair analysis include several hair qualities, including texture, porosity, and elasticity. You will also determine that effective scalp manipulation on a regular basis will stimulate the muscles and nerves of the scalp as well as increase the blood circulation in the scalp area.

Another important area of awareness is that of hair loss and how it affects over 63 million people in the United States. This particular malady can range from the most common type of hair loss, androgenetic alopecia, which is a result of progressive shrinking or miniaturization of certain scalp follicles, to postpartum alopecia, which is a temporary hair loss after pregnancy. The professional cosmetologist must also be able to identify various diseases and disorders of the hair and scalp since they are not allowed to treat certain conditions that must be referred to a medical professional for treatment.

Essential Experience

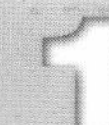

Hair Purpose

In your own words, explain the purpose of the two main types of hair found on the body: vellus and terminal hair.

Vellus: ____

____

____

____

____

____

____

____

Terminal: ____

____

____

____

____

____

____

2

Essential Experience

Hair Follicle Structure

Using the following key, label the cross-section of the hair.

arrector pili muscle	epidermis	hair shaft
bulb	hair follicle	sebaceous or oil glands
dermal papilla	hair root	

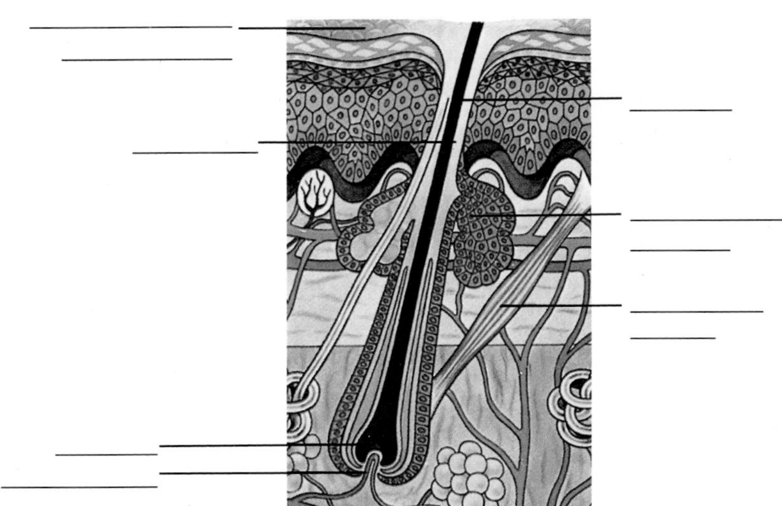

Essential Experience 3

Hair Structure

Using colored pencils or crayons, draw a cross-section of the hair and follicle depicting and labeling each of the following categories.

- Cortex
- Cuticle
- Medulla

4 Essential Experience

Hair Replacement and Growth

Hair growth occurs in cycles. Each complete cycle has three phases that are repeated over and over again throughout life. The three phases are anagen, catagen, and telogen. In your own words, please explain each phase.

Anagen: ____________________

____

____

____

____

____

Catagen: ____________________

____

____

____

____

____

____

Telogen: ____________________

____

____

____

____

____

Essential Experience 5

Directional Hair Growth

Find two individuals with distinct and different hair growth patterns. Using the following head outlines, diagram the growth patterns.

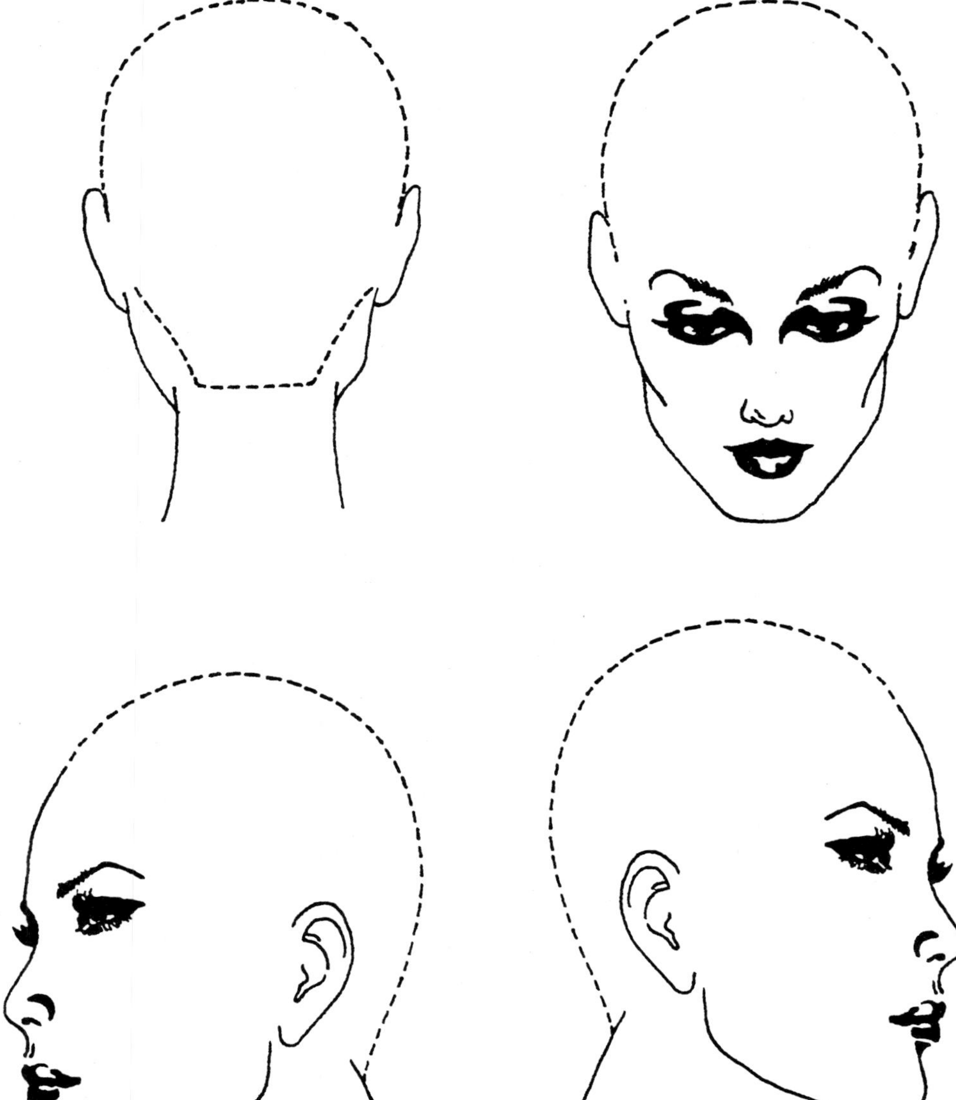

6 Essential Experience

Word Search

After determining the correct word from the clues provided, locate the words in the word search puzzle.

Word	Clue
________________	Abnormal hair loss
________________	Growth phase in the hair cycle in which new hair is created
________________	The lowest area or part of a hair strand
________________	The technical term for gray hair
________________	Inflammation of the subcutaneous tissue caused by *Staphylococci*
________________	Transitional phase of hair growth
________________	Outermost layer of hair
________________	The number of hairs per square inch (2.5 square cm) on the scalp
________________	Chemical side bond that joins the sulfur atoms of two neighboring cysteine amino acids to create cystine
________________	The ability of the hair to stretch and return to its original length
________________	Tube-like depression, or pocket, in the skin or scalp that contains the hair root
________________	Combined with crinium, it's the technical term for brittle hair
________________	Innermost layer of hair
________________	Technical term for beaded hair
________________	Dandruff
________________	The ability of the hair to absorb moisture
________________	The part of the hair structure found below the skin surface
________________	Skin disease caused by the mite
________________	Dry, sulfur-yellow, cuplike crusts on the scalp in tinea favosa or favus
________________	The portion of the hair that projects beyond the skin

Essential Experience continued 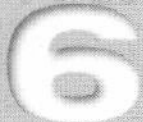

______________ The degree of coarseness or fineness of the hair

______________ Ringworm

______________ Hair that forms in a circular pattern, as on the crown

D C A D B Z J H Y A C W H O R L A E
E E A L I P A K W C T J T B A L L A
B I N T O S V V F P V O P L U C E N
N A B S A P U N T P A S B T I N E P
K O U F I G E L J Q N Z U T I G H I
E Q L X P T E C F H S C U T A Y G T
F U B U W N Y N I I S C X N T D Q Y
E T F G Y V C H T A D I A I N O V R
E F S S L P Z U Z F R E S H H L K I
L R P F M R K C A H O O B U Z I X A
A A G W J Q W L T S R L S O R I B S
S G D T J R L E E O T S L H N A E I
T I D E N U L I P R W E C I A D T S
I L R F D I T X T W H N X A C F I M
C I D E N I U W D G R I K T B L T D
I T M O N R W C U W Y S M C U I E O
T A M A K C M N S T I R O O T R E Y
Y S C C A R B U N C L E C W S Y E S

7 Essential Experience

Crossword Puzzle

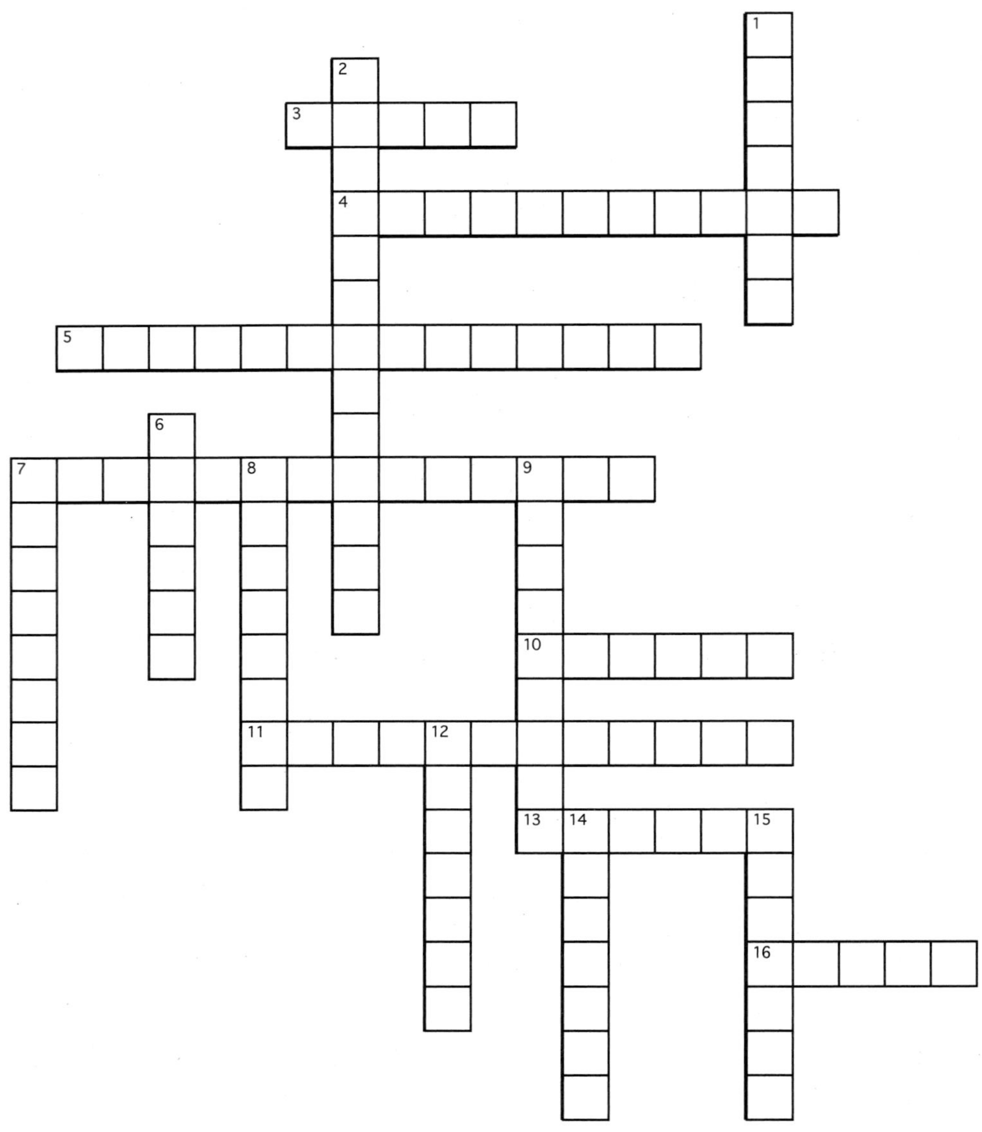

Across

Word	Clue
________________	**3.** Oily substance that lubricates the hair and skin
________________	**4.** Technical term for beaded hair
________________	**5.** Technical term for split ends
________________	**7.** Abnormal hair growth
________________	**10.** The middle layer of hair
________________	**11.** Involuntary muscle in the base of the hair follicle
________________	**13.** Hair flowing in the same direction
________________	**16.** Acids that are linked together end to end

Down

Word	Clue
________________	**1.** Chemical bond that links amino acids together
________________	**2.** Small, cone-shaped area located at the base of the hair follicle
________________	**6.** Short, fine, downy hair
________________	**7.** A weak physical side bond easily broken
________________	**8.** Long hair found on scalp, legs, arms, and bodies
________________	**12.** Tuft of hair that stands straight up
________________	**14.** Resting phase of hair cycle
________________	**15.** Pigment in the cortex, gives natural color to hair

8 Essential Experience

Grouping Properties of the Hair and Scalp by Category

Place the following terms or procedures into the appropriate category in the chart.

alopecia areata
anagen
androgenetic alopecia
arrector pili
bulb
canities
catagen
cortex
cowlick
cuticle
dandruff
density
dermal papilla
elasticity
fenasteride
fine
follicle
fragilitas crinium
hair root
hair stream
hypertrichosis
keratin
medulla
Minoxidil
monilethrix
pediculosis capitis
pityriasis
pityriasis capitis simplex
pityriasis steatoides
porosity
postpartum alopecia
scabies
telogen
texture
tinea capitis simplex
tinea
tinea favosa
trichorrhexis nodosa
trichoptilosis
vellus hair
whorl

Hair Distribution, Composition, and Structure

____

____

Hair Growth

____

Hair Analysis

____

Hair Loss

____

____

Essential Experience continued 8

Hair Disorders

Scalp Disorders

Essential Review

Using the following words, fill in the blanks below to form a thorough review of Chapter 11, Properties of the Hair & Scalp. Words or terms may be used more than once or not at all.

80 percent	**disulfide**	**polypeptide**
90 percent	**elasticity**	**porosity**
acidic	**eumelanin**	**round**
alkaline	**follicle**	**scabies**
amino acids	**hair bulb**	**scutula**
androgenetic alopecia	**hair root**	**sebaceous**
arrector pili	**hair shaft**	**sebum**
boil	**hair stream**	**simplex**
brittle	**healthy diet**	***Staphylcocci***
canities	**hydrogen**	**steatoides**
carbuncle	**hypertrichosis**	**swelling**
cells	**keratinization**	**terminal**
chemicals	**miniaturized**	**three**
cortex	**monilethrix**	**topical**
cuticle	**nodular**	**trichology**
dandruff	**one-half**	**trichoptilosis**
dermal papilla	**oval**	**unpigmented**
	pediculosis	**vellus**

1. The study of the hair is technically called____________.
2. The technical term for the hair found on the face is known as ____________.
3. One basic requisite for healthy hair is a ____________.
4. Full-grown human hair is divided into two principal parts which are known as the hair root and the ____________.
5. The two most common types of ______________ infections are furuncles and carbuncles.
6. The technical term for hair found on the head is ____________hair.
7. A tube-like depression or pocket in the skin or scalp that encases the hair root is called the ____________.
8. The thickened, club-shaped structure that forms the lower part of the hair root is known as the ____________.

Essential Review continued

9. The small involuntary muscle attached to the underside of the hair follicle is called the ____________.
10. Fear or cold causes the ____________ to contract, which makes the hair stand up straight, giving the appearance of goose bumps.
11. Oil glands which consist of a sac-like structure in the dermis are the ____________ glands.
12. An oily substance secreted from the sebaceous glands which keeps the skin surface soft and supple is ____________.
13. Hair is composed of cells arranged in ____________layers.
14. The outermost layer of the hair is called the ____________.
15. The cuticle layer of the hair can be raised by ____________.
16. The ____________ is the middle layer of the hair which gives elasticity.
17. The ____________ is that portion of the hair that projects beyond the skin.
18. The ____________is that portion of the hair that is located below the surface of the scalp.
19. The small cone-shaped area located at the base of the follicle is the ____________.
20. The average growth of healthy hair on the scalp is about __________________ inch (cm) per month.
21. Hair flowing in the same direction is known as ____________.
22. Cross-sections of straight hair tend to be ____________.
23. Hair is composed of protein that grows from cells originating within the hair follicle. They mature in a process called _____________.
24. Cross-sections of curly hair tend to be ____________.
25. Qualities by which human hair is analyzed are texture, density, __________, and __________.
26. The ability of the hair to stretch and return to its original form is _________.
27. The ability of the hair to absorb moisture is known as _________.
28. Hair is composed of protein that grows from ____________ originating within the hair follicle.
29. Hair is approximately ____________ protein.
30. The technical term for the most common type of hair loss is __________________.

Essential Review continued

31. Hair protein is made up of long chains of ____________, which are made up of elements.

32. A long chain of amino acids linked by peptide bonds is called a ____________ chain.

33. A ____________ bond is a physical side bond that is easily broken by water or heat.

34. Minoxidil is a ____________ medication applied to the scalp to stimulate hair growth.

35. The technical term for gray/unpigmented hair is ____________.

36. Salt bonds are easily broken by strong ____________ or ____________ solutions.

37. An abnormal development of hair on areas of the body that normally bear only downy hair is known as ____________ or hirsutism.

38. The technical term for split hair ends is ____________.

39. Trichorrhexis nodosa, or knotted hair, is the dry, brittle condition including formation of ____________ swellings along the hair shaft.

40. The technical term for beaded hair is ____________, which may be improved with scalp and hair treatments.

41. Fragilitas crinium is the technical term for ____________ hair that may split at any part of its length.

42. A ____________ bond joins the sulfur atoms of two neighboring amino acids.

43. Pityriasis is the medical term for ____________.

44. Two different types of melanin are ____________ and pheomelanin.

45. The two principal types of dandruff include pityriasis capitis ____________ (the dry type) and pityriasis ____________ (the greasy or waxy type).

46. Honeycomb ringworm is characterized by dry, sulfur-yellow, cup-like crusts on the scalp called ____________.

47. ____________ is a highly contagious, animal parasitic skin disease caused by the itch mite.

48. A contagious condition caused by the head louse is ____________ capitis.

49. A furuncle, or ____________, is an acute localized bacterial infection of a hair follicle.

50. A ____________ is the result of an acute staphylococci infection and is larger than a furuncle.

Essential Discoveries and Accomplishments

In the space below, jot some notes about what concepts of this chapter were hardest for you to understand or remember. Imagine finding yourself suddenly in the role of "teacher" and consider what you would tell your "students" about these concepts. Share your Essential Discoveries with some of the other students in your class and ask if they are helpful to them. You may want to revise your discoveries based on good ideas shared by your peers.

Discoveries:

List at least three things you have accomplished since your last entry that relate to your career goals.

Accomplishments:

CHAPTER 12

Basics of Chemistry

A Motivating Moment: "Never measure the height of a mountain until you have reached the top. Then you will see how low it was."

— Dag Hammarskjold

Essential Objectives

After studying this chapter and completing the Essential Companion components, you will be able to:

1. **Explain the difference between organic and inorganic chemistry.**
2. **Describe the different states of matter: solid, gas, and liquid.**
3. **Describe oxidation-reduction (redox) reactions.**
4. **Explain the difference between pure substances and physical mixtures.**
5. **Explain the difference among solutions, suspensions, and emulsions.**
6. **Explain pH and the pH scale.**

Essential Chemistry

Why is a basic knowledge of chemistry important to my career as a cosmetologist?

When you think about it, chemistry has an important role in every product you use, from the water you use to shampoo your hair, to the cosmetics applied when giving a facial, to the chemicals you apply to hair in styling or in chemical reformation. Many of the services you will provide actually change the hair, skin, and nails chemically as well as physically. Therefore, it is essential that you have a good working knowledge of chemistry in order to provide the safest and most effective services to your clients.

Cosmetologists should study and have a thorough understanding of chemistry because:

- Without an understanding of basic chemistry you would not be able to use professional products effectively and safely.
- Every product used in the salon and in cosmetology services contains some type of chemical.
- With an understanding of chemistry, you will be able to troubleshoot and solve common problems you may encounter with chemical services.

Essential Concepts

What do I need to know about basic chemistry in order to be successful and more effective as a professional cosmetologist?

Like anatomy and physiology, chemistry may be a somewhat scary subject to you. Think of it this way: chemistry is simply the study of matter, its composition, structure, properties, and the changes matter may undergo. You know that matter is anything that occupies space and has weight. Organic chemistry is the study of substances that contain the element carbon. All living things or things that were once alive, whether they are plants or animals, contain carbon. Organic substances that contain both carbon and hydrogen can burn, Inorganic chemistry, on the other hand, is the branch of chemistry that deals with all substances that do not contain carbon, such as water, air, iron, lead, minerals, and iodine. These are substances that will not burn and are usually soluble in water. Now, your goal in training as a cosmetologist is not to become a scientist, but to develop a comfort level with the basics and an ability to discuss chemistry in relation to your profession. This will increase your credibility significantly with your clients, especially during the consultation process.

Essential Experience 1

Organic versus Inorganic Chemistry

Use your knowledge of the difference between organic and inorganic substances to gather at least 10 items in each category. List your items in the space provided and explain what makes them either organic or inorganic.

Organic	Inorganic

2 Essential Experience

Product Research

Research a variety of shampoo and conditioning products available in your school, at local supply stores, or at home. Use the chart below to track your findings.

Product Name	Key Ingredients	Purpose of Each Ingredient	Prescribed for Which Hair Type?

Essential Experience 3

Matter

In the space below, list examples of how matter can change form. Be specific. For example, when you melt an ice cube (a solid), it becomes water (a liquid), and when you boil it, it becomes steam (a gas). Not all your examples will include taking on all three forms.

4 Essential Experience

Elements

An element is the basic unit of all matter. It is composed of a single part or unit and cannot be reduced to a more simple substance. There are 90 naturally occurring elements. Each element is identified by a letter symbol. The symbols for each element can be obtained by referring to the Periodic Table of Elements found in almost any chemistry textbook. Numbers are used with the elements to indicate how many parts are found in the substance. In the chart below, list the symbols for each substance and then explain its composition. (See the example for water.)

Substance	Symbol	Composition
Water		
Ammonia		
Hydrogen Peroxide		
Nitric Acid		
Sodium Hydroxide		
Sodium Chloride		
Hydrogen		
Sulfur		
Nitrogen		
Oxygen		
Carbon		
Iron		
Lead		
Silver		

Essential Experience 5

Litmus Paper Testing

Obtain a variety of products and test their acidity and alkalinity using litmus paper. List the products you are testing below and state the results. Also, brush one piece of litmus paper with hydrogen peroxide, and then brush one-half of the litmus paper with a haircolor product. You will actually be able to see the oxidation process take place.

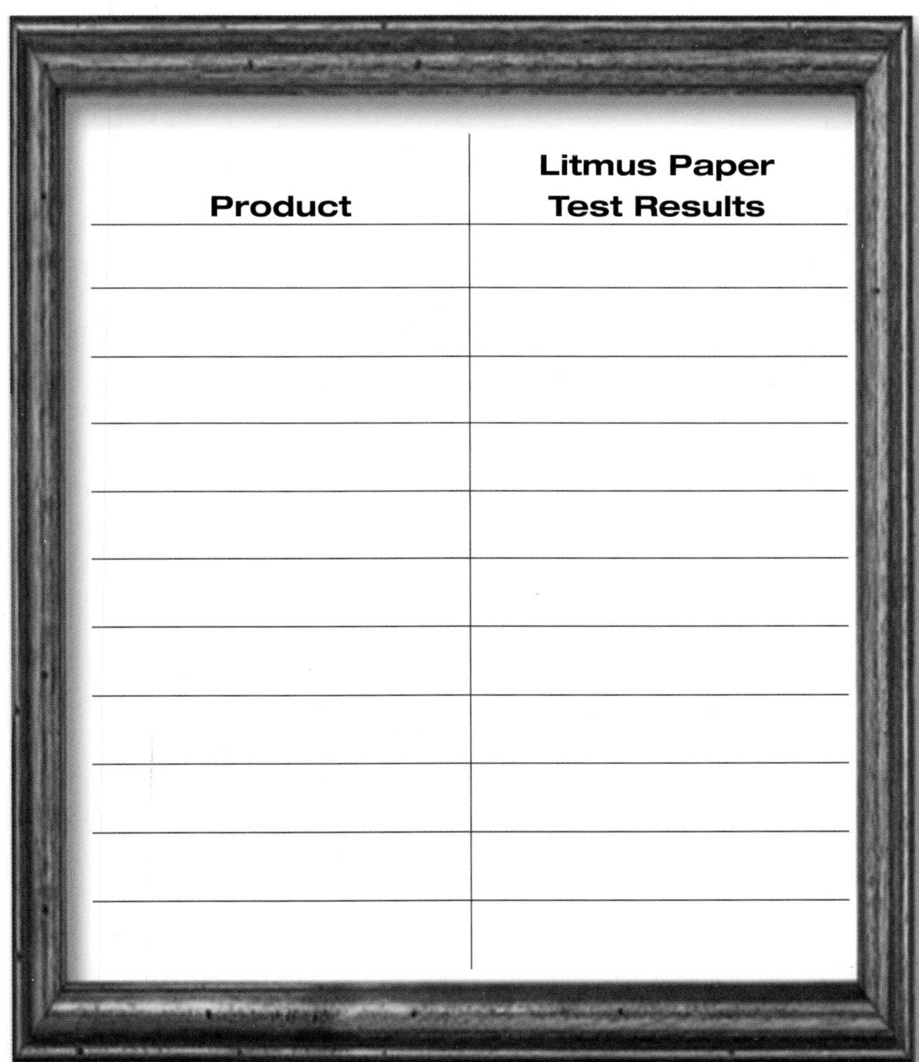

Product	Litmus Paper Test Results

6 Essential Experience

Crossword Puzzle

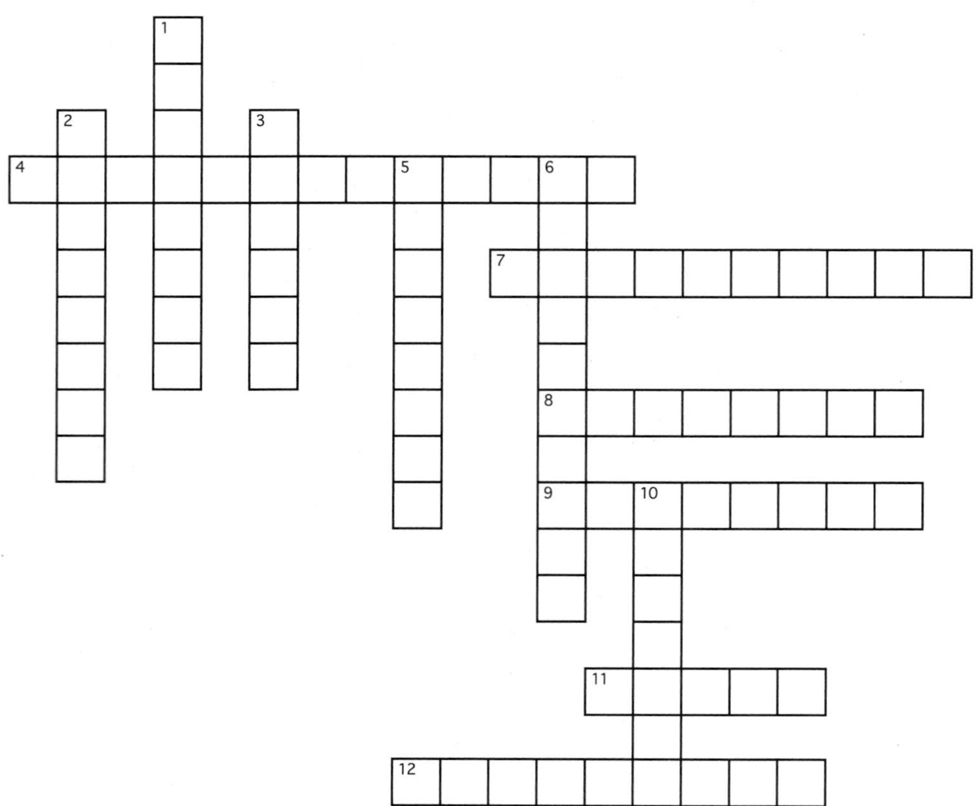

Clue

Across

4. Substances used to neutralize acids
8. Mixture of two or more immiscible substances
6. Chemical reaction that produces heat
2. Sweet, colorless, oily substance used as a moisturizing ingredient
7. The separation of an atom or molecule into positive and negative ions
9. Capable of being mixed with another liquid

Down

5. Two or more atoms joined chemically
11. Contraction for reduction-oxidation
12. The subtraction of oxygen from, or the addition of hydrogen to
3. The substance that is dissolved in a solution
10. The substance that dissolves the solute to form a solution
1. Easily evaporating

Essential Experience 7

Word Search

After determining the correct word from the clues provided, locate the words in the word search puzzle.

Word	Clue
______________	Solution having a pH below 7
______________	Solution having a pH above 7
______________	Colorless gas with pungent odor, composed of hydrogen and nitrogen
______________	The smallest particle of an element that retains the properties of that element
______________	Science that deals with the composition, structures, and properties of matter
______________	Rapid oxidation of a substance
______________	Chemical combination of two or more atoms of different elements
______________	The simplest form of matter
______________	Water-loving
______________	Not capable of being mixed
______________	Oil-loving
______________	Any substance that occupies space, has physical and chemical properties, and exists in the form of a solid, liquid, or gas
______________	The addition of oxygen to, or the subtraction of hydrogen from, a substance
______________	A stable mixture of two or more mixable substances
______________	Surface-active agent
______________	An unstable mixture of undissolved particles in a liquid

S	U	R	F	A	C	T	A	N	T	R	O	C	J	Y	S	A	I
J	S	P	Y	N	O	I	T	A	D	I	X	O	T	O	T	S	M
A	M	K	N	H	F	H	F	V	V	P	E	N	L	O	X	O	M
C	M	D	J	K	G	W	K	F	E	E	E	U	M	Q	W	I	I
U	O	M	V	X	I	B	L	N	P	M	T	C	O	V	E	A	S
B	Q	M	O	Y	G	K	R	V	E	I	I	T	P	D	U	Y	C
L	F	E	B	N	K	A	A	L	O	L	A	C	Y	O	V	A	I
W	N	A	L	U	I	I	E	N	I	D	P	Z	M	D	Y	U	B
V	D	A	Y	Y	S	A	K	H	V	L	P	I	O	B	R	C	L
J	Z	R	R	X	R	T	P	U	C	Y	U	H	Q	A	T	I	E
R	X	K	C	Z	R	O	I	D	B	C	B	V	E	E	S	L	P
Z	J	N	Z	E	R	C	A	O	N	I	W	T	T	Y	I	I	A
O	F	Z	T	D	J	J	J	F	N	U	L	C	O	X	M	H	C
Q	X	T	Y	Q	J	F	P	A	P	A	O	A	P	H	E	P	M
I	A	H	L	T	G	G	T	T	C	S	C	P	K	H	H	O	R
M	D	Y	F	I	K	X	X	Q	D	L	J	I	M	L	C	P	G
Y	F	D	E	Y	R	P	S	H	M	Y	Z	Y	D	O	A	I	X
T	K	I	O	A	N	O	I	S	N	E	P	S	U	S	C	L	D

Essential Experience 8

Matching Exercise

Match the following essential terms with their identifying phrases or definition.

______	**Chemical change**	**1.**	Special type of ingredients used in hair conditioners and as a water-resistant lubricant for the skin
______	**Acid**	**2.**	A sweet, colorless, odorless, oily substance used as a moisturizing agent
______	**Ammonia**	**3.**	The separation of an atom or molecule into positive and negative ions
______	**Physical change**	**4.**	Chemical reaction in which the oxidizing agent is reduced and the reducing agent is oxidized
______	**Atom**	**5.**	A change in the form or physical properties of a substance without the formation of a new substance
______	**Glycerin**	**6.**	A change in the chemical and physical properties of a substance by a chemical reaction that creates a new substance
______	**Chemistry**	**7.**	The smallest particle of an element that retains the properties of that element
______	**Ionization**	**8.**	A colorless liquid with a pungent odor composed of hydrogen and nitrogen
______	**Redox**	**9.**	Science that deals with the omposition, structures, and properties of matter
______	**Silicone**	**10.**	Having a pH below 7

Essential Review

Using the words provided, fill in the blanks below to form a thorough review of Chapter 12, Basics of Chemistry. Words or terms may be used more than once or not at all.

acid	**emulsions**	**organic**
alkali	**hydrophilic**	**oxidizing**
atom	**inorganic**	**physical**
chemical	**lipophilic**	**solvents**
chemistry	**liquids**	**surfactant**
compound	**matter**	**suspension**
density	**miscible**	**volatile organic compounds**
element	**molecule**	

1. A solution with a pH less than 7 has an ____________ pH, and a solution with a pH higher than 7 has an ____________ pH.
2. A ____________ change refers to a change in the form of a substance, without the formation of a new substance. A ____________ change is when a new substance is formed.
3. A ____________ is a substance that acts as a bridge to allow oil and water to mix or emulsify.
4. ____________________________ are substances containing carbon which evaporate quickly and easily.
5. An ____________ is the smallest particle of an element that is capable of showing the properties of an element.
6. Anything that occupies space is defined as ____________.
7. __________ are formed when two or more immiscible substances, such as oil and water, are united with the aid of a binder.
8. ____________ chemistry is the branch of chemistry that deals with all substances that do not contain carbon.
9. Matter exists in three forms: solids, ____________, and gases.
10. ____________ chemistry is the branch of chemistry that deals with all substances in which carbon is present.
11. ____________ agents are substances that readily release oxygen.
12. ____________ liquids are mutually soluble, meaning they can be mixed into stable solutions.

Essential Review continued

13. ____________ are any substances that are able to dissolve another substance.

14. Surfactant molecules have two ends:____________ and ________.

15. A ____________ is an unstable mixture of undissolved particles in liquid.

16. The basic unit of all matter is an ____________.

17. The science that deals with the composition, structure, and properties of matter is ____________.

18. Two or more atoms that are joined together chemically form a ____________.

19. When a substance is made up of two or more different elements chemically joined, it is a ____________.

Essential Discoveries and Accomplishments

In the space below, jot some notes about what concepts of this chapter were hardest for you to understand or remember. Imagine finding yourself suddenly in the role of "teacher" and consider what you would tell your "students" about these concepts. Share your Essential Discoveries with some of the other students in your class and ask if they are helpful to them. You may want to revise your discoveries based on good ideas shared by your peers.

Discoveries:

List at least three things you have accomplished since your last entry that relate to your career goals.

Accomplishments:

CHAPTER 13

Basics of Electricity

A Motivating Moment: "Now is a gift. That's why it is called the present. To be fully enjoyed, it must be unwrapped from the mistakes and guilt of the past and the worries of the future."

— Unknown

Essential Objectives

After studying this chapter and completing the Essential Companion components, you will be able to:

1. **Define the nature of electricity and the two types of electric current.**
2. **Define electrical measurements.**
3. **Understand the principles of electrical equipment safety.**
4. **Describe the main electric modalities used in cosmetology.**
5. **Describe other types of electrical equipment that cosmetologists use and describe how to use them.**
6. **Explain electromagnetic spectrum, visible spectrum of light, and invisible light.**
7. **Describe the types of light therapy and their benefits.**

Essential Electricity

Why is a basic knowledge of electricity important to my career as a cosmetologist?

Electricity is the primary source of energy needed, literally, to run the world and the salon where you will work. Electricity is essential for controlling and maintaining the professional environment in every professional establishment. It is responsible for such things as lighting, ventilation, temperature, and possibly even the hot water you will use. Electricity must be used intelligently and safely. As a professional, you must know how it works in order to maintain a safe environment for yourself, your coworkers, and your clients.

Electricity is critical in the salon for use with blowdryers, curling irons, lotion heaters, wax heaters, facial equipment, cash registers, telephones, computers, nail drills, and much more. While it is not necessary for you to become an electrical engineer, it is important that you have a working knowledge of how electricity is created and how it can be used safely in the salon.

Cosmetologists should study and have a thorough understanding of the basics of electricity because:

- Cosmetologists use and rely upon a variety of electrical appliances. Knowing what electricity is and how it works will allow you to use it wisely and safely.
- A basic understanding of electricity will enable you to properly use and care for your equipment and tools.
- Electricity and its use impact other aspects of the salon environment, such as lighting and the temperature of styling irons. Therefore, it impacts the services you offer your clients.

Essential Concepts

What do I need to know about basic electricity in order to be successful and more effective as a professional cosmetologist?

You need to be aware of the two types of electricity, how it is measured, and safety devices pertaining to electricity. You will need to have a working knowledge of the various types of currents that are used in the equipment found in the salon. It might help you to think of electricity in terms of the *flow* of an electric current. As a flow, an electric current is similar to a flow of water. It has a direction, requires a pathway, and can be stopped and started. While the flow of water can actually help create energy, the electric current *is* a flow of energy. It is this passage of energy that gives electricity powers than can be therapeutic or, if handled incorrectly, potentially dangerous and destructive.

The pathway for an electric current flowing through an appliance is called a circuit, which means that the current makes a kind of circle from its source through a conductor and back to its source again. If the current flows in a circuit constantly in one direction, it is called a *direct current* (DC). Most battery-operated devices use direct current. However, most appliances linked by a wall plug to a regional power system use *alternating current* (AC). In alternating current, the current changes direction in a circuit back and forth many times a second.

The flow of electricity can be stopped by simply breaking the circuit—by flipping a switch. When the switch is "on," the circuit is completed and electricity can flow. When the switch is "off," the circuit is broken and electricity cannot flow.

1 Essential Experience

Matching Exercise

Match each of the following essential terms with its definition or identifying term.

______ **Volt**	**1.** Measurement of how much electric energy is being used in one second
______ **Amp**	**2.** One-thousandth of an ampere
______ **Milliampere**	**3.** The unit of measurement for the amount of current running through a wire
______ **Ohm**	**4.** Unit for measuring the pressure that forces the electric current forward
______ **Watt**	**5.** The electricity in your house is measured in this manner
______ **Kilowatt**	**6.** This unit measures the resistance of an electric current

Essential Experience 2

Safety of Electrical Equipment

Fill in the blank for the selected safety precautions to be followed to avoid accidents and ensure greater client satisfaction.

1. All the electrical appliances you use should be ____________.
2. Read all ____________ before using any electrical equipment.
3. ____________ all appliances when not in use.
4. ____________ all electrical equipment regularly.
5. Keep all wires, plugs, and equipment in good ____________.
6. Use only one plug to each ____________.
7. You and your client should avoid contact with ____________ and metal surfaces when using electricity.
8. Do not leave your client unattended while ____________ to an electrical device.
9. Keep electrical cords off the ____________ and away from people's feet.
10. Do not attempt to ____________ around electric outlets while equipment is plugged in.
11. Do not touch two ____________ objects at the same time if either is connected to an electric current.
12. Do not step on or place ____________ on electrical cords.
13. Do not allow an electrical cord to become ____________ as it can cause a short circuit.
14. Disconnect appliances by pulling on the ____________, not the cord.
15. Do not attempt to ____________ electrical appliances unless you are qualified.

3 Essential Experience

Crossword Puzzle

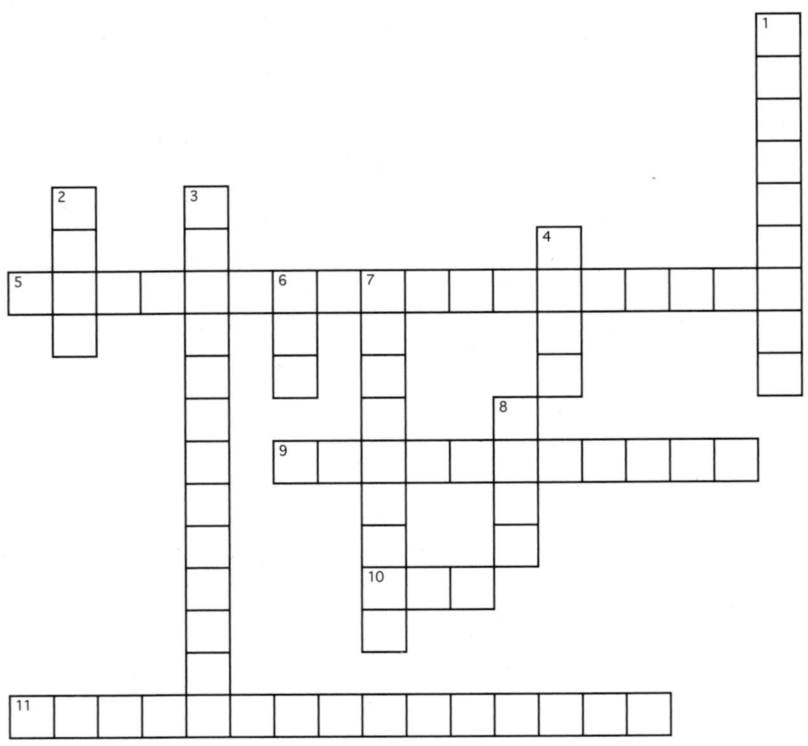

Across

Word	Clue
____________	**5.** A rapid and interrupted current, flowing first in one direction and then in the opposite direction
____________	**9.** One-thousandth of an ampere
____________	**10.** The unit that measures the resistance of an electric current
____________	**11.** The flow of electricity along a conductor

Essential Experience continued 3

Down

Word	Clue
__________________	**1.** Any substance that conducts electricity
__________________	**2.** The unit that measures the pressure or force that pushes the flow of electrons forward through a conductor
__________________	**3.** A constant, even-flowing current that travels in one direction only
__________________	**4.** A special device that prevents excessive current from passing through a circuit
__________________	**6.** The unit that measures the strength of an electric current
__________________	**7.** Or nonconductor is a substance that does not easily transmit electricity
__________________	**8.** A measurement of how much of how much electric energy is being used in one second

4 Essential Experience

Word Scramble

Using the clues provided, unscramble the terms below.

Scramble	**Correct Word**
tecdoelre	— — — — — — — — — *Clue:* An applicator for directing the electric current from the machine to the client's skin.
alpoytir	— — — — — — — — *Clue:* Indicates the negative or positive pole of an electric current.
dneao	— — — — — *Clue:* The positive electrode.
otdehac	— — — — — — — *Clue:* The negative electrode.
aismdloiet	— — — — — — — — — — *Clue:* The four main ones are galvanic, faradic, sinusoidal, and Tesla high frequency.
ngaciavl	— — — — — — — — *Clue:* A constant and direct current, producing chemical changes when it passes through the tissues and fluids of the body.
ostpohesirnio	— — — — — — — — — — — — — *Clue:* The process of introducing water-soluble products into the skin with the use of electric current.
aporsscthiae	— — — — — — — — — — — — *Clue:* Forces acidic substances into deeper tissue using galvanic current.
sipreahosna	— — — — — — — — — — — *Clue:* The process of forcing liquids into the tissues from the negative toward the positive poles.
oiuttidcsnerans	— — — — — — — — — — — — — — — *Clue:* The process used to soften and emulsify grease deposits and blackheads in the hair follicles.

Essential Experience 5

The Visible Spectrum

Color in the visible spectrum depicted in the diagram using colored pencils, crayons, or water colors.

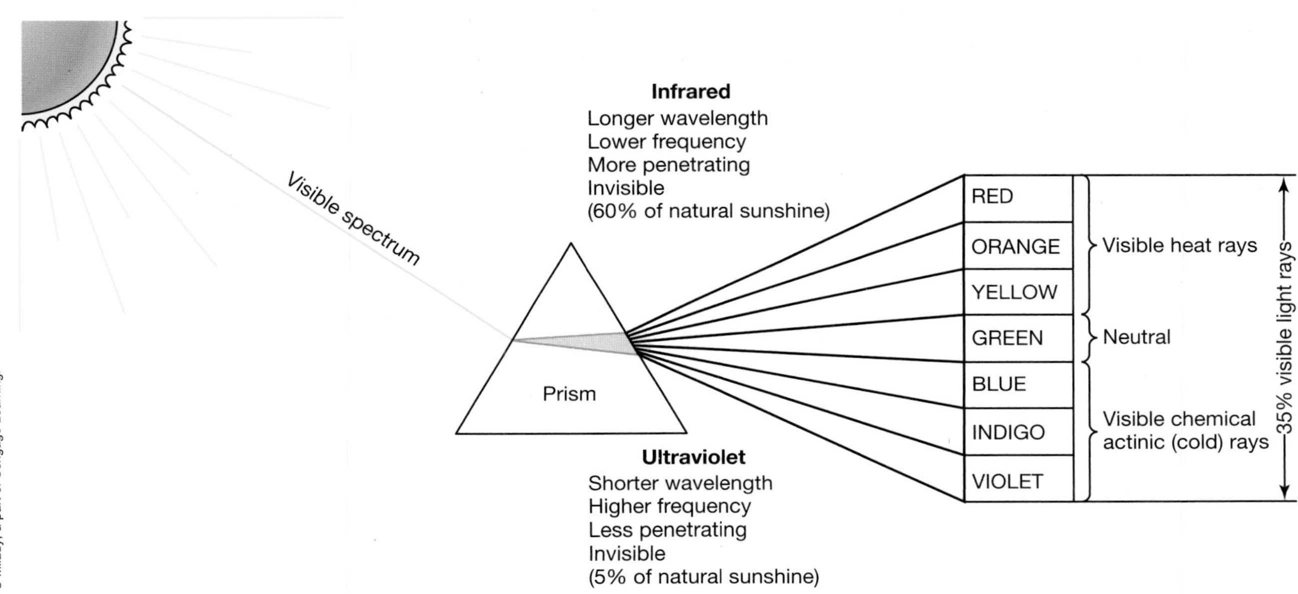

Essential Review

Using the following words, fill in the blanks below to form a thorough review of Chapter 13, Basics of Electricity. Words or terms may be used more than once or not at all.

alternating	**direct current**	**ohm**
ampere	**desincrustation**	**polarity**
anaphoresis	**electricity**	**radiant energy**
anode	**electrode**	**rectifier**
apparatus	**fuse**	**red**
blue	**galvanic**	**Tesla high frequency**
cathode	**heating cap**	**therapeutic**
circuit breaker	**infrared**	**vaporizer**
conductor	**infrared rays**	**visible light**
converter	**kilowatt**	**white**
direct	**modalities**	

1. ____________ is a form of energy that produces magnetic, chemical, and thermal effects.
2. A ____________ is a substance that permits electrical current to pass through it.
3. A steamer or ____________ produces moist, uniform heat that can be applied to the head or face.
4. A ____________ is used to change direct current into alternating current and a____________ is used to change alternating current to direct current.
5. A positive electrode is called a/an ____________ and a negative electrode is called a/an ____________.
6. A ____________ is a safety device that prevents excessive current from passing through.
7. An amp or ____________ is the unit of measurement for the amount of current running through a wire.
8. An ____________ is an applicator that directs the electric current from the machine to the client's skin.
9. ____________ is the process of forcing liquids into the tissues from the negative toward the positive pole.

Essential Review continued

10. Artificial light rays are produced by using an electrical ____________ called a therapeutic lamp.
11. ____________ current is a constant, even-flowing current traveling in one direction, while ____________ current is a rapid and interrupted current flowing first in one direction then in the opposite.
12. Do not use the negative ____________ current on skin with broken capillaries, pustular acne, or on a client with high blood pressure.
13. A switch that automatically interrupts or shuts off an electric circuit at the first indication of overload is a ______________.
14. ____________ rays make up 60 percent of natural sunlight.
15. The negative or positive state of electric current is ____________.
16. The process used to soften and liquefy grease deposits in the hair follicles and pores is _______________.
17. ____________ light contains fewer heat rays and has some germicidal and chemical benefits.
18. Another name for electromagnetic radiation is ______________.
19. The ____________________ current is a thermal or heat-producing current with a high rate of oscillation or vibration.
20. A uniform source of heat can be provided by a ____________.

Essential Discoveries and Accomplishments

In the space below, jot some notes about what concepts of this chapter were hardest for you to understand or remember. Imagine finding yourself suddenly in the role of "teacher" and consider what you would tell your "students" about these concepts. Share your Essential Discoveries with some of the other students in your class and ask if they are helpful to them. You may want to revise your discoveries based on any good ideas shared by your peers.

Discoveries:

____

____

____

____

____

____

____

____

____

____

____

List at least three things you have accomplished since your last entry that relate to your career goals.

Accomplishments:

____

____

____

____

____

CHAPTER 14

Principles of Hair Design

A Motivating Moment: "Nothing will be attempted if all possible objections must first be overcome."
— Samuel Johnson

Essential Objectives

After studying this chapter and completing the Essential Companion components, you will be able to:

1. **Describe the possible sources of hair design inspiration.**
2. **List the five elements of hair design.**
3. **List the five principles of hair design.**
4. **Understand the influence of hair type on hairstyle.**
5. **Identify different facial shapes and demonstrate how to design hairstyles to enhance or camouflage facial features.**
6. **Explain design considerations for men.**

Essential Design in Hairstyling

Why is understanding the basic elements of design so important to my success as a cosmetologist?

The answer is as simple as cooking! If you have ever created a masterpiece in the kitchen or even observed a great cook like your mother or grandmother in action, you know that it takes a great deal more than just knowing what ingredients to use. You must know exactly what quantity of each ingredient is needed. You must know at exactly what point each ingredient is added. You need to know things like cooking temperatures and how to use special kitchen tools such as knives or wire whisks. The exact same principles apply in hairstyling. You must attain a thorough knowledge of all the tools and implements required in creating a great design. In addition, you must know the principles of design and also understand how the client's face shape and features impact the chosen design. Once you have gained a solid working knowledge of all these parts, pieces, and principles, you will be able to provide quality services to each and every client.

As a cosmetologist, you should study and have a thorough understanding of the principles of hair design for the following reasons:

- You will be better able to understand why a particular hairstyle will or will not be the best choice for a client.
- The principles of design will serve as helpful guidelines to assist you in achieving your styling vision.
- You will be able to create haircuts and styles designed to help clients camouflage unattractive features while emphasizing attractive ones.

Essential Concepts

If there are so many key ingredients to hair design, where do I begin?

You must first gain an understanding of the five elements of design which are form, space, line, color, and texture. Then you must experiment with those five elements to create a variety of designs. You must also gain knowledge of the principles of hair design which include proportion, balance, rhythm, emphasis, and harmony, and how each affects the end result. Finally, you must learn about all the client's personal circumstances which will impact the overall design. These include the client's face shape, facial features, head shape, profile, and whether or not the client wears eyeglasses. All of these concepts will be contributing factors in providing the client with a complimentary and satisfactory hair design.

1 Essential Experience

The Elements of Design

Form

Take pictures of the same hairstyle on a client or another student from three different angles. Cut around the perimeter of the hairstyle for each angle. In the area provided below, outline the style in the Essential Companion. Discuss with fellow students how different the silhouette is from various angles. (If a camera is not available for your use, let your creative juices flow. Consider creating a silhouette on the chalkboard in the classroom by adjusting the overhead lighting and using a flashlight or spotlight. Once you have traced three different silhouettes on the chalkboard, copy a smaller version below.)

Space

In order to get a better grasp of what is meant by volume and how the same amount of volume can take on a variety of three-dimensional shapes and styles, try this project. At home in your kitchen, measure out exactly 8 ounces (236 ml) of water and pour it into a round plastic cup. Measure another 8 ounces of water and pour it into a square plastic container. Measure another 8 ounces of water and pour it into a rectangular-shaped plastic container. Place all three containers in the freezer. After they are frozen, remove the frozen masses from their respective containers and compare their shapes. Remember, each ice mold represents the exact same volume of water. (*Note:* You can use any size or shape of container for this experiment as long as it is freezer safe.)

Line

Curly, straight, or curved lines create the form, design, and movement of a hairstyle. Depict the following different lines by cutting pictures out of magazines and pasting them in the space provided below. Using a colored pen, emphasize the type of line the style depicts.

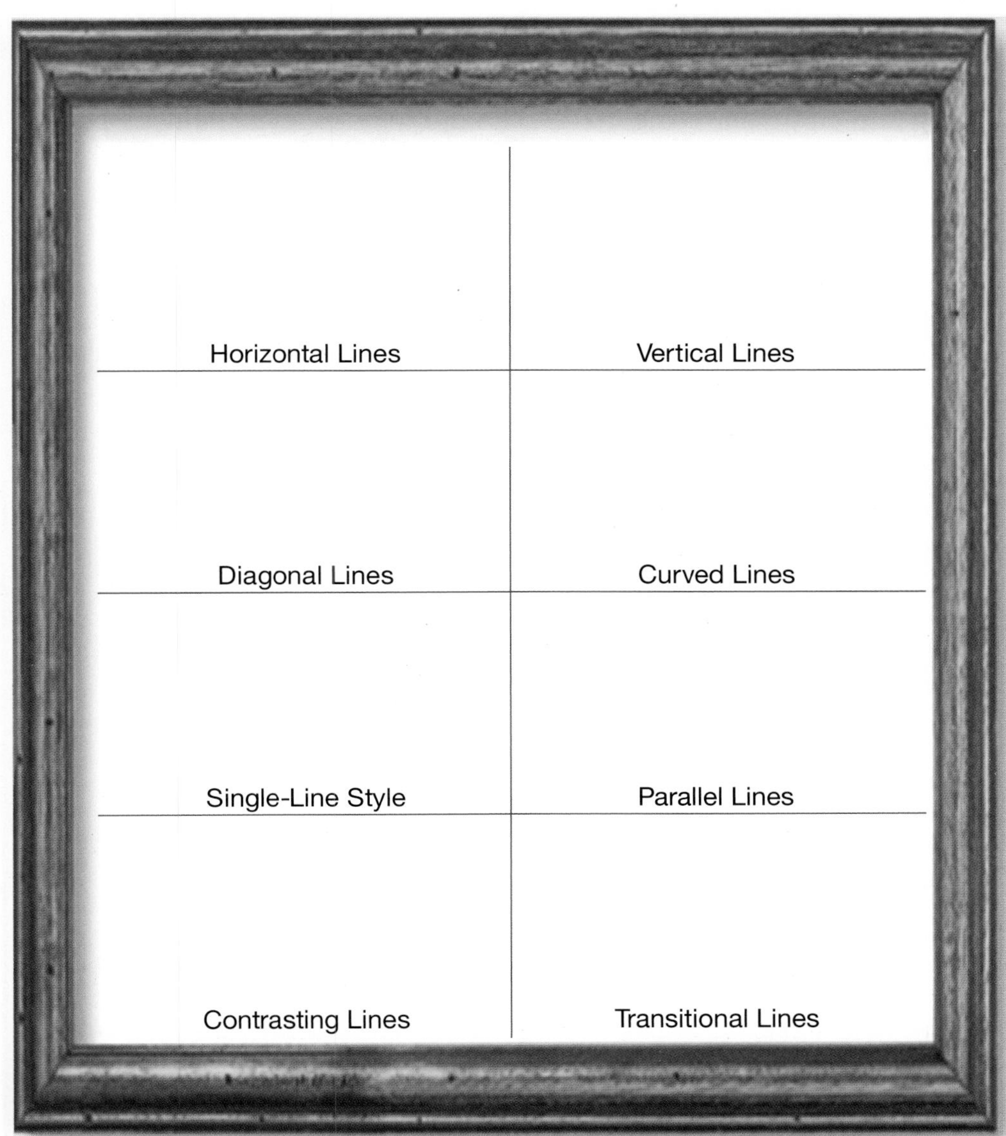

Color

You will learn to use color to bring dimension and finish to the style. Think about a living room that is painted dull beige with beige carpet and a light brown sofa. It likely appears to be rather dull. Imagine, however, what a difference you could make if you painted one wall a brighter contrasting color or added several throw pillows to the sofa in a variety of textures and colors, or added a brightly colored throw rug over the carpet. Imagine the difference any one of those changes would make to the room's overall appearance. The same principle applies to hair color. Again, using your favorite old magazines, select several pictures of different hairstyles and paste them below. Indicate which styles are improved because of color and which ones are just colored for the sake of color or to be different.

Essential Experience continued 1

Texture

All of us have a natural wave pattern. It may be straight, wavy, curly, or even extremely curly. When aiding our clients in selecting a hairstyle that will be the most flattering and easiest to maintain, we must take into consideration wave pattern. In this activity, you are being asked to search magazines for pictures that depict various types of wave patterns. Paste them in the spaces provided below and write a brief explanation about the look created by each wave pattern.

2 Essential Experience

The Principles of Design

Proportion

Proportion deals with the harmonious relationship of the parts of something to each other or to the whole. Have you ever seen something that is clearly out of proportion with its surroundings? Perhaps you have observed a cute, but extremely tiny, foreign car pull into the parking lot at the mall and then watched as a very large man about 6 feet and 6 inches tall, weighing around 230 pounds, hoists himself out of the vehicle. The man and the car are not really in harmony with each other. The same principle applies in hair design. To help you understand the importance of proportion with the face, features, head shape, and body size and shape, complete this exercise.

Using poster board or construction paper, paste pictures from magazines that depict the following proportional relationships.

- Someone whose hairstyle is much too large for their petite body.
- Someone whose hairstyle is much too small for their larger body frame.
- Someone whose hairstyle reflects classic proportions.

Essential Experience continued 2

Balance

When referring to balance, we mean that the hairstyle is equal in size or volume around the head. It can be both symmetrical and asymmetrical. Please complete the windowpane activity below.

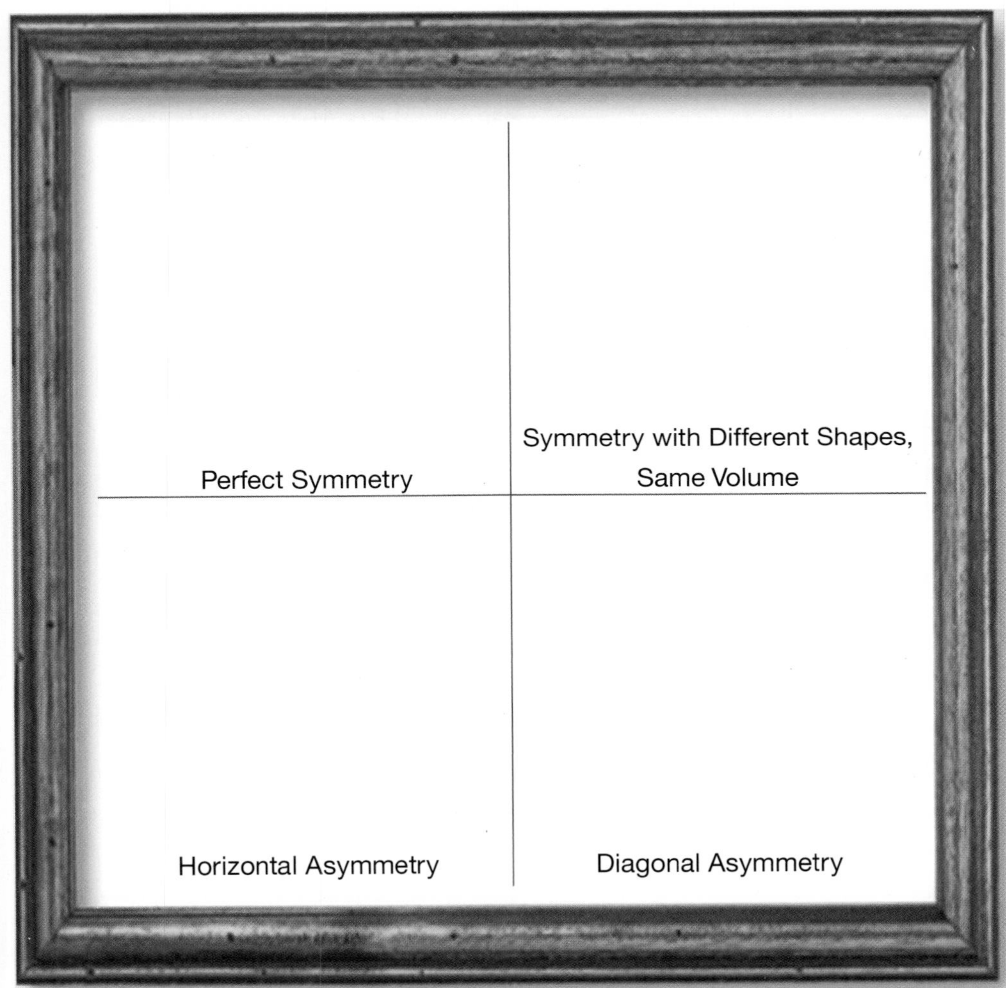

2 Essential Experience continued

Rhythm

When you think of someone having great rhythm, you are likely visualizing how they move on a dance floor. Rhythm means the same thing in a hairstyle. It means movement. Cut six different pictures out of magazines and paste them below. Indicate whether the style has a fast or slow rhythm.

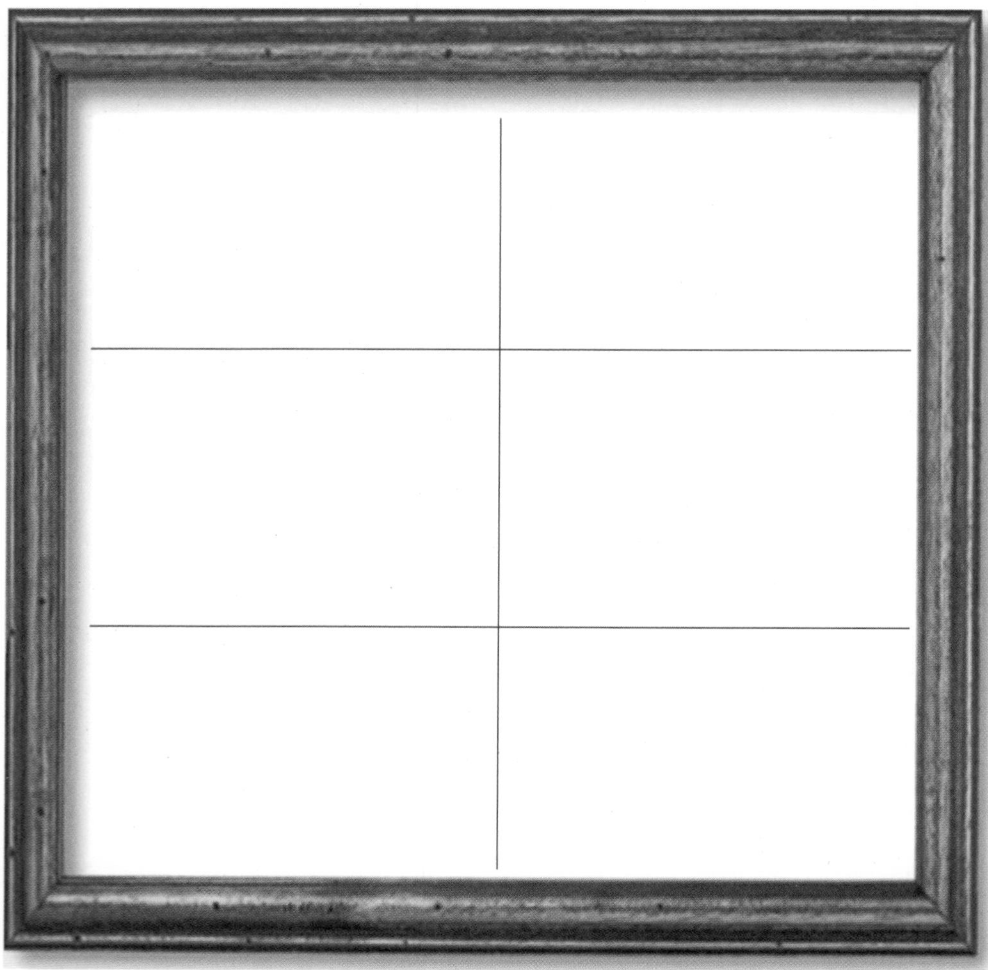

Essential Experience continued 2

Emphasis

Emphasis is the focal point or the point of prominence in the hairstyle. Our eyes tend to see this part of the style first. List a few ideas of how you can add emphasis to a hairstyle.

____

____

____

____

____

Harmony

Without harmony, none of the other principles of design will work. Harmony is what holds all the elements of the design together. Think about anyone you have known, a celebrity perhaps, who may have had great color or balance but the harmony just did not happen. List their names here and explain why there was no harmony.

____

____

____

____

____

3 Essential Experience

Windowpane Facial Types

Windowpaning is the process of transferring key elements, points, or steps in a lesson into visual images that are hand sketched into the squares or *panes* of a matrix. Look through magazines and find pictures that depict the face shapes indicated below. Let your mind think in pictures and sketch the essential concepts printed in each of the following windowpanes.

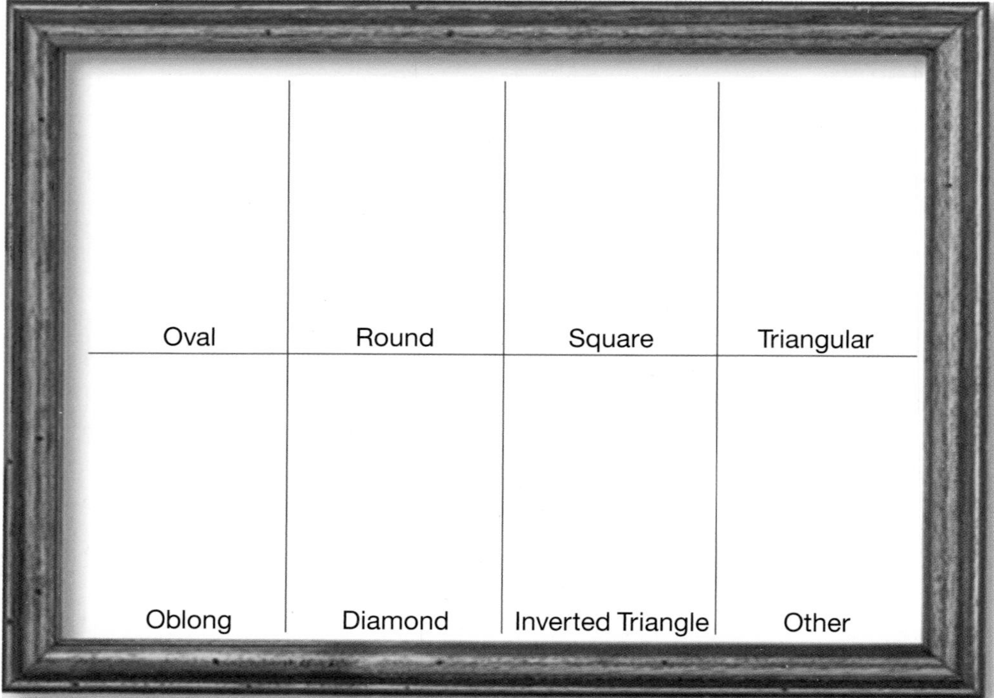

On a separate sheet of paper, describe the appropriate hairstyle for each of the face shapes listed in the matrix. For the magazine pictures, explain why the hairstyle works or doesn't work.

Essential Experience 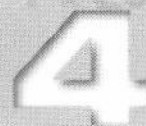

Matching Exercise

Special Considerations A

Match the following essential terms with their identifying terms or phrases.

______	**Wide forehead**	**1.**	Asymmetrical, off-center style is best
______	**Close-set eyes**	**2.**	Use curved lines at the jaw line
______	**Crooked nose**	**3.**	Direct hair forward over the sides of the forehead
______	**Square jaw**	**4.**	A receding forehead and chin
______	**Long jaw**	**5.**	Use bangs with little or no volume
______	**Convex profile**	**6.**	Hair should be full and fall below the jaw
______	**Large forehead**	**7.**	Direct hair back and away from the face at the temples
______	**Prominent nose**	**8.**	Bring hair forward at forehead with softness around face
______	**Small chin**	**9.**	Hair should be longer or shorter than chin
______	**Large chin**	**10.**	Move hair up and away from face along chin line

4 Essential Experience continued

Special Considerations B

Match the following essential terms with their identifying terms or phrases.

______	**Narrow forehead**	**1.**	Use straight lines at the jaw line
______	**Wide-set eyes**	**2.**	Direct bangs over the forehead with outward directed volume
______	**Wide, flat nose**	**3.**	Hair should sweep off the face, creating a line from nose to ear
______	**Round jaw**	**4.**	A prominent forehead and chin
______	**Straight profile**	**5.**	Direct hair away from the face at the forehead
______	**Concave profile**	**6.**	Use a higher half bang to create length in the face
______	**Receding forehead**	**7.**	Direct hair forward in the chin area
______	**Small nose**	**8.**	Draw hair away from face, use center part
______	**Receding chin**	**9.**	Ideal profile

Essential Experience 5

Crossword Puzzle

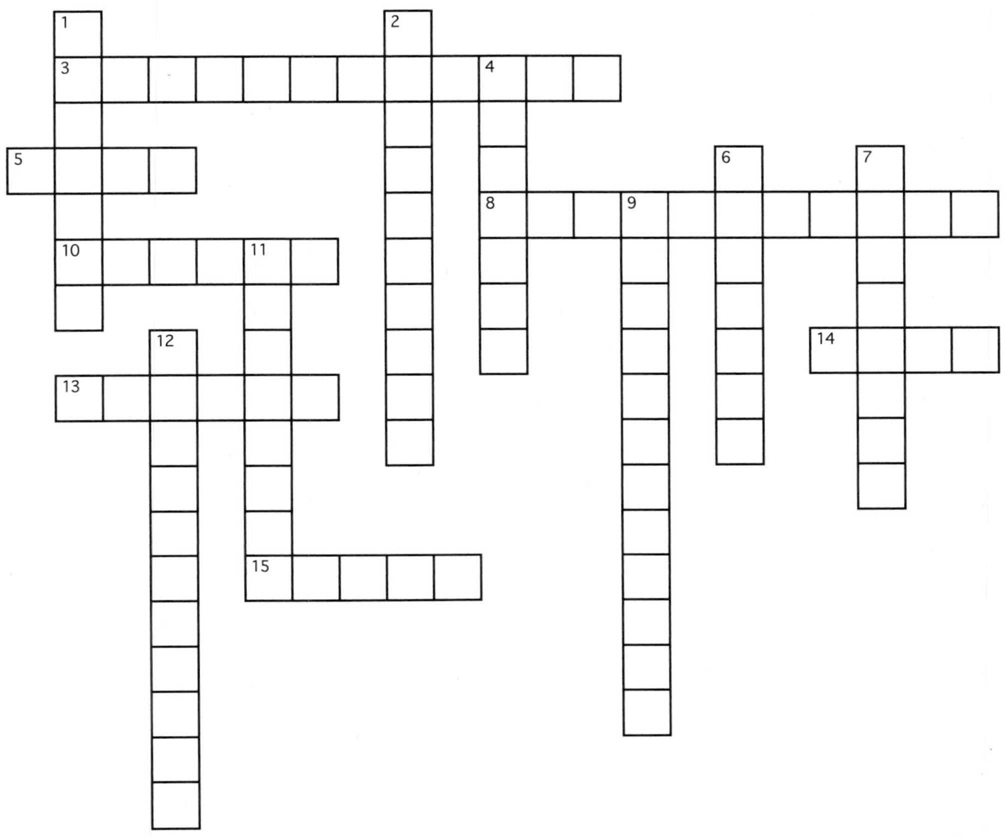

Across

Word	Clue
______________	**3.** Unequal proportions designed to balance facial features
______________	**5.** Triangular section that begins at the apex and ends at the front corners
______________	**8.** Horizontal and vertical lines that meet at a 90-degree angle
______________	**10.** Curving outward
______________	**13.** Regular, recurrent pattern of movement
______________	**14.** Outline of the overall hairstyle
______________	**15.** The area surrounding the form or the area the hairstyle occupies

Down

Word	Clue
______________	**1.** Establishing equal or appropriate proportions to create symmetry
______________	**2.** Harmonious relationship between parts
______________	**4.** Curving inward
______________	**6.** Orderly and pleasing arrangement of shapes and lines
______________	**7.** Lines positioned between horizontal and vertical
______________	**9.** Curved lines used to blend and soften
______________	**11.** Place in a hairstyle where the eye is drawn first
______________	**12.** Hairstyle design that is similar on both sides of the face

Essential Review

Complete the following review of Chapter 14, Principles of Hair Design, by circling the correct answer to each statement.

1. The outline or silhouette of a hairstyle is known as the ____________.

   a) space b) line
   c) form d) design

2. The shape, design, and movement of the hairstyle is created by the ____________.

   a) space b) lines
   c) form d) design

3. The area surrounding the form or the area the hairstyle occupies is called ____________.

   a) space b) lines
   c) form d) design

4. Lines that are parallel to the floor are known as ____________.

   a) vertical b) diagonal
   c) horizontal d) curved

5. Lines used to soften a design are ____________.

   a) vertical b) diagonal
   c) horizontal d) transitional

6. Lines used to make a hairstyle appear longer and narrower are ____________.

   a) vertical b) diagonal
   c) horizontal d) curved

7. Lines positioned between horizontal and vertical and which are used to create interest are ____________.

   a) vertical b) diagonal
   c) horizontal d) curved

8. An example of a line that is found in the one-length or blunt cut hairstyle is the ____________ line.

   a) single b) contrasting
   c) transitional d) repeating

Essential Review continued

9. Lines that meet at a 90-degree angle and create a hard edge are called ____________ lines.

a) single
b) contrasting
c) transitional
d) repeating

10. Curved lines used to soften and blend horizontal or vertical lines are known as ____________ lines.

a) vertical
b) contrasting
c) transitional
d) repeating

11. Lighter and warmer colors are used to create the illusion of ____________.

a) subtlety
b) repetition
c) volume
d) closeness

12. Dark and cool colors move forward or toward the head and create the illusion of less ____________.

a) volume
b) height
c) width
d) strength

13. When choosing haircolor, it should be compatible with the client's ____________.

a) eye color
b) skin tone
c) family's choice
d) childhood dreams

14. Texture can be natural or created with styling techniques, chemical changes, curling irons, or ____________.

a) client's desire
b) stylist's desire
c) hair brushing
d) hot rollers

15. Curly hair can be permanently straightened with ____________.

a) curling irons
b) hair relaxers
c) pressing irons
d) crimping irons

16. Curly and extremely curly hair does not reflect much light and could be ____________ to the touch.

a) soft
b) smooth
c) limp
d) coarse

17. The five principles of hair design are proportion, balance, rhythm, emphasis, and ____________.

a) symmetry
b) asymmetry
c) harmony
d) diagonal

18. ____________ wave patterns accent the face and are particularly useful when you wish to narrow a round head shape.

a) Rough
b) Busy
c) Smooth
d) Numerous

19. Establishing equal or appropriate proportions to create symmetry is known as ____________.

a) balance
b) harmony
c) rhythm
d) emphasis

20. The pattern that creates movement in a hairstyle is known as ____________.

a) balance
b) harmony
c) rhythm
d) emphasis

21. ____________ is considered the most important of the principles of hair design.

a) Balance
b) Harmony
c) Rhythm
d) Emphasis

22. The ____________ in a hairstyle is the place the eyes see first.

a) balance
b) harmony
c) rhythm
d) emphasis

23. Generally, the ideal face shape is said to be the ____________ shape.

a) square
b) round
c) oval
d) pear

24. The face is divided into ____________ zones.

a) one
b) two
c) three
d) four

25. The aim of creating the illusion of width in the forehead would be best for the ____________ face shape.

a) round
b) triangular
c) oblong
d) diamond

26. The aim of reducing the width across the cheekbone line is best for the ____________ face shape.

a) round
b) triangular
c) oblong
d) diamond

Essential Review continued

27. The aim of making the face appear shorter and wider is best for the ____________ face shape.

a) round
b) pear
c) oblong
d) diamond

28. Using a higher half bang to create length in the face would be best for ____________.

a) a wide forehead
b) close-set eyes
c) a narrow forehead
d) wide-set eyes

29. Directing the hair forward over the sides of the forehead is best for ____________.

a) a wide forehead
b) close-set eyes
c) a narrow forehead
d) wide-set eyes

30. Asymmetrical, off-center styles are best for ____________.

a) narrow forehead
b) close eyes
c) long jaw line
d) crooked nose

31. The profile which has a receding forehead and chin is called the ____________ profile.

a) convex
b) concave
c) straight
d) curved

32. The profile which has a prominent forehead and chin is called the ____________ profile.

a) convex
b) concave
c) straight
d) curved

33. Bangs with little or no volume should be used for a ____________.

a) receding forehead
b) large forehead
c) low forehead
d) small forehead

34. A part that helps develop height on top and make thin hair appear fuller is the ____________ part.

a) center
b) side
c) diagonal
d) zigzag

35. The ____________ part should be used to create width or height in a hairstyle.

a) triangular
b) diagonal
c) side
d) zigzag

Essential Review continued

36. The ___________ part is used to create a dramatic effect.

a) triangular
b) diagonal
c) side
d) zigzag

37. The ___________ part is considered to be the basic parting for the bang section.

a) triangular
b) diagonal
c) side
d) zigzag

38. The ___________ part is used to direct hair across the top of the head.

a) triangular
b) diagonal
c) side
d) center

39. The ___________ part is considered to be the classic part and is usually used for an oval face, but can be used to create the illusion of oval for a round or wide face.

a) curved
b) side
c) center
d) diagonal

40. The __________ part is used for a receding hairline or high forehead.

a) curved
b) side
c) center
d) diagonal

Essential Discoveries and Accomplishments

In the space below, jot some notes about what concepts of this chapter were hardest for you to understand or remember. Imagine finding yourself suddenly in the role of "teacher" and consider what you would tell your "students" about these concepts. Share your Essential Discoveries with some of the other students in your class and ask if they are helpful to them. You may want to revise your discoveries based on any good ideas shared by your peers.

Discoveries:

____

____

____

____

____

____

____

____

____

____

List at least three things you have accomplished since your last entry that relate to your career goals.

Accomplishments:

____

____

____

____

CHAPTER 15

Scalp Care, Shampooing, & Conditioning

A Motivating Moment: "Do not go where the path may lead; go instead where there is no path and leave a trail."
— Ralph Waldo Emerson

Essential Objectives

After studying this chapter and completing the Essential Companion components, you will be able to:

1. **Explain the two most important requirements for scalp care.**
2. **Describe the benefits of scalp massage.**
3. **Treat scalp and hair that are dry, oily, or dandruff ridden.**
4. **Explain the role of hair brushing to a healthy scalp.**
5. **Discuss the uses and benefits of the various types of shampoo.**
6. **Discuss the uses and benefits of the various types of conditioner.**
7. **Demonstrate the appropriate draping for a basic shampooing and conditioning, and draping for a chemical service.**
8. **Demonstrate the Three-Part Procedure and explain why it is useful.**

Essential Shampooing and Conditioning

Why are shampooing and conditioning so important to my training when they seem to be such insignificant services?

Just because you have been shampooing and conditioning your own hair for a number of years does not mean that you have the appropriate knowledge to deliver a professional shampoo and conditioning service to your clients. It is necessary to understand that the procedures and products that you have used at home are likely not professional grade and may not be client-oriented. In fact, it is not uncommon for people to choose their shampoo or conditioning treatment based on its fragrance or because talented marketing managers suggest it is beneficial for their hair.

Your ability to provide a thorough and pleasing shampoo to your clients is essential. It is generally the first service you provide a client and it allows you to begin building a positive client relationship. More importantly, the shampoo service is the most repeated service you will provide to your clients. In most cases, a thorough shampoo will precede a haircut, a style, a color treatment, and any chemical reformation. You can be sure that how well you perform the shampoo service will greatly influence the client's perception of how well you will perform other services they desire. And remember, when you give a good shampoo with a relaxing scalp massage, you lay the groundwork for selling the client many more services both today and in the future!

Cosmetologists should study and have a thorough understanding of scalp care, shampooing, and conditioning because:

- The shampoo service is the first opportunity to reinforce your position as a professional who attends to the specific, individual needs of your client.
- You will be able to examine, identify, and address hair and scalp conditions that do not require a physician's care and be able to refer clients to a physician if a more serious issue is identified.
- A thorough knowledge of hair care products will assist you in determining the best preparation for other services to be performed.
- A successful home-care regimen recommendation will keep your work looking its best for all to see.

Essential Concepts

What do I need to know about shampooing, rinsing, and conditioning in order to provide a quality service?

It may help you to understand some history about cleansing the hair. The word shampoo is derived from the Hindu word *champna,* which means to press, knead, or shampoo. History tells us that humankind has found many ways to cleanse the body in order to prevent disease. Natural ingredients were used to accomplish this, including soapwort, which is a plant that produces lather in water. Near the middle of the twentieth century, however, scientists created chemical ingredients to replace natural ones. Chemists became aware of the pH (potential hydrogen) level of hair and recognized that products should be created which would maintain the natural pH of the hair.

As a professional, you need to know how important proper brushing is before the shampoo service. You will then need to practice and master the shampoo procedure. Once you have accomplished this, you will want to achieve a keen understanding of the chemistry of shampoos, rinses, and conditioning treatments and the effects these products and their chemicals have on the hair. You, as a professional cosmetologist, actually become the client's hair physician. Therefore, your knowledge of the effects of various products on the hair will be critical in your role as a professional consultant who prescribes treatment for the hair.

1 Essential Experience

Partner Research Shampoo Products

Find a partner and conduct a research project on the various shampoo products used in your school. You may want to expand your project by researching the shampoo products used at home by both partners. Use the following chart to list each type of shampoo, the type of hair they are created for, and the ingredients found in each. After you have collected the data, make a determination regarding any common ingredients in the products. Finally, obtain some litmus paper and test each product to determine the pH level (level of acidity and alkalinity) of each product.

Product Name	Recommended for Which Hair Type	Ingredients	pH Level

After identifying the common ingredients, write a brief explanation of why you believe these ingredients are used in so many shampoo products.

____

____

____

____

____

Essential Experience 2

The pH Levels of Shampoos

Using the pH scale provided below, label the pH levels of the shampoos you researched in Essential Experience 1.

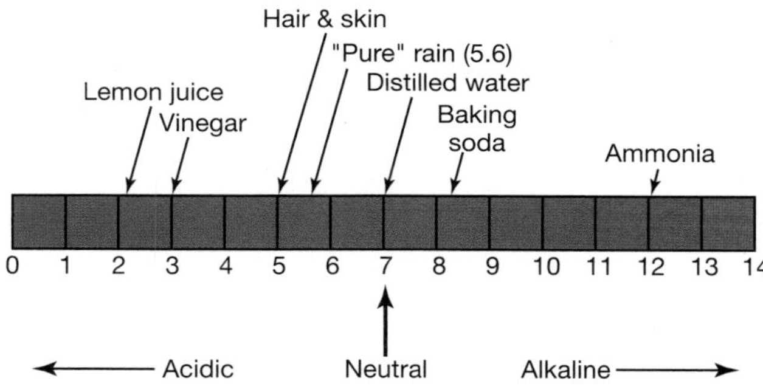

3 Essential Experience

Shampoo Hair Swatches

Collect hair swatches for various types of hair including normal, color-treated, relaxed, and permed. Shampoo the swatches at least five times with one available shampoo product, using a different shampoo for each swatch. Report the effects of the shampoo on each swatch. Then divide each swatch in half and condition one half. Report on the effects of each shampoo on each swatch. Report on the results after half the swatch has been reconditioned. Tape the swatches into the box provided.

Swatch Type	Shampoo Used	Results	Conditioned Swatch	Results
Normal				
Color-treated				
Relaxed				
Permed				

Make recommendations for the ideal shampoo for each hair type and explain why others are not appropriate.

____

____

____

Essential Experience 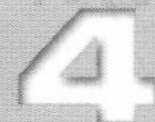

Soft and Hard Water Analysis

Arrange to have both soft and hard water available for use in this experiment. Using the different water types and a professional shampoo product, compare the product's lathering ability, cleansing ability, and the appearance of the hair afterward. Record your results below.

5 Essential Experience

Pre-Service Steps

Number the following pre-service steps in the order they should occur.

_______ Reviewed schedule

_______ Wore gloves

_______ Greeted client

_______ Cleaned tools

_______ Rinsed and dried tools

_______ Eliminated distractions

_______ Immersed implements

_______ Cleaned station

_______ Removed implements

_______ Stored implements

_______ Washed hands

_______ Filled disinfectant container

_______ Collected implements

_______ Reviewed intake form

_______ Prepared self

_______ Washed hands

_______ Cleared head

Essential Experience 6

Hair Brushing Steps

Number the following hair brushing steps in the order they should occur.

_______ Laid brush (held in right hand) with bristles down on hair close to scalp

_______ Repeated three times on each strand

_______ Made client comfortable

_______ Removed hair ornaments

_______ Examined scalp

_______ Subsectioned hair 1 inch (2.5 cm) from front hairline to crown

_______ Removed jewelry and glasses

_______ Used half-head parting

_______ Held strand of hair in nondominant hand between thumb and fingers

_______ Rotated brush by turning wrist slightly and sweeping bristles full length of hair shaft

_______ Continued brushing until entire head had been brushed

_______ Draped client for a shampoo

Essential Rubrics

Rubrics are used in education for organizing and interpreting data gathered from observations of student performance. It is a clearly developed scoring document used to differentiate between levels of development in a specific skill performance or behavior. A rubric is provided in this study guide as a self-assessment tool to aid you in your behavior development.

Rate your performance according to the following scale.

(1) Development Opportunity: There is little or no evidence of competency; assistance is needed; performance includes multiple errors.

(2) Fundamental: There is beginning evidence of competency; task is completed alone; performance includes few errors.

(3) Competent: There is detailed and consistent evidence of competency; task is completed alone; performance includes rare errors.

(4) Strength: There is detailed evidence of highly creative, inventive, mature presence of competency.

Space is provided for comments to assist you in improving your performance and achieving a higher rating.

SCALP MASSAGE PROCEDURE ASSESSMENT

Performance Assessed	**1**	**2**	**3**	**4**	**Improvement Plan**
Cupped client's chin in left hand					
Placed right hand at base of skull					
Rotated head gently					
Reversed hand positions and repeated					
Placed fingertips on each side of head					
Slid hands firmly upward					
Spread fingertips till they met at top of head					
Repeated four times					
Placed fingertips on each side of head 1 inch (2.5 cm) back					

Essential Rubrics continued

Performance Assessed	1	2	3	4	Improvement Plan
Slid hands firmly upward					
Spread fingertips until they met at top of head					
Rotated and moved client's scalp					
Repeated four times					
Held back of client's head with left hand					
Placed stretched thumb and fingers on forehead					
Moved hand slowly and firmly upward to 1 inch (2.5 cm) past hairline					
Repeated four times					
Placed palms firmly against scalp					
Lifted scalp in rotary movement above client's ears					
Lifted scalp in rotary movement at front and back of head					
Placed fingers of both hands at client's forehead					
Massaged around hairline by lifting and rotating					
Dropped back 1 inch (2.5 cm) and repeated movement					
Placed fingers of each hand on sides of client's head					
Manipulated scalp with thumbs working toward crown					
Repeated four times					
Repeated manipulation working toward center back of head					

Essential Rubrics continued

Performance Assessed	1	2	3	4	Improvement Plan
Placed left hand on client's forehead					
Massaged from right ear to the left ear along base of skull with heel of hand					
Rotated from base of client's neck along shoulder and back across shoulder blade to spine					
Slid hand up client's spine to base of neck					
Repeated on opposite side					
Placed both palms at base of neck					
Used rotary movement, catching muscles in palms					
Massaged along shoulder blades to point of shoulders and back again					
Massaged from shoulders to spine and back again					
Massaged from base of client's skull down spine with rotary movement					
Used firm finger pressure and brought hand slowly to client's skull					

Essential Rubrics continued

BASIC SHAMPOO PROCEDURE ASSESSMENT

Performance Assessed	1	2	3	4	Improvement Plan
Made client comfortable					
Draped client for shampoo					
Removed hair ornaments					
Removed jewelry and glasses					
Examined scalp					
Brushed hair thoroughly					
Adjusted water temperature					
Saturated hair with warm water					
Applied shampoo and lathered					
Began at front hairline and worked to top of head					
Continued to back of head, shifting fingers back 1 inch (2.5 cm) at a time					
Lifted client's head with dominant hand					
With nondominant hand, started at top of right ear using back and forth movement, worked to back of head					
Dropped fingers down about 1 inch (2.5 cm), repeated process until right side of head had been massaged					
Began at left ear and repeated the prior two steps on the left side of head					
Allowed client's head to relax and worked around hairline with thumbs in a rotary movement					

Essential Rubrics continued

Performance Assessed	1	2	3	4	Improvement Plan
Repeated all steps until scalp has been thoroughly massaged					
Removed excess lather by squeezing hair gently					
Rinsed hair thoroughly					
Used strong spray, lifted hair at crown and back with fingers of left hand; permitted spray to rinse hair thoroughly					
Cupped hand along nape line and patted the hair, forcing spray against base scalp area					
Shampooed and rinsed again if needed					
Gently squeezed excess water from hair; applied conditioner avoiding base of hair near scalp					
Gently combed conditioner through, distributing it with a wide-tooth comb					
Left conditioner on for recommended time; rinsed thoroughly and finished with a cool water rinse to seal cuticle					
Massaged scalp					
Placed plastic cap					
Rinsed hair thoroughly					
Removed excess moisture from hair at shampoo bowl					
Towel-dried hair					
Cleaned shampoo bowl					
Combed hair beginning at nape					
Changed drape if needed					

Essential Review

Using the following words, fill in the blanks to form a thorough review of Chapter 13, Shampooing, Rinsing, & Conditioning. Words or terms may be used more than once or not at all.

0 to 6.9	**H_2O**	**powder**
4.5 to 5.5	**H_2O_2**	**protein**
7.1 to 14	**hard**	**scales**
acid	**humectants**	**shampooing**
astringent lotions	**hydrogen**	**shampoos**
blood	**ingredients**	**skin**
brittle	**medicated**	**soft**
chemical service	**natural**	**stimulating**
citric acid	**nonstripping**	**tangles**
condition	**oily**	**temperature**
dry	**polymers**	**volume**

1. An important preliminary first step for a variety of hair services is ____________.
2. To be effective, a shampoo must remove all dirt, oils, cosmetics, and ____________ debris without adversely affecting either the scalp or hair.
3. ____________ hair should be shampooed more often than other types.
4. Hair can usually be characterized as oily, ____________, normal, or chemically treated.
5. Rainwater or water that has been chemically treated is known as ____________ water.
6. ____________ water contains certain minerals that lessen the ability of the shampoo to lather readily.
7. ____________ bristles are recommended for hair brushing.
8. Select the shampoo according to the ____________ of the client's hair.
9. A high-pH shampoo can leave the hair dry and ____________.
10. You should not brush the hair prior to giving a ________________.
11. Brushing stimulates the ____________ circulation to the scalp and helps remove dust, dirt, and hair spray buildup from the hair.

Essential Review continued

12. Moisturizing treatments soften and loosen ____________ from the scalp.
13. The inner side of your wrist is used to test the water ____________.
14. Biotin and protein are conditioning agents that restore moisture and elasticity, strengthen the hair shaft, and add ____________.
15. ____________ cleanse the hair and scalp prior to a service.
16. The key to determining which shampoo will leave the hair shiny and manageable is the ____________ list.
17. The amount of ____________ in a solution determines whether it is more alkaline or more acid.
18. Shampoos that are more acid will fall in the range of ____________ on the pH scale.
19. Shampoos that are more alkaline will fall in the range of ____________ on the pH scale.
20. An acid-balanced shampoo will fall in the range of ____________ on the pH scale.
21. ____________ shampoos contain special chemicals that are effective in reducing excessive dandruff.
22. Most conditioners contain silicone along with moisture-binding ____________ that absorb moisture or promote the retention of moisture.
23. Penetrating conditioners that are left on the hair for ten to twenty minutes restore ____________ and moisture.
24. Scalp ________________ remove oil accumulation from the scalp and are used after a scalp treatment.
25. Products that do not remove artificial color from the hair are known as ____________.

Essential Discoveries and Accomplishments

In the space below, jot some notes about what concepts of this chapter were hardest for you to understand or remember. Imagine finding yourself suddenly in the role of "teacher" and consider what you would tell your "students" about these concepts. Share your Essential Discoveries with some of the other students in your class and ask if they are helpful to them. You may want to revise your discoveries based on any good ideas shared by your peers.

Discoveries:

List at least three things you have accomplished since your last entry that relate to your career goals.

Accomplishments:

CHAPTER 16

Haircutting

A Motivating Moment: "Courage is the first of human virtues because it makes all others possible."
— Aristotle

Essential Objectives

After studying this chapter and completing the Essential Companion components, you will be able to:

1. Identify reference points on the head form and understand their role in haircutting.
2. Define angles, elevations, and guidelines.
3. List the factors involved in a successful client consultation.
4. Explain the use of the various tools of haircutting.
5. Name three things you can do to ensure good posture and body position while cutting hair.
6. Perform the four basic haircuts.
7. Discuss and explain three different texturizing techniques performed with shears.
8. Explain what a clipper cut is.
9. Identify the uses of a trimmer.

Essential Haircutting

I really want to specialize in hair design, so why is it so important for me to master the art of haircutting?

Haircutting is a technique that requires many hours of practice and a vivid imagination. It is an extremely important skill that must be mastered because the cut serves as the basis for every hairstyle. It may not be done as frequently as a shampoo or style, but it is certainly completed more frequently than chemical services. If you want to ensure that the style you provide your client is the most attractive and will look good even when he or she styles his or her own hair, you must deliver a quality haircut. The way to accomplish this is with frequent practice, repetitive exercises, timed procedures, and a strong desire to become an accomplished haircutter.

Cosmetologists should study and have a thorough understanding of haircutting because:

- Haircutting is a basic, foundational skill upon which all other hair design is built.
- Being able to rely on your haircutting skills and techniques when creating a haircut is what will build confidence, trust, and loyalty between a cosmetologist and her clients.
- The ability to duplicate an existing haircut or create a new haircut from a photo will build a stronger professional relationship between stylist and client.
- A good haircut that is easy to style and maintain will make clients happy with their service and build repeat services.

Essential Concepts

What are the most important techniques and procedures I should learn to become a good haircutter?

Haircutting is actually more than just reducing length and bulk from the hair. It begins with using quality tools, and there are many to aid you in achieving a dynamic haircut. You will want to practice techniques with shears, razors, clippers, thinning shears, and all the ancillary tools such as combs and brushes. You will want to work with all these tools until you have complete control and can handle them with ease. You will need to become familiar with all the terms used in haircutting. It is important to remember that terminology in our industry constantly changes. Do not let yourself get sidetracked because one instructor or one book calls a specific cut one thing and another calls it something else. It is the end result that matters, not what the technique, procedure, or style is named.

Your instructor will take you through steps of sectioning for various types of cuts. You will find that proper sectioning is extremely important, especially until you have learned to manage and control larger amounts of hair. You will learn about angles and elevations and how to combine them to create a wide variety of hairstyles. It is highly recommended that you style every haircut you complete while learning. This allows you to see the results of your efforts. If, for example, you are unable to achieve the desired style after the cut, it may be because you have not yet mastered that particular haircut. Just remember that no one performs a perfect haircut the first time. Good haircutting takes practice and commitment—so don't give up.

Essential Experience 1

Identify the Tools

Using the photos found below, label each tool using the following terms (some terms may be used more than once).

Back	Barber comb	Blade
Finger grip	Finger tang	Finger rest
Handle	Head	Heel
Pivot	Pivot screw	Point
Shoulder	Still blade	Styling comb
Tang	Thinning shears	Edge
Wide-tooth comb	Haircutting shears	Moving blade
Shank	Tail comb	

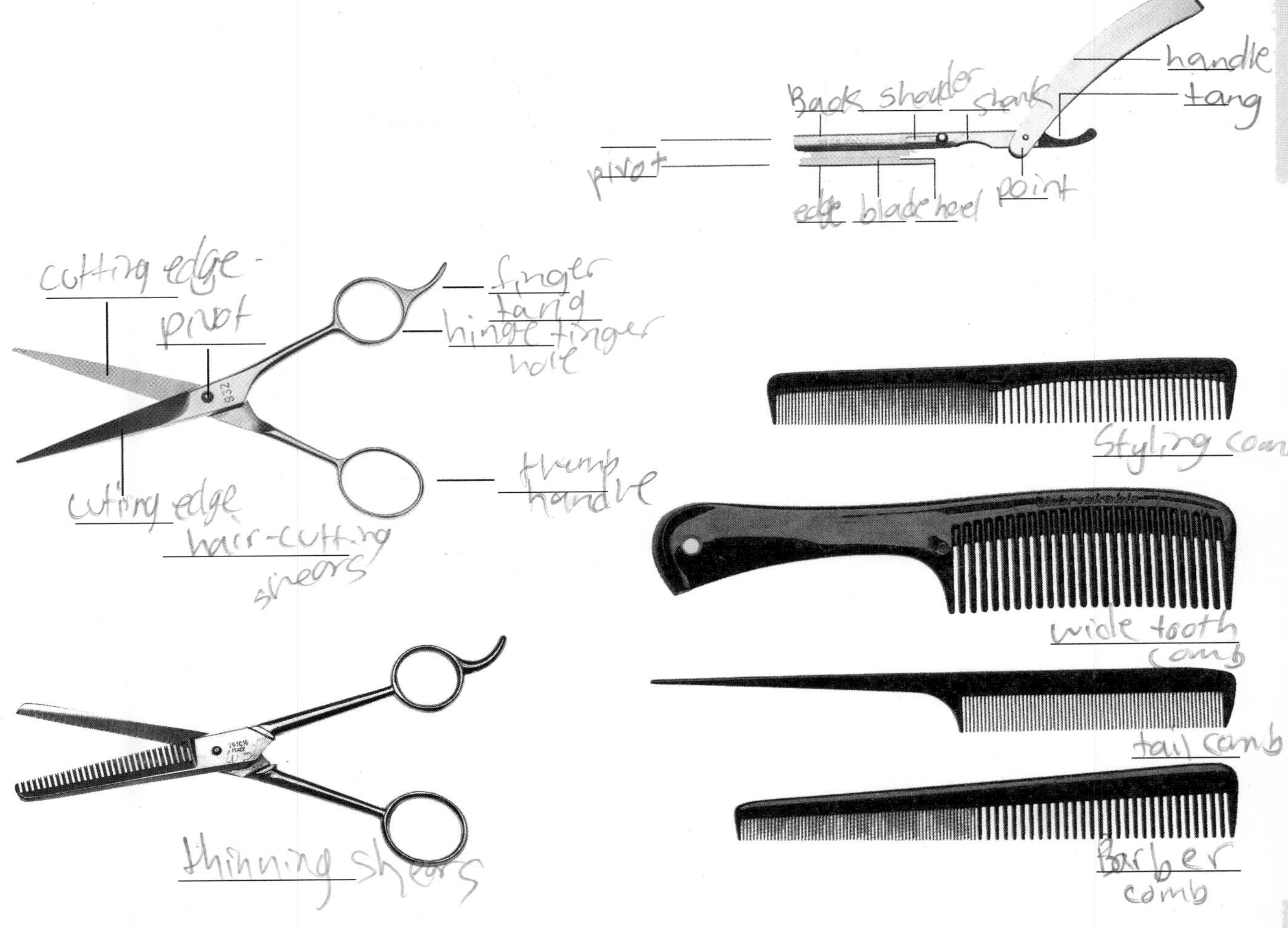

2 Essential Experience

Windowpane Concepts A

Windowpaning is the process of transferring key elements, points, or steps in a lesson into visual images that are hand sketched into the squares or *panes* of a matrix. Let your mind think in pictures and sketch the essential concepts printed in each of the following windowpanes. Do not be concerned with your artistic ability. Use lines and stick figures to depict each concept.

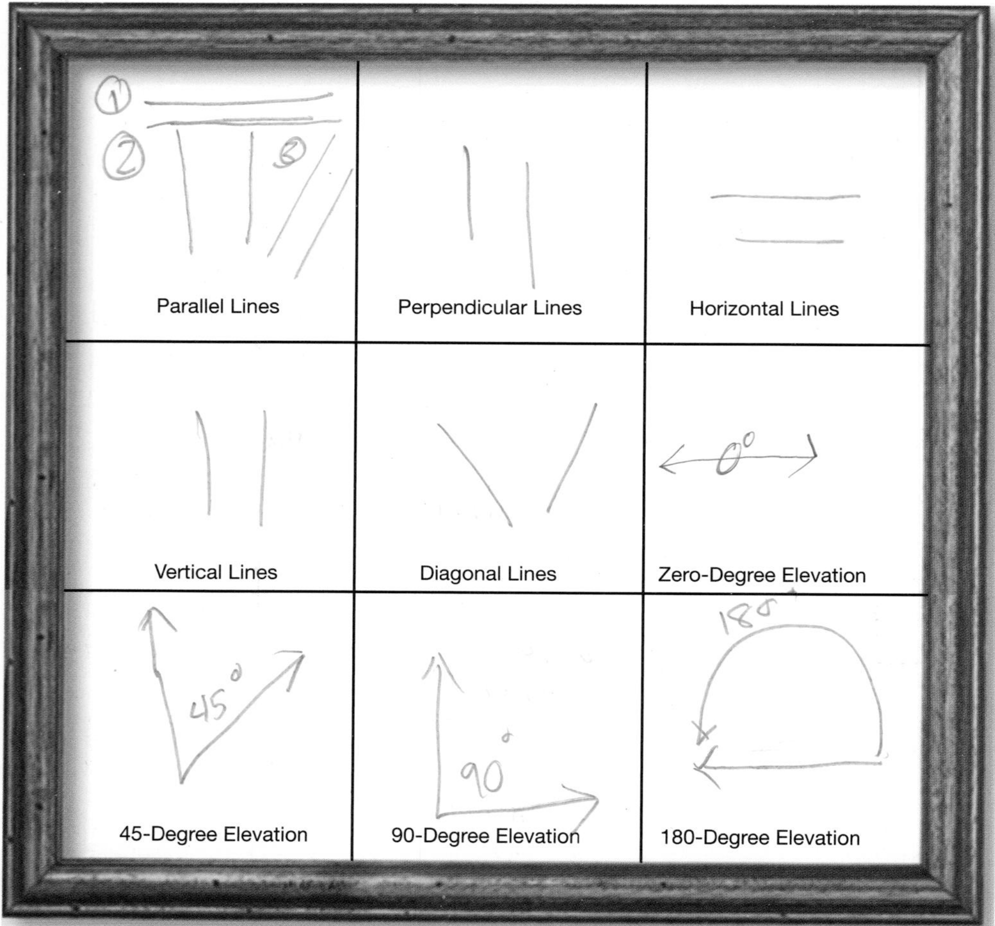

Essential Experience 3

Matching Exercise

Terms A

Match the essential terms with their identifying terms or phrases.

Answer	Term	Definition
10	**Beveling**	**1.** Lines between horizontal and vertical
9	**Haircutting shears**	**2.** Outer line
5	**Thinning shears**	**3.** Used to remove superfluous hair and to create clean lines around ears and neckline
4	**Razor**	**4.** Used to create very short tapers quickly
3	**Clippers**	**5.** Usually used to cut a blunt straight line; can be used to thin hair by slithering
8	**Edgers**	**6.** Lines that are parallel to the floor; used in low elevation haircuts
7	**Angle**	**7.** Space between two lines that intersect
2	**Perimeter**	**8.** Used to remove bulk from the hair
6	**Horizontal**	**9.** Used to cut hair with a softer edge than shears
1	**Diagonal**	**10.** Cutting the ends of the hair at a slight taper

3 Essential Experience continued

Terms B

Match the essential terms with their identifying terms or phrases.

J	**Blunt cut**	**1.** Cutting with the points of the shears to create texture in the hair ends
K	**Elevation**	**2.** This shape has a stacked area around the exterior and is cut at low to medium elevations
B	**Graduated**	**3.** Graduated effect achieved by cutting the hair with elevation or overdirection
D	**Guideline**	**4.** Section of hair that determines the length the hair will be cut
C	**Layering**	**5.** Level at which a blunt cut falls; where the ends of the hair hang together
A	**Notching or point cutting**	**6.** Line dividing the hair to create subsections
F	**Parting**	**7.** How tightly the hair is pulled before cutting
J	**Sections**	**8.** Lines that are perpendicular to the floor
G	**Tension**	**9.** Cutting the hair straight across the strand; all hair hangs to one level, forming a weight line
E	**Weight line**	**10.** Divisions of the hair made before cutting
H	**Vertical**	**11.** Angle at which the hair is held away from the head for cutting

Essential Experience 4

Windowpane Concepts B

Windowpaning is the process of transferring key elements, points, or steps in a lesson into visual images that are hand sketched into the squares or *panes* of a matrix. Let your mind think in pictures and sketch the essential concepts printed in each of the following windowpanes. Do not be concerned with your artistic ability. Use lines and stick figures to depict the concepts requested.

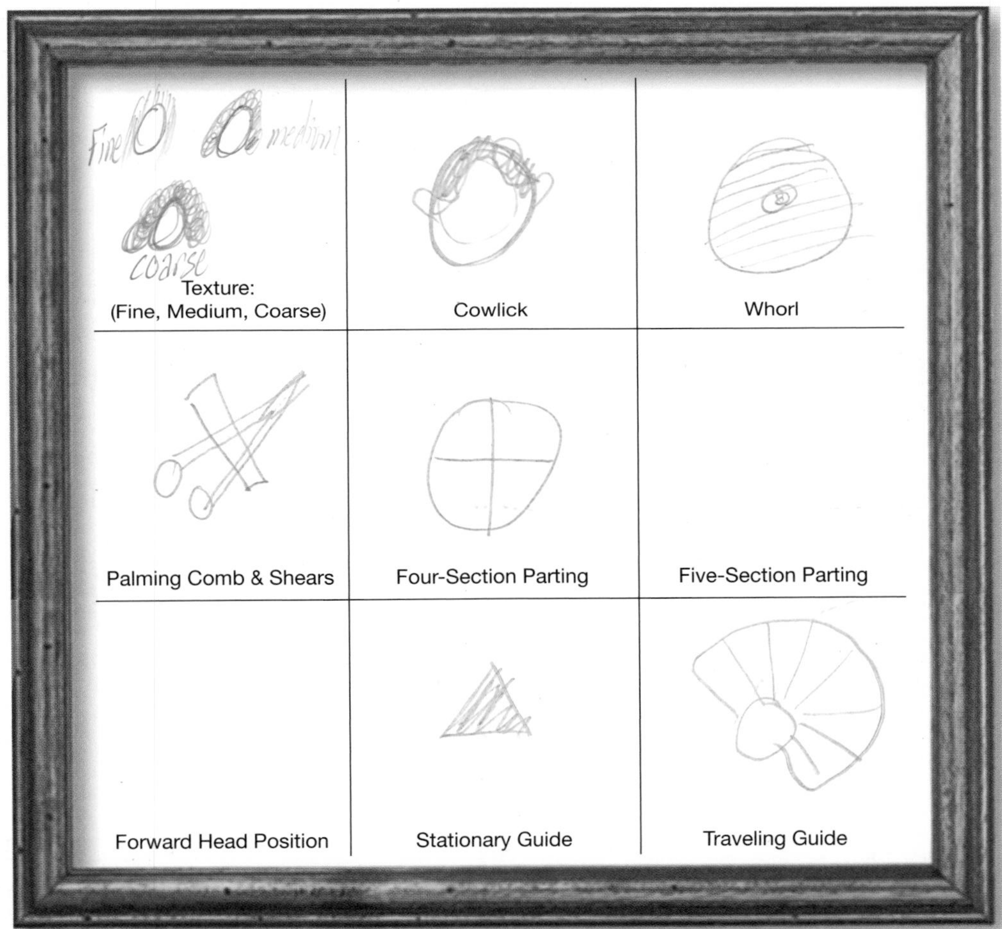

5 Essential Experience

Style Analysis for Techniques, Angles, and Elevations

As a professional stylist you will have numerous clients who bring in photographs because they want to achieve the same or similar look. Therefore, learning how to evaluate a style and determine how it was achieved will be of great benefit to you. With that in mind, look through various magazines and select three particular cuts that appeal to you. Paste them on the chart below in the left column. In the right column, diagram and/or explain the techniques, angles, and elevations you would use to create this particular haircut and style.

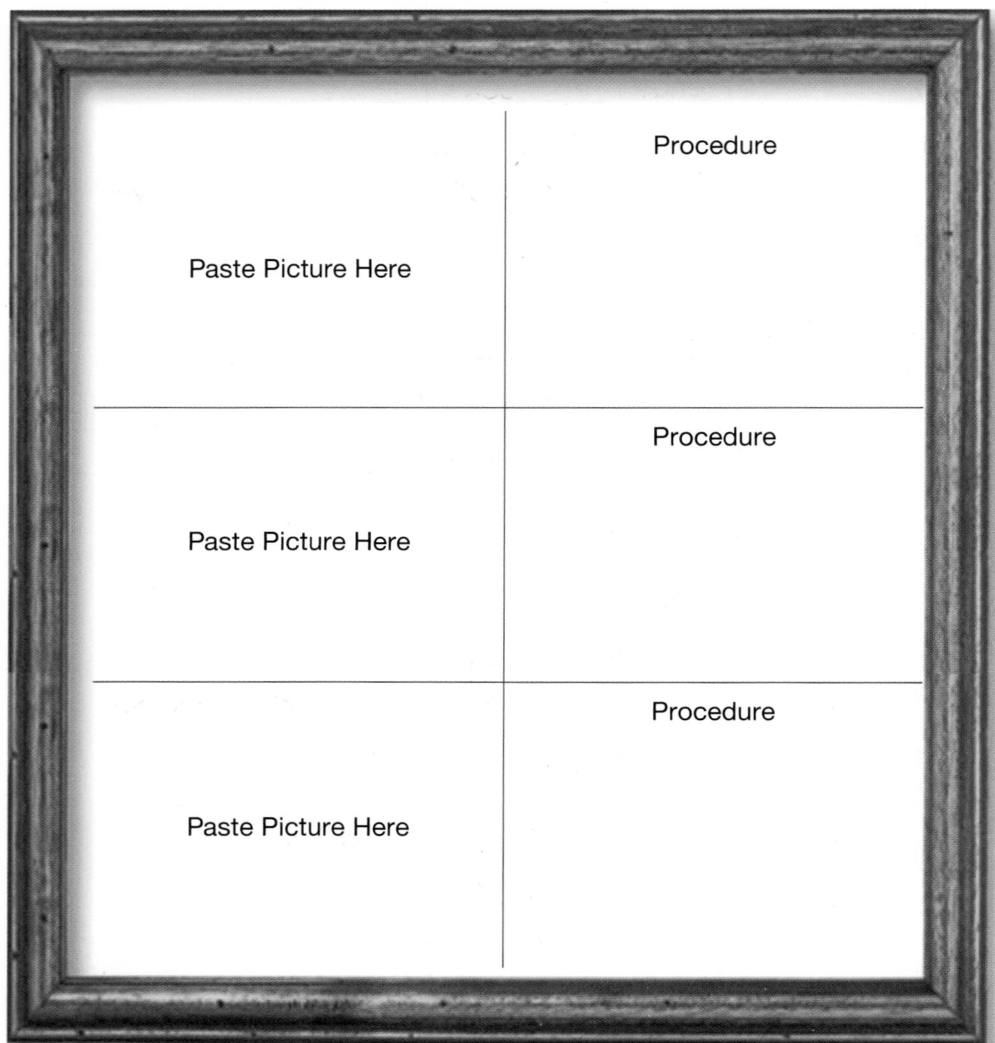

Paste Picture Here	Procedure
Paste Picture Here	Procedure
Paste Picture Here	Procedure

Essential Experience 6

Word Scramble

Using the clues provided, unscramble the terms below.

Scramble	Correct Word
ntlub uct	blunt cut *Clue:* Cut straight across.
adterudga	graduated *Clue:* A wedge or stack.
nergif	fringe *Clue:* Triangular section that begins at apex and ends at front corners.
egrynial	Layering *Clue:* Cutting the hair with elevation or overdirection.
iseontcs	sections *Clue:* Divisions in hair before cutting.
ladnioag	diagonal *Clue:* Between horizontal and vertical.
lenaigvrt	traveling *Clue:* Moving.
liavctre	vertical *Clue:* Perpendicular to the floor.
diew hotot	wide tooth *Clue:* Comb used to create softer edge when cutting with shears.
sderge	edgers *Clue:* Remove superfluous hair.
utsenoicsb	subsection *Clue:* Partings.
hrlwo	whorl *Clue:* Requires extra length.
zroar	razor *Clue:* Cuts hair with softer edge.

7 Essential Experience

Word Search A

After determining the correct word from the clues provided, locate the words in the word search puzzle.

Word	Clue
______________	Used for close tapers
______________	Holding the shears at an angle other than 90 degrees to the hair strand
______________	A cut that is short on the bottom and long on the top
______________	Cheaters
______________	Found in the hairline or the interior of the hair
______________	Slithering
______________	The angle at which the hair is held away from the head
______________	Section of hair that determines the length
______________	90-degree haircut
______________	Lines that are parallel to the floor

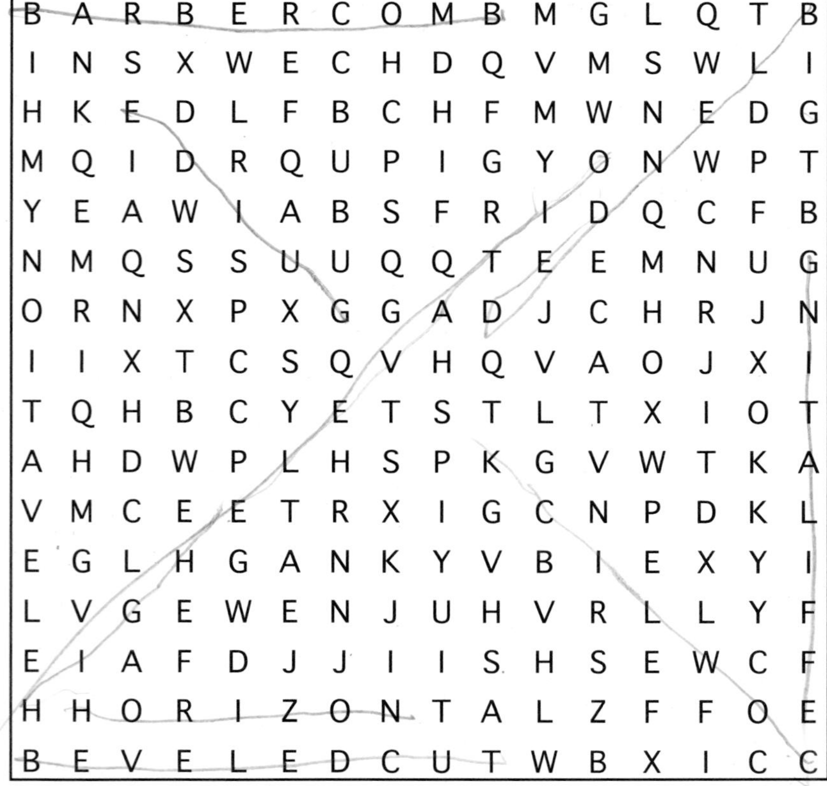

Essential Experience 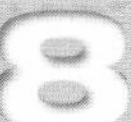

Haircut Procedures and Techniques

In your own words, explain the purpose of the following procedures.

Checking a Haircut

[One possible response follows]

cross checking the haircut is sperding the hair routin. the opasite way you can cut. it to check for precision of line and shape. If you use vertical partings in a haircut, cross-check the lengths with horizontal partings

Slide Cutting

[One possible response follows]

used for cutting or thinning the hair in which the fingers and shears glide along the edge of the hair to remove length

Shears-Over-Comb Technique

[One possible response follows]

benning technique that has crossed ove into cosmetology, hold the hair in place with the comb. while using the tips of the shears to remove length

9 Essential Experience

Word Search B

After determining the correct word from the clues provided, locate the words in the word search puzzle.

Word	Clue
______________	Traveling
______________	Also known as pointing
______________	Lines that never meet in space
______________	Subsections
______________	A popular barbering technique
______________	Used to cut a blunt straight line across the hair
______________	Stable
______________	How tightly the hair is pulled when cutting
______________	Removing bulk without removing length
______________	Level at which the blunt cut falls

P	Y	Q	R	X	X	M	X	G	O	M	K	F	T	S	N	Z	I
M	A	G	S	U	R	G	M	X	G	A	Y	A	T	O	D	H	Q
X	E	R	K	Q	Y	E	T	S	U	Y	O	A	I	I	A	S	U
S	W	U	T	B	M	H	A	Q	B	K	T	S	H	W	V	Z	N
C	F	A	S	I	M	F	E	S	T	I	N	B	V	I	C	Z	V
G	F	Q	Y	R	N	O	A	E	O	E	C	K	P	O	P	J	H
I	R	H	V	S	P	G	C	N	T	G	Y	P	G	R	L	K	C
S	K	Q	E	A	G	N	A	R	P	S	C	J	R	A	V	S	F
D	Z	B	N	N	E	R	G	E	E	A	D	E	O	W	V	I	G
Z	F	T	W	P	Y	N	G	Q	N	V	R	M	N	U	A	M	L
Q	N	S	D	G	I	N	S	H	W	I	O	A	N	Q	X	D	J
M	P	B	U	H	I	U	K	S	S	Q	L	S	L	M	Y	M	R
M	O	I	C	N	Z	U	N	T	S	Q	V	T	R	L	K	R	O
H	D	T	N	D	U	X	D	B	P	D	P	M	H	A	E	C	Z
E	O	I	D	L	W	A	T	Q	T	S	E	A	H	G	E	L	A
N	H	R	I	G	I	H	C	F	J	D	H	Z	P	L	I	H	R
T	G	C	Z	A	B	J	A	X	Y	U	J	X	F	G	E	E	S
M	O	V	I	N	G	K	W	E	J	L	J	Q	H	J	T	O	W

Essential Rubrics

Rubrics are used in education for organizing and interpreting data gathered from observations of student performance. It is a clearly developed scoring document used to differentiate between levels of development in a specific skill performance or behavior. A rubric is provided in this study guide as a self-assessment tool to aid you in your behavior development.

Rate your performance according to the following scale.

(1) Development Opportunity: There is little or no evidence of competency; assistance is needed; performance includes multiple errors.

(2) Fundamental: There is beginning evidence of competency; task is completed alone; performance includes few errors.

(3) Competent: There is detailed and consistent evidence of competency; task is completed alone; performance includes rare errors.

(4) Strength: There is detailed evidence of highly creative, inventive, mature presence of competency.

Space is provided for comments to assist you in improving your performance and achieving a higher rating.

BLUNT HAIRCUT PROCEDURE ASSESSMENT

Performance Assessed	1	2	3	4	Improvement Plan
Detangled the hair with wide-tooth comb					
Combed the hair back and away from the face to find the natural part or parted the hair the way the client will be wearing it					
Took a center parting from the front hairline to the nape, dividing the head in two halves					
Found the apex of the head, took a parting from the apex to the back of the ear on both sides and clipped, resulting in four sections					

Essential Rubrics continued

Performance Assessed	1	2	3	4	Improvement Plan
Began at the nape, on the left side, took a horizontal parting ¼ to ½ inch (0.6 to 1.25 cm) from the hairline					
With client's head upright, combed the subsection in a natural fall from scalp to ends					
With dominant hand, combed the subsection again, stopping just above the cutting line					
Made sure comb was horizontal and just above cutting line (desired line)					
Cut subsection straight across, kept shears horizontal and parallel to the floor					
Repeated prior step on the right side, using the length of first subsection as a guide					
Checked to make sure cutting line was straight before moving on					
Returned to left side, took another horizontal parting, creating a subsection the same size as previous subsection allowing view of the guideline through the new subsection					
Combed hair down in a natural fall, and cut the length to match the guide					
Repeated on the right side					
Continued working up the back of the head, alternating from left section to right section, using subsections					

Essential Rubrics continued

Performance Assessed	1	2	3	4	Improvement Plan
Combed hair into its natural falling position, and cut with little or no tension to match the guide					
Began on left side, took a horizontal parting and parted off a portion from the back area to match					
Held comb parallel to floor, cut hair straight across just below the comb, connecting the line to the back					
Repeated step on right side of head					
Cut right side in same manner as left side					
Checked both sides for evenness					
Made any needed adjustments					
Continued working on left side with horizontal partings until all hair had been cut to match the guide					
Made sure hair fell on the side, not the face, when cutting hair along the face					
Repeated procedure on right side					
Swept up cut hair from the floor and disposed of properly					
Blowdry haircut using very little lift off scalp					
After drying hair, had client stand and checked line in mirror					
Cleaned up any hair at neckline and checked where hair fell when dry					

GRADUATED HAIRCUT PROCEDURE ASSESSMENT

Performance Assessed	1	2	3	4	Improvement Plan
Parted hair into six sections according to procedure					
Established guideline by first cutting the center of the nape section to the desired length					
Used a horizontal cutting line parallel to the fingers					
Cut the right and left sides of the nape section the same length as the center guideline					
Worked upward in the left back section, measured and parted off the first horizontal section approximately 1-inch (2.5 cm) wide					
Began at the center part, established a vertical subsection approximately ½-inch (1.25 cm) wide					
Extended the subsection down to include the nape guideline and combed the subsection smooth at a 45-degree angle to the scalp					
Held fingers at a 90-degree angle to the strand and cut					
Proceeded to cut the entire horizontal section by parting off vertical subsections and cutting in the same manner as before					
Checked each section vertically and horizontally throughout the haircut					
Each completed section served as a guideline for the next section					
Parted off another horizontal section approximately 1-inch (2.5 cm) wide					

Essential Rubrics continued

Performance Assessed	1	2	3	4	Improvement Plan
Began at the center, created another vertical subsection that extended down and included the previously cut strands					
Combed the hair smoothly at a 45-degree elevation to the head					
Held the fingers and shears at a 90-degree angle to the subsection and cut					
Cut the entire horizontal section in the same manner					
Made sure the second section blended evenly with the previously cut section					
Continued taking horizontal sections throughout the left and right back sections and followed the same cutting procedure					
The hair gradually became longer as it reached the apex					
Maintained the length in the upper crown by holding each vertical subsection throughout the crown area at a 90-degree angle while cutting					
After checking the back and crown for even blending, proceeded to the left-side section					
Established a narrow guide section on the left side at the hairline approximately ½-inch (1.25 cm) wide					
Moved to the right side of the head and established a matching guideline					
Established a ½-inch (2.5 cm) side section that curved and followed the hairline above the ear back to the nape section					

Essential Rubrics continued

Performance Assessed	1	2	3	4	Improvement Plan
Smoothly combed the section, including the side guideline and part of the nape section					
Held the hair with little or no tension and cut the hair from the nape guide to the side guide					
Established a horizontal section on the left side taking into account the protrusion of the ear					
Starting at the ear, parted a ½-inch (1.25 cm) vertical subsection included the underlying guideline and a small portion of the nape section					
Continued the same cutting procedure previously followed					
Took vertical subsections, combed smoothly, elevated at a 45-degree angle from the head, held the fingers at a 90-degree angle to the strand					
Cut the section even with the side guideline and nape section					
Held the vertical subsections straight out from the head at 45 degrees					
Continued establishing horizontal sections on the left side of the head and followed the same cutting procedure					
Checked each section horizontally to ensure the ends were evenly blended					

Essential Rubrics continued

Performance Assessed	1	2	3	4	Improvement Plan
Added strands from the back section when checking to ensure that the two sections were uniform in length					
When the left side section was completed, the strands in the uppermost part of the section were the same length as those in the upper crown area					
In the final 1-inch (2.5 cm) section, combed the vertical subsections and held them at a 90-degree angle to the head					
Positioned fingers at 90 degrees to the strand and cut parallel to the fingers					
Checked the completed section horizontally to make sure the ends were even					
Moved to the right side of the head and cut the hair in the same manner as on the left side, using the previously established guide					
Once the back and both sides were complete, moved to the fringe and top areas					
Created a fringe guide section along the hairline about ½-inch (1.25 cm) wide					
Started at the center part and worked on the left side of the forehead, cut to the desired length					
Combed the fringe section, including the center guide strand and a small portion of the side area					
Connected the two guidelines to determine the angle of the cut					

Essential Rubrics continued

Performance Assessed	1	2	3	4	Improvement Plan
Cut fringe section at a low elevation					
Checked the cut for evenness and accuracy					
Cut ½-inch (1.25 cm) section					
Brought down another ½-inch (1.25 cm) section and cut this subsection of the bang section at a low elevation to the guideline					
Took a vertical parting along hairline that connects the guideline from the bang and the guideline from in front of the ear					
Slid hand slowly, kept both guidelines in grasp, and stopped with about ¼ inch (0.6 cm) of both guidelines in hand					
Used the guideline established in the previous step and took ½-inch (1.25 cm) subsections and cut the top section at a 45-degree angle, blending with the sides					
Finished the top section by taking ½-inch (1.25 cm) vertical subsections parallel to the center part.					
Held the hair up from the head at a 90-degree angle including the hair from the crown and bang areas and cut to blend the section with the two precut sections					
Continued cutting in this manner until the remainder of the top section is cut					
Held the hair up from the head at a 90-degree angle and checked the completed cut					
Trimmed any uneven ends					

Essential Rubrics continued

UNIFORM-LAYERED HAIRCUT PROCEDURE ASSESSMENT

Performance Assessed	1	2	3	4	Improvement Plan
Sectioned hair into five sections					
Took two partings ½-inch (1.25 cm) apart, creating a section that ran from the front hairline to the bottom of the nape					
Combed all other hair out of the way					
Began at the crown, combed the section straight out from the head					
Kept fingers parallel to the head form, and cut to the desired length					
Continued working forward to the front hairline, making sure to stand to the side of the client					
Continued cutting the guideline from the crown to the nape, rounding off corners and kept fingers parallel to the head form					
Separated the sides from the back by parting the hair from the apex to the back of the ear					
Worked through the back area first					
The parting pattern was wedge-shaped, and each section began at the same point in the crown and was slightly wider at the bottom of the nape					
Worked through the right side first					

Essential Rubrics continued

Performance Assessed	1	2	3	4	Improvement Plan
Took a vertical parting that began at the crown and connected with the guideline, creating a vertical section that ended at the hairline					
Kept the sections small to maintain control					
Began at the crown and used previously cut guideline					
Combed the new section to the guide, and elevated the hair straight out from the head, with no overdirection					
Cut the line by keeping fingers parallel to the head and matching the guide, working from top to bottom					
Continued working with a traveling guideline to the back of the ear					
Repeated on opposite side					
Blended top with side section					
Connected previously cut sections to crown					
Cross-checked hair in crown area					
Cross-checked top section					
Cut sides and connected to previous section at back of ear and top					
Repeated on the opposite side					
Cross-checked side sections					
Completed the blended haircut					

LONG-LAYERED (180-DEGREE) HAIRCUT PROCEDURE ASSESSMENT

Performance Assessed	1	2	3	4	Improvement Plan
Sectioned hair into five sections					
Began at top of the crown by taking a ½-inch (1.25 cm) subsection across the head					
Combed hair straight up from the head form and cut straight across					
Worked to the front of the top section by taking a second ½-inch (1.25 cm) subsection					
Directed the first subsection (guideline) to the second one and cut to the same length					
Continued, using the previously cut subsection as the guideline to cut a new ½-inch (1.25 cm) subsection throughout the top section					
On the left front section, used ½-inch (1.25 cm) horizontal subsections					
Combed the hair straight up and matched to the previously cut hair (guideline) in the top section					
Continued working down the side, using ½-inch (1.25 cm) subsections until the hair no longer reached the guide					
Repeated on the right side					
Completed the back sections					
Continued cutting using ½-inch (1.25 cm) horizontal subsections, working from top to bottom until hair no longer reached guide					
Ensured side lengths were even					

Essential Rubrics continued

MEN'S BASIC CLIPPER CUT PROCEDURE ASSESSMENT

Performance Assessed	1	2	3	4	Improvement Plan
Made a horseshoe parting about 2 inches (5 cm) below the apex of the head, beginning and ending at the front hairline					
Combed the hair above the part forward					
Starting in nape area, placed the haircutting comb against scalp, teeth up					
Angled comb against scalp from 0 to 45 degrees, allowing for the natural contour of the head					
Cut the hair that extended through the teeth of the comb					
Repeated step 2 while moving up back of head					
Blended lengths over the curve of the head by cross-cutting horizontally, from side to side					
Shaped back center area first, from nape to parietal ridge					
Using the clipper-over-comb technique, cut both sides of the back, from ear to ear					
Carefully blended lengths over the curve of the head by cross-cutting					
Using a low number attachment on the clipper, cut up each side from the sideburn to the parietal ridge					

Essential Rubrics continued

Performance Assessed	1	2	3	4	Improvement Plan
Measured distance between eyebrows and natural hairline to establish an appropriate guideline for length in crown area					
Cut a narrow guideline at crown end of horseshoe parting					
Determined the length by the forehead measurement					
Began at crown end, cut top area with clipper to the exact length of initial crown guideline					
While moving toward forehead, overdirected hair toward guideline in order to increase length at forehead					
Using clipper and attachment, shortened and shaped hair around ears and sideburns					
Continued to cut hair until shape of head and length of hair were in harmony					
Used a clipper or trimmer to blend or outline perimeter					

Essential Review

Complete the following review of Chapter 16, Haircutting, by circling the correct answer to each statement.

1. Cutting all the hair to one length is a/an ____________ cut.
   a) elevation b) blunt
   c) graduated d) beveled

2. A cut that has a stacked area around the exterior and is cut at low to medium elevations is a/an ____________ cut.
   a) elevation b) blunt
   c) graduated d) beveled

3. Cutting with the points of the shears to create texture is known as ____________.
   a) layering b) undercutting
   c) elevation d) notching

4. Subdivisions of a section, used for control when cutting are known as ____________.
   a) subsections b) guides
   c) sections d) tension

5. If the hair is cut partially wet and partially dry, the results will be ____________.
   a) even b) perfect
   c) uneven d) curly

6. The tools also known as trimmers that are used to clean necklines and around the ears are ____________.
   a) clippers b) edgers
   c) razor d) shears

7. A tool used to cut blunt straight lines is called the ____________.
   a) clippers b) edgers
   c) razor d) shears

8. The tool used to cut hair with a softer edge is known as the ____________.
   a) clippers b) edgers
   c) razor d) shears

Essential Review continued

9. The comb used for close tapers in the nape and sides is the ____________ comb.

   a) styling b) barber
   c) wide-tooth d) tail

10. The comb used mainly to detangle the hair is the ____________ comb.

   a) styling b) barber
   c) wide-tooth d) tail

11. ____________ points are points on the head that mark where the surface of the head changes or the behavior of the hair changes, such as the ears, jawline, occipital bone, or apex.

   a) Parietal b) Crown
   c) Elevation d) Reference

12. ____________ lines are parallel to the floor.

   a) Horizontal b) Perpendicular
   c) Diagonal d) Vertical

13. Lines that are perpendicular to the floor are ____________ lines.

   a) parallel b) perpendicular
   c) diagonal d) vertical

14. A haircutting technique that is measured in degrees is ____________.

   a) carving b) elevation
   c) clipper-over-comb d) traveling

15. Lines that are used for blending and stacking are ____________ lines.

   a) parallel b) perpendicular
   c) diagonal d) vertical

16. A stable guide that does not move is also known as a ____________ guide.

   a) moving b) traveling
   c) stationary d) mobile

Essential Review continued

17. When the hair is cut at 90 degrees and higher, the result is a ____________ haircut.

a) blunt
b) layered
c) graduated
d) blended

18. A 180-degree haircut is also known as a ____________.

a) low elevation cut
b) combined elevation cut
c) long layered haircut
d) blended elevation cut

19. A 0-degree haircut is also known as a ____________ elevation.

a) low
b) high
c) reverse
d) blended

20. A barbering technique that has become popular with cosmetologists is the ____________ -over-comb method.

a) clipper
b) razor
c) trimmer
d) shears

21. A/an ____________ is a thin continuous mark used as a guide.

a) angle
b) line
c) elevation
d) section

22. Gliding the fingers and shears along the edge of the hair to remove length is called ____________ cutting.

a) point
b) slide
c) notching
d) razor

23. The process of thinning with scissors is known as ____________.

a) effilating
b) shaving
c) sliding
d) trimming

24. ____________ guides are used mostly in blunt (one-length) haircuts or when using overdirection to create a length or weight increase in a haircut.

a) Traveling
b) Movable
c) Stationary
d) Portable

25. ______________ is used mostly in graduated and layered haircuts, and in those situations where a length increase in the design is desired.

a) Effilating
b) Trimming
c) Elevating
d) Overdirection

Essential Discoveries and Accomplishments

In the space below, jot some notes about what concepts of this chapter were hardest for you to understand or remember. Imagine finding yourself suddenly in the role of "teacher" and consider what you would tell your "students" about these concepts. Share your Essential Discoveries with some of the other students in your class and ask if they are helpful to them. You may want to revise your discoveries based on any good ideas shared by your peers.

Discoveries:

List at least three things you have accomplished since your last entry that relate to your career goals.

Accomplishments:

CHAPTER 17

Hairstyling

A Motivating Moment: "If you are looking for a big opportunity, find a big problem."
— Unknown

Essential Objectives

After studying this chapter and completing the Essential Companion components, you will be able to:

1. Demonstrate finger waving, pin curling, roller setting, and hair wrapping.
2. Demonstrate various blowdry styling techniques.
3. Demonstrate the proper use of thermal irons.
4. Demonstrate various thermal iron manipulations and explain how they are used.
5. Describe the three types of hair pressing.
6. Demonstrate the procedures for soft pressing and hard pressing.
7. Demonstrate three basic techniques of styling long hair.

Essential Wet Hairstyling

What roles will wet hairstyling, thermal hairstyling, and hair pressing play in my success as a cosmetologist?

Hairstyles, like fashions, are cyclical. Just as you have seen the bell-bottom pants of the late 1960s come into fashion again, hairstyles, such as those that were popular in the 1920s, surface from time to time in our society. History has shown that all societies have cut and arranged hair to modify its natural state. The pages of our history books depict great diversity from decade to decade. They show the blond wigs of Roman matrons, the gray wigs of English barristers, and the black wigs of Japanese geisha. We also see the sleek, waved look worn by the flappers in the 1920s and the trend toward informality and individualism in the twenty-first century.

Recent surveys of today's modern salons indicate that the new stylists joining their teams must be skilled in many styling techniques, including thermal styling and curling. History shows us that thermal or heat techniques have been used for centuries to create certain looks. The heat from the sun was used to speed up the processing of hair lighteners, permanent waves, and hair color. Hair was wrapped around reeds and sticks and sun-dried for certain looks. Fortunately, the tools and implements have improved drastically since those primitive times.

Marcel Grateau developed the thermal iron technique in 1875, which is still called Marcel waving today. The use of blowdrying and curling irons became really popular in the late 1960s with the first *bob* cut and has become increasingly popular into the twenty-first century as more women have entered the business world and time is so critical. These techniques are used for what are called *quick services* in the salon. However, the same care must be taken with these techniques as with wet hairstyling.

Hair pressing is both a popular and profitable service that is used in many of today's professional establishments. Overly curly hair comes in a variety of colors, textures, and ethnic forms. We have all heard the expression, "The grass looks greener on the other side of the fence." Accordingly, we human beings always seem to want something that we do not have. If we have straight hair, we want it to be curly; therefore we seek out chemical texture services to add curl to our hair. If we have naturally curly hair, we want it to be straight; therefore we seek out either pressing or chemical services to remove the curl. All those desires contribute to your success as a professional cosmetologist.

Essential Wet Hairstyling continued

Once you become a professional cosmetologist, you will hold your license or certification for many years to come, hopefully over several decades. You must be prepared to address your client's desires and needs regardless of prevailing styles. Therefore, it is essential that you learn the basics of hairstyling in order to be proficient in providing the client's desired style.

Cosmetologists should study and have a thorough understanding of hairstyling because:

- Hairstyling is an important, foundational skill that allows the professional to articulate creativity and deliver a specific outcome desired by the client.
- Clients rely on you to teach them about their hair and how to style it so they can have a variety of options based on their lifestyle and fashion needs. You are the expert!
- The client looks to you for that special style desired for that special day.
- Hairstyling skills will enable you to help clients to be as contemporary as they would like to be, allowing them to keep up with the trends.

Essential Concepts

What are the most important elements in hairstyling that I need to know?

Hairstyling is an art form; hair is the medium and you are the artist. Hairstyling results from a detailed set of principles, elements, tools, and implements. You will need to learn to master the use of the tools and implements used in hairstyling as well as how to properly prepare the hair for the styling service. You will become familiar with a variety of styling aids which do just that—aid you in creating the desired look or style. You will learn that finger waving is the art of shaping and directing the hair into alternate parallel waves with well-defined ridges using the fingers, combs, waving lotion, hairpins, or clips.

You will learn how the concept of waves evolved into the concept of curls, including pin curls and roller curls. There are a variety of techniques for creating pin curls and roller sets that will allow you to work your magic as an artist in the medium of hair. You will master several brushing and combing procedures that will give the finished look to the style you have designed.

In addition, thermal styling is the art of drying, waving, and curling hair by means of heat, using special manipulative techniques. It includes drying and styling the hair, curling or waving the hair, and straightening the hair. Each piece of equipment used in thermal styling is designed for a specific styling technique. The essential techniques that you must master are the use of the blowdryer and the curling iron. You will need to know how each piece of equipment functions and how to create a variety of looks with each.

You will need to learn about the three types of hair pressing techniques: the soft press, the medium press, and the hard press. It is essential that you understand which type of press is used on which type of hair. Of course, you will also need to master each of the techniques. Learning about special problems with pressing and fine tuning all the safety measures that must be followed will also contribute to your success.

Essential Experience 1

Mind Map of Wet Hairstyling

Mind mapping simply creates a free-flowing outline of material or information with the central or key point being located in the center. The key point of this mind map is wet hairstyling. Diagram the different tools, implements, and elements or categories of wet hairstyling. Use terms, pictures, and symbols as desired. Using color will increase the mind's retention and memory of the material. Keep your mind open and uncluttered and do not worry about where a line or word should go as the organization of the map will usually take care of itself.

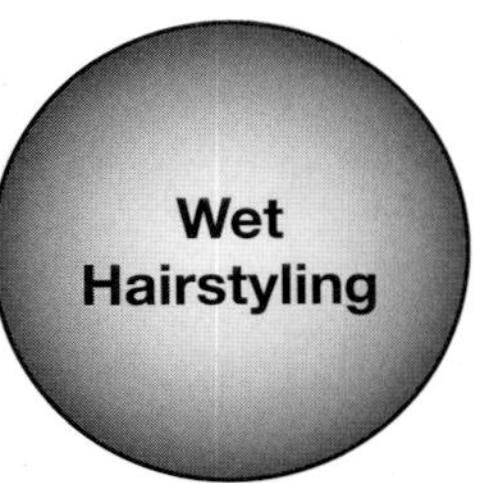

2 Essential Experience

Windowpane Pin Curls

Windowpaning is the process of transferring key elements, points, or steps in a lesson into visual images that are hand sketched into the squares or *panes* of a matrix. Let your mind think in pictures and sketch the essential concepts printed in each of the following windowpanes. Do not be concerned with your artistic ability. Use lines and stick figures to depict the concepts indicated.

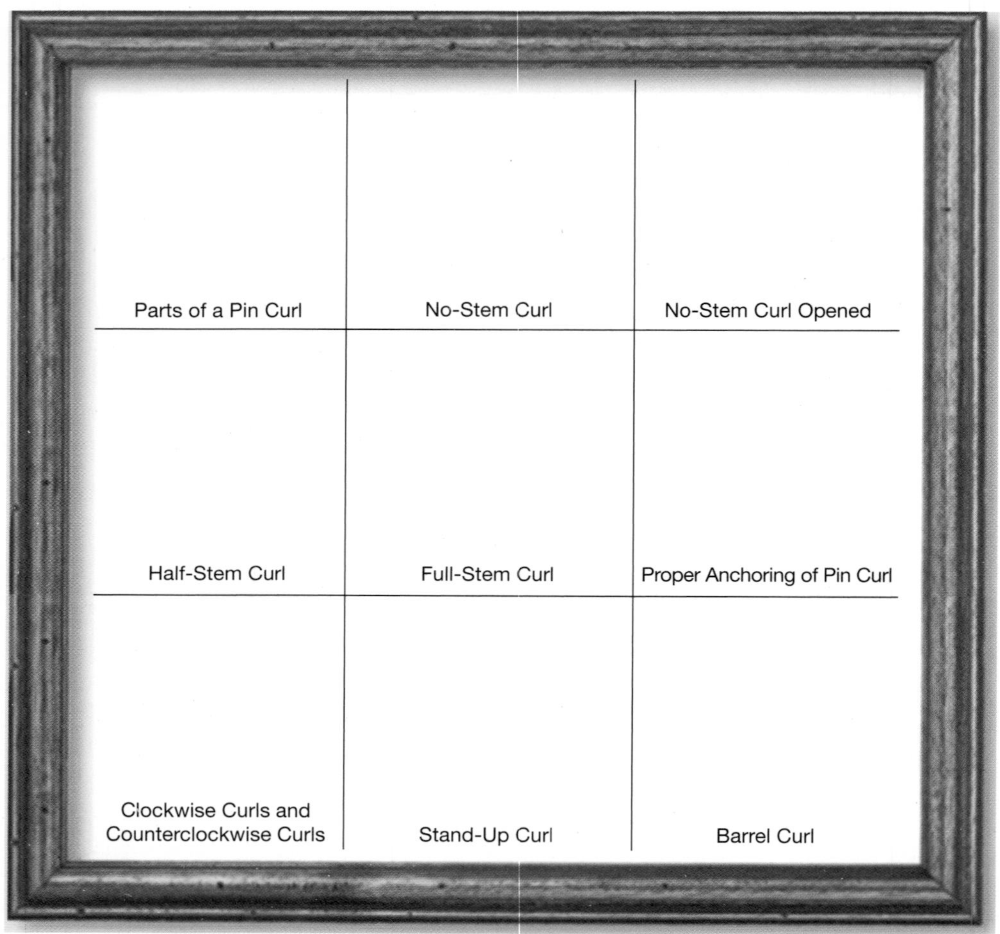

Follow-up Activity: Perform each of the following curls or movements on a mannequin for a grade from your instructor.

____ No-Stem Curl	___ Half-Stem Curl	___ Full-Stem Curl
____ Clockwise Curl	___ Stand-Up Curl	___ Barrel Curl

Essential Experience 3

Matching Exercise

Match each of the following essential terms with their identifying phrase or definition.

______	**Circular**	**1.**	Pin curls sliced from a shaping and formed without lifting the hair from the head
______	**Oblong**	**2.**	Pie-shaped with the open end smaller than the closed end; in a wave pattern, the direction is alternated
______	**Shaping**	**3.**	Recommended along the front or facial hairline to avoid breaks or splits in the finished style
______	**Ridge curl**	**4.**	Remains the same width throughout the shaping
______	**Spiral curl**	**5.**	Used for even construction suitable for curly hairstyles without much volume or lift
______	**Carved curls**	**6.**	Also known as the *half-moon* or *c-shaped base*
______	**Closed**	**7.**	Recommended at front hairline for a smooth upsweep effect
______	**Rectangular**	**8.**	Section of hair molded in a circular motion
______	**Triangular**	**9.**	Pin curls that produce waves that get smaller toward the end
______	**Arc base**	**10.**	Pin curls placed behind or below a ridge to form a wave
______	**Square base**	**11.**	Forcing the strand through the comb while applying pressure with the thumb on the back of the comb to create tension
______	**Ribboning**	**12.**	Method of curling hair by winding strand around the rod

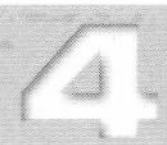

Essential Experience

Windowpane Roller Placement

Windowpaning is the process of transferring key elements, points, or steps in a lesson into visual images that are hand sketched into the squares or *panes* of a matrix. Let your mind think in pictures and sketch the essential concepts printed in each of the following windowpanes. Do not be concerned with your artistic ability. Use lines and stick figures to depict the concepts indicated.

Roller Curl Base
Roller Curl Stem
Roller Curl
Proper Roller Clipping
Cylinder Roller
Tapered Roller
Roller On Base
Roller Half Base
Roller Off Base

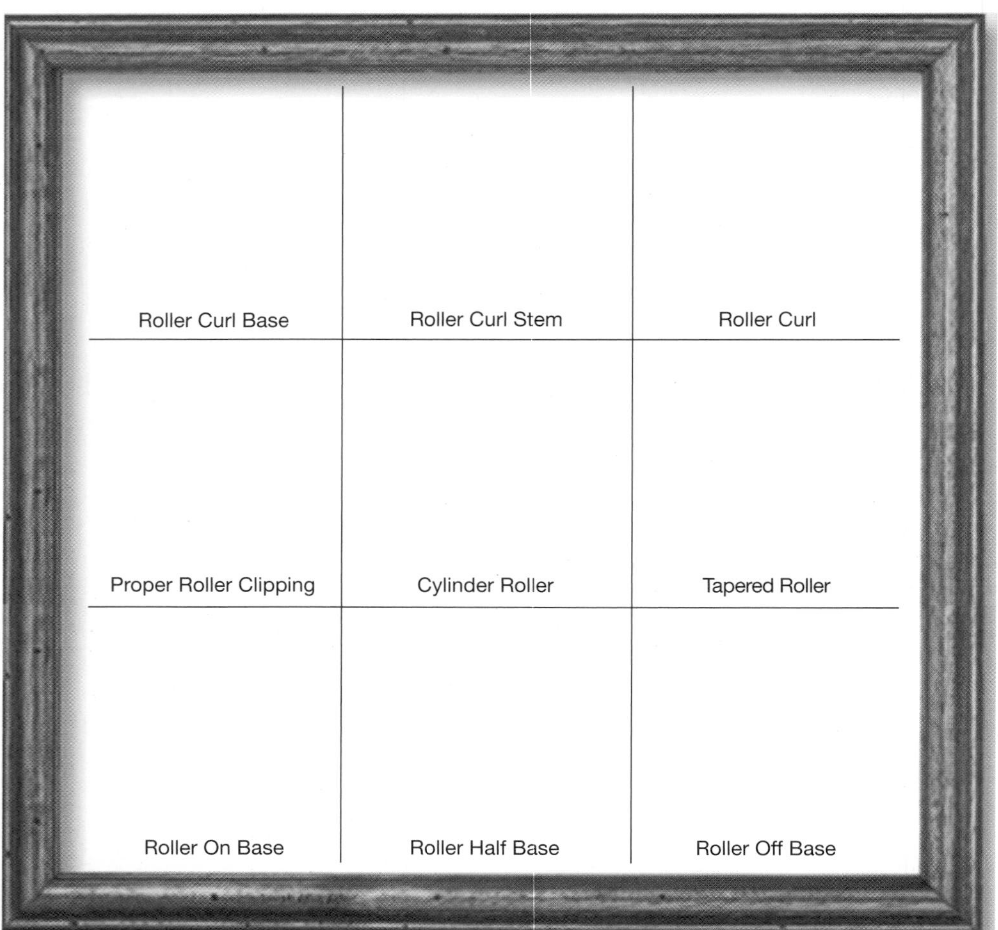

Essential Experience 5

Word Search

After determining the correct word from the clues provided, locate the words in the word search puzzle.

Word	Clue
________________	Also called *ruffing*
________________	Pin curls with large openings; fastened to head in a standing position on a rectangular base
________________	Pin curls sliced from a shaping and formed without lifting the hair from the head
________________	Nozzle attachment that directs the air flow
________________	Blowdryer attachment that causes air to flow more softly
________________	Technique of passing a hot curling iron through the hair before performing a hard press
________________	Produces a strong curl with full volume
________________	Removes 100 percent of the curl by applying the pressing comb twice on each side of the hair
________________	Curl placed directly on its base
________________	Forces hair between the thumb and back of comb to create tension
________________	Pin curls placed immediately behind or below a ridge to form a wave
________________	Round, solid prong of a thermal iron
________________	Part of thermal irons in which rod rests when irons are closed
________________	Two rows of ridge curls, usually on the side of head
________________	Method of curling the hair by winding a strand around the rod
________________	Also called *cascade curls*
________________	Section of pin curl between the base and first arc
________________	Hairstyle arranged up and off the shoulders
________________	Type of gel that makes hair pliable for finger waving

S	L	R	U	C	L	E	R	R	A	B	S	T	G	M
L	R	U	C	L	A	R	I	P	S	B	G	N	N	K
R	E	S	N	O	I	T	O	L	G	N	I	V	A	W
U	S	L	D	S	M	T	R	G	I	H	U	Q	K	Q
C	U	R	W	O	I	O	O	N	S	S	S	U	M	X
P	F	U	S	M	U	O	O	U	N	S	W	S	M	B
U	F	C	B	L	P	B	R	S	H	E	L	L	E	U
-	I	D	M	D	B	B	L	Q	W	R	A	F	T	R
D	D	E	H	I	-	J	D	E	U	P	D	O	S	H
N	O	V	R	K	V	X	Y	C	P	D	F	E	-	T
A	X	R	C	O	N	C	E	N	T	R	A	T	O	R
T	L	A	E	P	H	G	N	I	C	A	E	R	N	N
S	B	C	J	J	D	F	O	K	J	H	D	S	H	B
Z	R	S	K	I	P	W	A	V	E	S	Z	H	S	Q
I	T	J	R	E	S	A	B	-	L	L	U	F	S	T

Essential Experience 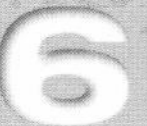

Iron Manipulations

Using a cold thermal iron, a mannequin, and other required implements practice the textbook exercises for manipulating thermal irons.

Exercise 1: Since it is important to develop a smooth rotating movement, practice turning the irons while opening and closing them at regular intervals. Practice rotating the irons downward toward you and upward away from you.

Exercise 2: Practice releasing the hair by opening and closing the irons in a quick, clicking movement.

Exercise 3: Practice guiding the hair strand into the center of the curl as you rotate the irons. This exercise will ensure that the end of the strand is firmly in the center of the curl.

Exercise 4: Practice removing the curl from the irons by drawing the comb to the left and the rod to the right. Use the comb to protect the scalp from burns.

After completing the exercises, please explain any difficulties you may have had with the exercises in the space below. Discuss these difficulties with your instructor.

____

____

____

____

____

____

____

____

____

7 Essential Experience

Safety Precautions

In the space provided, explain why the following safety precautions are necessary in the use of thermal waving and curling.

1. Irons should not be overheated.

____

2. The temperature of the irons must be tested before applying to hair.

____

3. Irons should be handled carefully.

____

4. Irons should be placed in a safe place to cool.

____

____

5. Handles should not be placed too close to the heater when heating the irons.

____

6. Irons should be properly balanced when placed in the heater.

____

7. **Celluloid combs or metal combs cannot be used.**

____

8. **Combs with broken teeth must not be used.**

____

9. **Comb must be placed between scalp and thermal iron when curling or waving.**

____

10. Hair ends must not be allowed to protrude over the irons.

____

Essential Experience continued

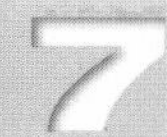

11. Thermal irons are generally not used on chemically straightened hair.

____

12. A first aid kit must be readily available.

____

8 Essential Experience

Thermal Curling Preparation

List the five general steps used in preparing for an electric or stove-heated thermal curling iron procedure. Bear in mind that these methods may be changed by your instructor.

1. ______________________________

2. ______________________________

3. ______________________________

4. ______________________________
____
____
____

5. ______________________________

Essential Experience

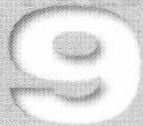

Windowpaning Thermal Curling

Windowpaning is the process of transferring key elements, points, or steps in a lesson into visual images that are hand sketched into the squares or *panes* of a matrix. Let your mind think in pictures, and sketch the essential concepts printed in each of the following windowpanes. Do not be concerned with your artistic ability. Use lines and stick figures to depict the concepts requested.

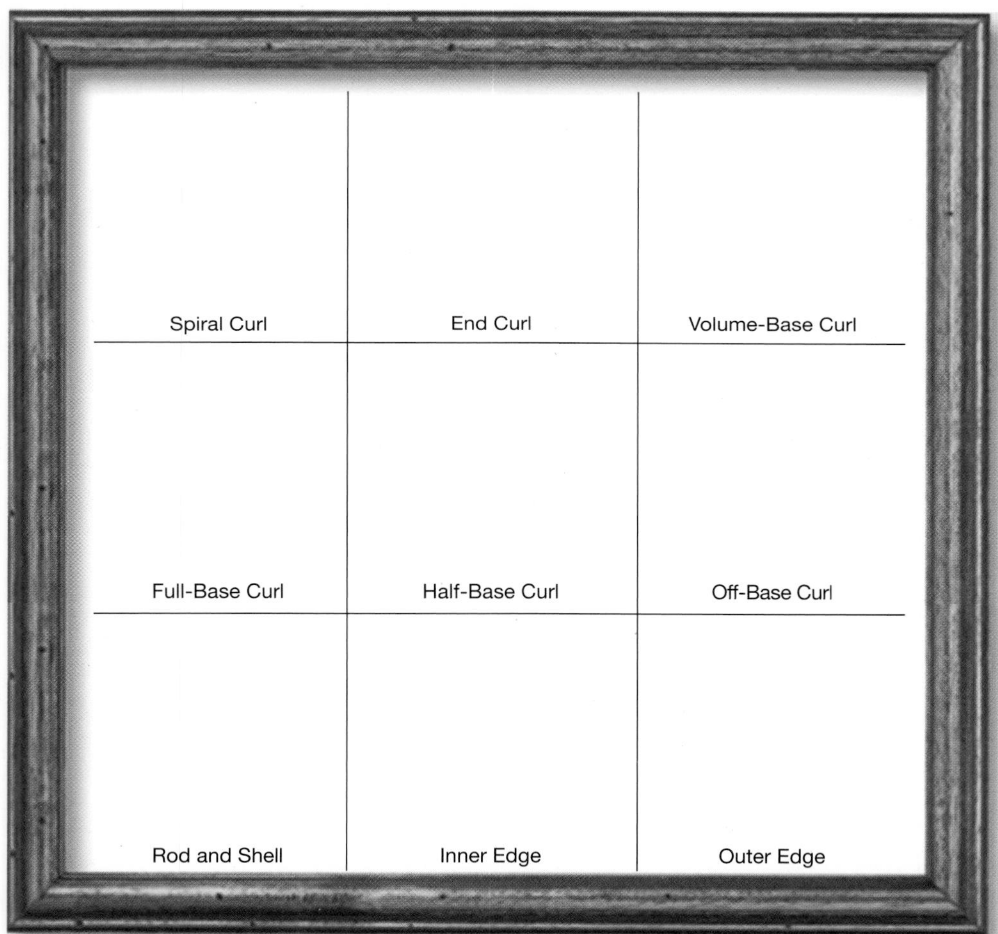

10 Essential Experience

Thermal Waving With Conventional Thermal Irons

List below the equipment, implements, and materials used in thermal waving with a conventional thermal (Marcel) iron.

____

____

In your own words, list the basic procedural steps which can be used to create a style with a conventional thermal (Marcel) iron for a left-going wave.

1. ____

2. ____

____

3. ____

____

____

____

4. ____

____

____

____

5. ____

____

6. ____

____

____

____

7. ____

____

Essential Experience continued 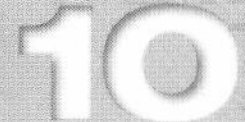

8. ______________________________

9. ______________________________

10. ______________________________

11. ______________________________

12. ______________________________

11 Essential Experience

Types of Hair Pressing

In your own words in the space provided, explain what is meant by each type of pressing technique and how each is accomplished.

Soft Press: ______________________________

____

____

Medium Press: ______________________________

____

____

Hard Press: ______________________________

____

____

____

Essential Experience 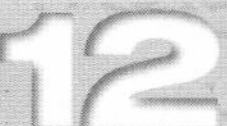

Product Knowledge

Research a variety of pressing oils or creams available in your school and found at local supply stores. Use the chart below to track your findings.

Product Name	Key Ingredients	Purpose	Benefits	Directions for Use

13 Essential Experience

Hair and Scalp Analysis

List the eight points that should be thoroughly covered in the hair and scalp analysis before proceeding with a hair pressing service.

1. ______________________________
2. ______________________________
3. ______________________________
4. ______________________________
5. ______________________________
6. ______________________________
7. ______________________________
8. ______________________________

List at least five reminders and hints on soft pressing.

1. ______________________________
2. ______________________________
3. ______________________________
____
4. ______________________________
5. ______________________________
6. ______________________________
____
____
7. ______________________________
____

Essential Experience 14

Jeopardy

As in the game Jeopardy, write questions which would be correctly answered.

Hair Pressing for $100.

1. To temporarily straighten overly curly or unruly hair.

____

2. A series of conditioning treatments.

____

____

3. Soft, medium, hard.

____

Hair Pressing for $200.

1. Double press.

____

2. Breakage.

____

3. Medium hair.

____

Hair Pressing for $300.

1. Scalp abrasions, contagious scalp condition, scalp injury, chemically treated hair.

____

____

2. Wiry, curly hair.

____

3. Regular and electric.

____

14 Essential Experience continued

Hair Pressing for $400.

1. Carbon.

____

____

2. Apply less pressure to the hair near the ends.

____

Essential Rubrics

Rubrics are used in education for organizing and interpreting data gathered from observations of student performance. It is a clearly developed scoring document used to differentiate between levels of development in a specific skill performance or behavior. A rubric is provided in this study guide as a self-assessment tool to aid you in your behavior development.

Rate your performance according to the following scale.

(1) Development Opportunity: There is little or no evidence of competency; assistance is needed; performance includes multiple errors.

(2) Fundamental: There is beginning evidence of competency; task is completed alone; performance includes few errors.

(3) Competent: There is detailed and consistent evidence of competency; task is completed alone; performance includes rare errors.

(4) Strength: There is detailed evidence of highly creative, inventive, mature presence of competency.

Space is provided for comments to assist you in improving your performance and achieving a higher rating.

HORIZONTAL FINGER-WAVING PROCEDURE

Performance Assessed	1	2	3	4	Improvement Plan
After shampooing the hair, parted it, combed it smooth, and arranged it according to the planned style					
Using wide teeth of comb allowed hair to move more easily					
Followed natural growth pattern when combing and parting the hair					
Applied waving lotion with an applicator bottle to the side of the hair while damp					
Combed lotion throughout the section					

Essential Rubrics continued

Performance Assessed	1	2	3	4	Improvement Plan
Began first wave on right side of head					
Used index finger of left hand as a guide, shaped top hair with comb into the beginning of the S-shaping, using circular movement					
Started at hairline, worked toward crown in 1½- to 2-inch (3.7 to 5 cm) sections until crown was reached					
To form first ridge, placed index finger of left hand above position for first ridge					
With comb teeth pointing slightly upward, inserted comb directly under index finger and drew comb forward about 1 inch (2.5 cm) along fingertip					
With teeth still inserted in ridge, flattened comb against head in order to hold ridge in place					
Removed left hand from head and placed middle finger above ridge and index finger on teeth of comb					
Drew out the ridge by closing the two fingers and applying pressure to head					
Did not try to increase height or depth of ridge by pinching or pushing with fingers					
Without removing comb, turned teeth downward and combed hair in right semicircular direction to form a dip in hollow part of the wave					

Performance Assessed	1	2	3	4	Improvement Plan
Followed this procedure, section by section, until crown was reached, where ridge phased out					
The ridge and wave matched evenly without showing separation in ridge and hollow part of wave					
To form the second ridge, began at the crown area; movements were reverse of those followed in first ridge; comb was drawn from tip of index finger toward base of index finger					
All movements were followed in reverse pattern until hairline is reached completing the second ridge					
Movements for the third ridge closely followed those used to create the first ridge					
Third ridge was started at the hairline and extended back toward the back of the head					
Continued alternating directions until the side of the head was completed					
Used the same procedure for the left (light) side of the head as used for the right (heavy) side of the head					
First, shaped the hair by combing it in the direction of the first wave					
Starting at hairline, formed the first ridge, section by section, until the second ridge of the opposite was reached					

Essential Rubrics continued

Performance Assessed	1	2	3	4	Improvement Plan
Both the ridge and the wave blended without splits or breaks, with the ridge and wave on the right side of the head					
Started with ridge and wave in back of head and proceeded, section by section, toward left side of face					
Continued working back and forth until entire side was completed					
Placed net over hair, secured if necessary, and safeguarded client's forehead and ears while under dryer with cotton, gauze, or paper protectors					
Adjusted dryer to medium heat and allowed hair to dry thoroughly					
Removed client from under dryer and let hair cool down					
Removed clippies and hairnet from hair					
Combed out and reset waves into soft, waved hairstyle					
Added a finishing spray for hold and shine					

CARVED OR SCULPTED CURLS PROCEDURE

Performance Assessed	1	2	3	4	Improvement Plan
Parted hair appropriately for design					
Formed the first shaping					
Created first curl by starting curls at the open end of the shaping					
Pointed nondominant index finger down and held the strand in place					

Performance Assessed	1	2	3	4	Improvement Plan
Ribboned the strand					
Wound curl forward, keeping the hair ends inside the center of the curl					
Anchored curl with clip					
Placed clip in the circle parallel to stem					
Did not pin across circle					
Placed cotton between clip and skin if necessary					

WET SET WITH ROLLERS PROCEDURE

Performance Assessed	1	2	3	4	Improvement Plan
Combed shampooed hair in direction of setting pattern					
Starting at front hairline, parted off section the same length and width as roller					
Chose type of base according to desired volume					
Combed the hair out from the scalp to the ends using the fine teeth of the comb					
Repeated several times to make sure that the hair was smooth					
Held hair with tension between thumb and middle finger of left hand					
Placed the roller below the thumb of left hand					
Did not converge ends of hair					
Wrapped ends of hair smoothly around roller until hair caught and did not release					
Placed thumbs over the ends of roller and rolled hair firmly to scalp					

Performance Assessed	1	2	3	4	Improvement Plan
Clipped roller securely to scalp hair					
Placed client under hood dryer set at a comfortable temperature					
When hair was dry, allowed it to cool, then removed the rollers					
Combed out and styled hair as desired					

BLOWDRYING SHORT, LAYERED, CURLY HAIR PROCEDURE

Performance Assessed	1	2	3	4	Improvement Plan
Distributed styling product through the hair with fingers and combed through with a wide-tooth comb					
Using the comb, molded hair into the desired shape while still wet					
For volume and lift, used a small round brush					
Applied mousse or spray volumizer at the base					
Sectioned and parted hair according to size of curl desired					
Inserted round brush at the base of the curl					
Using roller setting technique, dried each section either full base or half base					
For maximum lift, inserted brush on base and directed hair section up at a 125-degree angle					
Rolled hair down to base with medium tension					

Performance Assessed	1	2	3	4	Improvement Plan
Directed the stream of air from blowdryer over curl in back-and-forth motion					
When section was completely dry, depressed cooling button and cooled down the section to strengthen the curl formation					
Released the brush by unwinding section from the brush; for less lift at scalp, began by holding section at a 90-degree or 70-degree angle, following the same procedure					
Made sure scalp and hair were completely dry before combing out the style					
Finished with hair spray					

THERMAL WAVING PROCEDURE

Performance Assessed	1	2	3	4	Improvement Plan
Dried client's hair completely					
Re-draped client for a dry hair service					
Heated iron					
Combed hair in general desired shape					
With the comb, picked up a strand of hair about 2 inches (5 cm) in width					
Inserted iron in hair with the groove facing upward					
Closed iron and gave it a ¼ turn forward					
At the same time, drew the hair with the iron about ¼ inch (0.6 cm) to the left, and direct the hair ¼ inch (0.6 cm) to the right with the comb					

Performance Assessed	1	2	3	4	Improvement Plan
Rolled the iron one full turn forward					
Kept hair uniform with the comb for a few seconds to heat throughout					
Reversed movement by unrolling hair from iron					
Opened iron and placed it just below the ridge or crest and closed it					
Keeping the iron perfectly still, directed the hair with the comb upward about 1 inch (2.5 cm) forming a half circle					
Without opening the iron, rolled it half-turn forward and away keeping comb still and unchanged					
Slid iron down about 1 inch (2.5 cm) by opening the iron slightly, gripping it loosely, and then sliding it down the strand					
Began second ridge for a right-moving ridge					
Picked up next strand in the comb and included a small section of the waved strand as a guide					
Continued until finished waving achieved					

SOFT PRESSING PROCEDURE

Performance Assessed	1	2	3	4	Improvement Plan
Placed pressing comb in heater					
Unclipped one section at a time and subdivided into small subsections					

Essential Rubrics continued

Performance Assessed	1	2	3	4	Improvement Plan
Began at right side of head, worked from front to back					
If necessary, applied pressing oil evenly and sparingly over small hair sections					
Tested temperature of heated pressing comb on white cloth or white paper to determine heat intensity before placing it on the hair					
Lifted the end of a small hair section with index finger and thumb of left hand and held it upward away from scalp					
Held pressing comb in right hand, and inserted teeth of comb into top side of hair section					
Drew out pressing comb slightly and made a quick turn so hair strand wrapped itself partly around comb					
Back rod of comb did the pressing					
Pressed comb slowly through hair strand until the ends of hair passed through the teeth of the comb					
Brought each completed hair section over to the opposite side of the head					
Continued steps on both sections on right side of head					
Repeated same procedure on both sections of left side of head					

Performance Assessed	1	2	3	4	Improvement Plan
Applied a little pomade to hair near the scalp and brushed it through the hair; if desired, thermal roller or croquignole curling was given at this time					
Styled and combed hair according to client's wishes					

KNOT PROCEDURE

Performance Assessed	1	2	3	4	Improvement Plan
Applied styling product and blew hair dry					
Set hair					
Using grooming bristle brush, parted on desired side					
Brushed into a low ponytail at the nape					
Secured ponytail with elastic(s), keeping hair as smooth as possible					
Used sides of bristle brush to smooth hair					
Placed two bobby pins onto band and spread them apart					
Placed one bobby pin in the base					
Locked the two pins together					
Took a small section of hair from the underside of the ponytail, wrapped it around the ponytail to cover the elastics and secured it with a bobby pin underneath					

Essential Rubrics continued

Performance Assessed	1	2	3	4	Improvement Plan
Smoothed out ponytail and held with one hand and backbrushed from underneath ponytail with other hand					
Gently smoothed out the ponytail after backbrushing, using sides of bristles					
Rolled hair under and toward the head to form the chignon					
Secured on left and right undersides of the roll with bobby pins					
Fanned out both sides by spreading the chignon with fingers					
Secured with hairpins, pinning close to head					
Used bobby pins if more hold was needed					
Finished with a strong finishing spray					
Added ornamentation if desired					

Essential Review

Using the following words, fill in the blanks below to form a thorough review of Chapter 17, Hairstyling. Words or terms may be used more than once or not at all.

anchored	**flattering**	**rectangular**
arc	**full-stem**	**ribboning**
backcombing	**gel**	**ridge**
barrel	**hairpins**	**rollers**
base	**horizontal**	**ruffing**
c-shaped	**indentation**	**shallow**
carved	**invisible**	**silicone**
circle	**karaya**	**smooth**
circular	**no-stem**	**square**
clockwise	**oblong**	**stand-up**
counterclockwise	**off**	**stem**
curls	**on**	**tapered**
cylinder	**pinching**	**tension**
decrease	**pin curls**	**unpigmented**
direction	**pins**	**vertical**
drying	**pliable**	**visible**
finger waving	**pomade**	
finishing	**pushing**	

1. A stylist's goal is to create a style that is both ____________ and easy to manage.
2. Open-center curls produce even, ____________ waves and uniform curls.
3. In ____________ finger waving, ridges are parallel around the head.
4. One complete turn around the roller will create a ____________ curl.
5. The art of shaping and directing the hair into alternate parallel waves and designs is ____________.
6. The three parts of a pin curl are the ____________, ____________, and ____________.
7. The finished result will be determined by the ____________ you place the stem of the curl.

Essential Review continued

8. Curls formed in the opposite direction of the movement of the hands of a clock are known as ______________.
9. Forcing a strand of hair through a comb while applying pressure with the thumb on the back of the comb to create tension is called ___________.
10. ___________ are used to create many of the same effects as stand-up pin curls.
11. Two and a half turns around the roller will create ___________.
12. Curls formed in the same direction as the movement of the hands of a clock are known as ___________.
13. The most commonly shaped base you will use is the ___________ base.
14. Cascade or ___________ curls are used to create height.
15. For the least volume, the roller sits ___________ base.
16. Tools and implements required in wet hairstyling include rollers, clips, combs, brushes, and ___________.
17. Waving lotion makes the hair ___________ and keeps it in place during the finger-waving procedure.
18. A ___________ curl allows for the greatest mobility.
19. Waving lotion is applied to one side of the head at a time to prevent ___________.
20. ___________ provide the bases for patterns, lines, waves, curls, and rolls that you can use to create hairstyles.
21. Closed-center curls produce waves that ___________ in size.
22. Do not try to increase the height or depth of a ridge by ___________ or ___________ with the fingers.
23. Waving lotion is made from ___________ gum.
24. A loose roller will lose its ___________ and result in a weak set.
25. Secure net over finger waves with ___________ or clippies if needed.
26. In ___________ finger waving, ridges run up and down the head.
27. Backbrushing is also known as ___________.
28. ___________ is a firm-bodied and usually clear or transparent product that comes in a tube or bottle and has a strong hold.
29. To ensure that the curl holds firmly, it should be ___________ correctly.

30. Pin curls recommended at the side front hairline for a smooth upsweep effect are ____________ bases.

31. Pin curls sliced from a shaping without lifting hair from the head are referred to as ____________ curls.

32. For full volume, the roller sits ____________ base.

33. Large stand-up pin curls on a rectangular base with large center openings are known as ____________ curls.

34. Teasing, ratting, matting, or French lacing are also known as ____________.

35. ____________ or wax adds considerable weight to the hair by causing strands to join together.

36. A ____________ curl produces a tight, firm, long-lasting curl.

37. ____________ adds gloss and sheen to the hair while creating textural definition.

38. A ____________ curl is a wave behind the ridge.

39. The most widely used hairstyling product is hair spray or ____________ spray.

Complete the following by circling the correct answer.

40. When blowdrying, determine the size of the brush to be used by the desired style and ______________ of the hair.

    a) elasticity
    b) texture
    c) length
    d) porosity

41. The styling parts of the thermal iron are comprised of the rod and the ______________.

    a) groove
    b) handle
    c) shell
    d) clamp

42. The temperature of the heated thermal iron is tested on ______________.

    a) wax paper
    b) hair strand
    c) damp cloth
    d) tissue paper

43. Curling with two loops is also known as ______________ curling.

    a) end
    b) spiral
    c) figure-eight
    d) half-base

Essential Review continued

44. The technique of waving and curling the hair known as Marcel waving is also called ______________.

a) blowdrying
b) thermal waving
c) heat rolling
d) finger waving

45. Combs for thermal curling should be made of ______________.

a) celluloid
b) hard rubber
c) plastic
d) soft rubber

46. To give a finished appearance to hair ends, use ______________ curls.

a) figure-eight
b) loop
c) figure-six
d) end

47. For successful blowdry styling, the air should be directed from the scalp to the ______________.

a) floor
b) ceiling
c) face
d) ends

48. When the blowdry style is complete, the scalp must be ______________.

a) oily
b) moist
c) damp
d) dry

49. Overheated irons are often ruined because the metal loses its ______________.

a) color
b) balance
c) temper
d) strength

50. Electric vaporizing irons should not be used on pressed hair because they cause the hair to ______________.

a) break
b) dry
c) straighten
d) revert

51. ______________ hair withstands less heat in a thermal styling service than normal hair.

a) Lightened
b) Healthy
c) Coarse
d) Curly

Essential Review continued

52. A conventional thermal iron is ______________ heated.

a) electric b) self
c) coal d) stove

53. ______________ hair, as a rule, can tolerate more heat than fine hair.

a) Red b) Coarse
c) Oily d) Short

54. Spiral curls are hanging curls that are suitable for ______________ hairstyles.

a) short b) clipped
c) long d) straight

55. Until dexterity is achieved and ease of manipulation is mastered, it is best to ______________ practice with irons.

a) cold b) hot
c) warm d) rigid

56. How long does a hair press last?

a) a week b) till the next haircut
c) overnight d) till the next shampoo

57. The types of hair pressing are soft, medium, and ______________.

a) light b) hard
c) extreme d) heavy

58. The temperature of the pressing comb and the amount of pressure used are adjusted based on the ______________ of the hair.

a) texture b) length
c) style d) cleanliness

59. Which type of hair requires the most pressure and heat?

a) fine b) medium
c) normal d) wiry

60. Which type of hair requires less pressure and heat than any other type?

a) fine b) medium
c) coarse d) wiry

Essential Review continued

61. When pressing gray hair, use moderate heat and ______________.

a) more pressing oil b) moderate pressure
c) less pressure d) a larger pressing comb

62. Applying a heated comb twice on each side of the hair is known as a ______________.

a) regular press b) hard press
c) soft press d) comb press

63. Test the temperature of a pressing comb on ______________.

a) inner wrist b) terry cloth towel
c) light paper d) dark paper

64. Burnt hair strands ______________.

a) need extra pressing oil b) occur in hard presses
c) cannot be straightened d) cannot be conditioned

65. Using excess heat on gray, tinted, or lightened hair may ______________ the hair.

a) discolor b) highlight
c) strengthen d) curl

66. Failure to correct dry and brittle hair can result in hair ______________ during hair pressing.

a) curling b) discoloration
c) strengthening d) breakage

67. Hair pressing treatments between shampoos are called ______________.

a) re-presses b) re-do's
c) touch-ups d) soft press

68. Before performing a hair press, the hair should be sectioned into ______________ main sections.

a) 3 b) 4
c) 5 d) 9

69. Carbon may be removed from the pressing comb by rubbing with a _______________.

a) wet towel
b) pressing oil
c) strong alcohol
d) fine steel wool

70. In a hair pressing procedure, the actual pressing or straightening of the hair is accomplished with the comb's _______________.

a) back rod
b) wide teeth
c) warm handle
d) narrow tail

71. After cleaning the comb's surface, immerse the comb in a hot _______________ solution for about one hour to give the metal a smooth and shiny appearance.

a) 70 percent alcohol
b) baking soda
c) soapy water
d) clear ammonia

72. When pressing _______________ hair, use a moderately heated pressing comb applied with light pressure.

a) coarse
b) thick
c) long
d) unpigmented

73. Pressing combs should be constructed of good-quality stainless steel or _______________.

a) zinc
b) rubber
c) brass
d) plastic

74. In pressing coarse hair, more heat is required because it has the greatest _______________.

a) elasticity
b) length
c) porosity
d) diameter

75. Handles of pressing combs are usually made of _______________.

a) wood
b) steel
c) carbon
d) brass

Essential Discoveries and Accomplishments

In the space below, jot some notes about what concepts of this chapter were hardest for you to understand or remember. Imagine finding yourself suddenly in the role of "teacher" and consider what you would tell your "students" about these concepts. Share your Essential Discoveries with some of the other students in your class and ask if they are helpful to them. You may want to revise your discoveries based on good ideas shared by your peers.

Discoveries:

List at least three things you have accomplished since your last entry that relate to your career goals.

Accomplishments:

CHAPTER 18

Braiding & Braid Extensions

A Motivating Moment: "Everyone has his burden. What counts is how you carry it."
— Merle Miller

Essential Objectives

After studying this chapter and completing the Essential Companion components, you will be able to:

1. **Explain how to prepare the hair for braiding.**
2. **Demonstrate the procedure for cornrowing.**

Essential Braiding

Why do I need to learn about braiding when I am not interested in providing these services?

Long hair styles with braids are becoming more and more popular across cultures, generations, and ethnic backgrounds. The fact is that many licensed cosmetologists do not offer these types of services. This can present a problem for clients desiring them. On the other hand, however, it can present an opportunity for those professionals who are expert in these services and readily available to provide them. By offering total hair care services to all clients, you will build a solid client base more readily and will never need to refer a client to another stylist or salon. In the end, you will reap the benefits of increased income and satisfied clients.

Cosmetologists should study and have a thorough understanding of the importance of a braiding and braid extensions because:

- These services are very popular and consumers are interested in wearing styles specific to their hair texture.
- These techniques provide an opportunity for stylists to express their artistic abilities and to add another high-ticket service to their current service menu!
- All professional cosmetologists should be prepared to work with every type of hair and hairstyle trends within every culture.
- Working with braid extensions exposes cosmetologists to the fundamental techniques of adding hair extensions, which is another lucrative service for the stylist and the salon.

Essential Concepts

What do I need to know about braiding in order to provide a quality service?

In order to be properly prepared to offer quality braiding services, the first step you have to perfect is the client consultation. As with any service, learning to communicate with the client and truly listen to his or her desires, interests, and requests will be key in the success of the service. You will need to learn the important steps in preparing textured hair for braiding and/or hair extension services. Finally, you will need to be able to demonstrate masterful techniques for a wide variety of braids, including invisible, rope, fishtail, and single braids. You will want to perfect your skills in single braids and cornrowing, both with and without extensions. Once you have mastered these skills, you will have taken the first step in establishing a sound braiding business.

Essential Experience

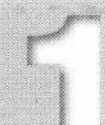

Preparing Textured Hair for Braiding

Number the following steps in their proper procedural order.

_______ Drape client

_______ Section hair

_______ Complete pre-service procedure

_______ Comb hair applying detangling solution as needed

_______ Ear to ear parting

_______ Divide section into two equal parts and twist together to the end

_______ Shampoo the hair

_______ Twist remaining sections until entire head is sectioned

_______ Complete post-service procedure

_______ Open one combed section and apply blowdrying cream from scalp to ends

_______ Dry for five to ten minutes under medium-heat dryer

_______ Blowdry using pick attachment on blowdryer

_______ Gently towel-dry hair

2 Essential Experience

The Developmental Stages of Locks

In the space provided, list all five phases in the development of locks in the left column. In the right column, thoroughly explain each phase.

PHASE	DEVELOPMENT

Essential Experience 3

Procedure for Basic Cornrows

Number the following steps in their proper procedural order.

______ **Dry hair.** Gently towel dry the hair, then blowdry it completely.

______ **Perform Pre-Service Procedure.**

______ **Determine size of base and apply oil.** Depending on desired style, determine the correct size and direction of the cornrow base. With tail comb, part hair into 2-inch (5 cm) sections, and apply a light essential oil to the scalp. Massage oil throughout scalp and hair.

______ **Take two even partings.** Start by taking two even partings to form a neat row for the cornrow base. With a tail comb, part the hair into a panel, using butterfly clips to keep the other hair pinned to either side.

______ **Continue picking up strands with each revolution.** As you move along the braid panel, pick up a strand from the scalp with each revolution, and add it to the outer strand before crossing it under, alternating the side of the braid on which you pick up the hair.

______ **Divide the panel into three even strands.** To ensure consistency, make sure that strands are the same size. Place fingers close to the base. Cross the left strand (1) under the center strand (2). The center strand is now on the left and the former left strand (1) is the new center.

______ **Braid next panel.** Braid the next panel in the same direction and in the same manner. Keep the partings clean and even.

______ **Begin underhand cornrow.** Cross the right strand (3) under the center strand (1). Passing the outer strands under the center strand this way creates the underhand cornrow braid.

______ **Braid to ends and finish.** Simply braiding to the ends can finish the cornrow; small rubber bands can be used to hold the ends in place. Other optional finishes, such as singeing (heat sealing), are considered advanced methods and require special training.

______ **Pick up new strand with each revolution.** With each crossing under or revolution, pick up from the base of the panel a new strand of equal size and add it to the outer strand before crossing it under the center strand.

3 Essential Experience continued

_____ **Shampoo hair.** Shampoo, rinse, apply conditioner, and rinse thoroughly.

_____ **Complete Post-Service Procedure.**

_____ **Drape client.** Drape the client for a shampoo. If necessary, comb and detangle the hair before shampooing.

_____ **Braid to the end.** As new strands are added, the braid will become fuller.

_____ **Repeat until all the hair is braided, and apply oil sheen for shine.**

Essential Experience 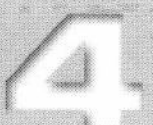

Word Search

After identifying the correct word from the clues provided, locate the words in the word search puzzle.

Word	Clue
________________	Occurs after several years of maturation of a lock
________________	Another name for cornrows
________________	Narrow rows of visible braids that lie close to the scalp
________________	Flat leather pads with close and fine teeth
________________	Another name for locks
________________	Simple two-strand braid in which hair is picked up from the sides and added to the strands as they are crossed over each other
________________	Stage when a bulb can be felt at the end of each lock
________________	A board of fine upright nails
________________	Another name for visible braid
________________	Three-strand braid produced by overlapping the strands of hair on top of each other
________________	A manufactured synthetic fiber similar to coiled hair types
________________	Beautiful wool fiber from Africa
________________	Natural textured hair that is intertwined and meshed together to form a single or separate network.
________________	Phase of lock development when the lock is totally closed on the end
________________	Method of locking that takes advantage of the hair's natural ability to coil
________________	Stage of development when hair is soft and coiled into spiral configurations
________________	Braid made with two strands that are twisted around each other
________________	Free-hanging braids, with or without extensions; can be executed either underhand or overhand

4 Essential Experience continued

_______________ Development of lock stage where hair begins to interlace and mesh

_______________ Refers to the hair diameter, feel, and wave pattern

_______________ Three-strand braid made by the underhand technique

_______________ Strong fiber from ox

I	L	R	D	D	A	G	N	I	W	O	R	G	X	Y
N	S	P	R	O	U	T	I	N	G	L	S	F	S	H
V	U	R	A	B	A	S	L	V	A	W	I	I	F	P
I	U	E	O	D	V	E	O	E	O	S	N	N	T	O
S	L	-	B	D	R	H	E	R	H	G	Q	O	J	R
I	M	L	G	X	Y	E	N	T	L	R	C	L	C	T
B	A	O	N	X	D	R	A	E	B	P	Z	A	A	A
L	T	C	I	W	O	I	B	D	U	P	U	K	N	L
E	U	K	W	C	L	R	A	B	L	H	M	E	E	W
B	R	S	A	B	A	E	F	R	H	O	Y	N	R	W
R	A	I	R	I	N	N	H	A	B	A	C	A	O	M
A	T	A	D	O	G	P	Z	I	K	E	C	K	W	H
I	I	S	P	T	I	S	M	D	J	X	P	K	S	E
D	O	I	M	Y	I	B	P	A	L	M	R	O	L	L
N	N	S	I	O	P	Y	G	T	E	X	T	U	R	E

Essential Experience 5

Research and Design

Contact various salons in your area and interview them by asking the following questions.

- Does your salon offer braiding and/or extensions as a service?
- If yes, what braiding services do you offer?
- What braids are the most popular in your salon?
- What is the average time it takes your stylists to complete a full head of cornrows?
- What is the price structure your salon charges for braiding services?
- Do you have any specific advice for a newly licensed professional with respect to offering braiding services?

- Look through various style magazines and locate at least three different braided styles. Recreate these styles on a mannequin or a model.

- Use your imagination and the skills you have mastered in braiding to create a special-effects braid. Stylists have created such looks as hats, flowers, baskets, or bird cages with braids. Tap into your creative abilities and design your own special look.

Essential Rubrics

Rubrics are used in education for organizing and interpreting data gathered from observations of student performance. It is a clearly developed scoring document used to differentiate between levels of development in a specific skill performance or behavior. A rubric is provided in this study guide as a self-assessment tool to aid you in your behavior development.

Rate your performance according to the following scale:

(1) Development Opportunity: There is little or no evidence of competency; assistance is needed; performance includes multiple errors.

(2) Fundamental: There is beginning evidence of competency; task is completed alone; performance includes few errors.

(3) Competent: There is detailed and consistent evidence of competency; task is completed alone; performance includes rare errors.

(4) Strength: There is detailed evidence of highly creative, inventive, mature presence of competency.

Space is provided for comments to assist you in improving your performance and achieving a higher rating.

PREPARING TEXTURED HAIR FOR BRAIDING PROCEDURE

Performance Assessed	1	2	3	4	Improvement Plan
Draped the client for a shampoo					
Combed and detangled the hair					
Shampooed, applied conditioner, and rinsed thoroughly					
Gently towel dried the hair					
Parted damp hair from ear to ear across crown					
Used butterfly clips to separate front section from back section					
Parted the back of head into four to six sections					
Separated the sections with clips					

Performance Assessed	1	2	3	4	Improvement Plan
Beginning on left section in the back, combed the ends of the hair first, working up to the base of the scalp					
Divided section into two equal parts and twisted them together to hold the section in place					
Continued sectioning					
Placed client under a medium-heat hood dryer for five to ten minutes to remove excess moisture					
Opened one of the combed sections					
Applied blowdrying cream to hair from scalp to ends					
Using a pick nozzle attachment on a blowdryer, held hair down and away from client's head to dry					
Used comb-out motion with the pick					
Used moderate tension, and directed air flow down the hair shaft to smooth and seal the cuticle					

ROPE BRAID PROCEDURE

Performance Assessed	1	2	3	4	Improvement Plan
Draped the client for a shampoo					
Shampooed, applied conditioner, and rinsed thoroughly					
Gently towel dried the hair, then blowdried completely					

Essential Rubrics continued

Performance Assessed	1	2	3	4	Improvement Plan
Took a triangular section of hair from the front. If client/model had bangs, began behind the bangs					
Divided the section into two equal strands					
Crossed the right strand over the left strand					
Placed strands in right hand					
Place index finger in between and your palm facing upward					
Twisted the left strand two times clockwise (toward the center)					
Picked up a 1-inch (2.5 cm) section from the left side					
Added this section to the left strand					
Put both strands in left hand with the index finger in between and palm up					
Pick up a 1-inch (2.5 cm) section from the right side and add it to the right strand					
Put both strands in right hand with index finger in between and palm up					
Twisted toward the left (toward the center) until palm was facing down					
Worked toward the nape until the style was complete					
Secured with a rubber band					
Created a rope ponytail with the remaining hair					
Repeated steps until the end of the hair was reached for all sections					
Secured ends with a rubber band					

FISHTAIL BRAID PROCEDURE

Performance Assessed	1	2	3	4	Improvement Plan
Draped the client for a shampoo					
Shampooed, applied conditioner, and rinsed thoroughly					
Gently towel dried the hair, then blowdried completely					
Took a triangular section from the front					
Divided section into two equal strands					
Crossed the right strand over the left strand					
Placed both strands in the right hand, index finger in between and palm up					
Crossed section over the left strand and added it to the right strand					
Placed two outer strands in the left hand, index finger in between strands with palm up					
Crossed this section over the right strand and added it to the left strand					
Put both strands in the right hand					
Moved hand down toward the nape with each new section picked up					
Secured the hair with an elastic band to hold					

Essential Rubrics continued

INVISIBLE BRAID PROCEDURE

Performance Assessed	1	2	3	4	Improvement Plan
Draped the client for a shampoo; if necessary, comb and detangle the hair					
Shampooed, applied conditioner, and rinsed thoroughly					
Gently towel dried the hair and blowdried completely					
At crown of head, took a triangular section of hair and placed it in left hand					
Divided the section into three equal strands, two in left hand, and one in right hand					
Crossed right strand over center strand.					
Placed fingers close to the scalp for a tight stitch					
Crossed right strand (1) over center strand (2)					
Crossed left strand (3) over center section and placed it in right hand					
Placed all three strands in left hand with fingers separating the strands					
With right hand, picked up a 1" × 1" (2.5 × 2.5 cm) section of hair on the right side and added to strand 2 in left hand					
Took combined strands in right hand and crossed them over the center strand					
Placed all the strands in right hand					
With left hand, picked up a 1-inch (2.5 cm) section on the left side					

Performance Assessed	1	2	3	4	Improvement Plan
Added this section to the left outer strand (1) in right hand					
Took the combined strands and crossed them over the center strand					
Placed all three sections in left hand, picked up right side, and added to outer strand (3)					
Continued movements until the braid was complete					
Secured braid					

SINGLE BRAIDS WITHOUT EXTENSIONS PROCEDURE

Performance Assessed	1	2	3	4	Improvement Plan
Draped the client for a shampoo					
Shampooed, applied conditioner, and rinsed thoroughly					
Gently towel dried hair, then blowdried completely					
Applied a light essential oil to the scalp and massaged the oil into the scalp and hair					
Divided hair in half by parting from ear to ear across the crown					
Clipped aside the front section					
Determined the size and direction of the base of the braid					
Parted a diagonal section in the back of the head about 1-inch (2.5 cm) wide, taking into account the texture and length of the client's hair					
Divided the section into three even strands					

Essential Rubrics continued

Performance Assessed	1	2	3	4	Improvement Plan
Placed fingers close to the base					
Crossed left strand under the center strand and cross the right strand under					
Passed the outer strands under the center strands, moving down the single braid to the end					
Secured the end as desired					
Moved to the next subsection or braid and repeated braiding movement					
Moved across the back, and took the next diagonal parting					
Continued procedure until the entire back is completed					
Moved to the front and repeated the procedure in the front section					
Rubber bands were used to secure each braid					
Applied an oil sheen product for a shiny finished look					

BASIC CORNROWS PROCEDURE

Performance Assessed	1	2	3	4	Improvement Plan
Draped the client for a shampoo					
Shampooed, applied conditioner, and rinsed thoroughly					
Gently towel dried the hair, then blowdried completely					
Determined size of base and applied oil					
With tail comb, parted hair into 2-inch (5 cm) sections					

Essential Rubrics continued

Performance Assessed	1	2	3	4	Improvement Plan
Applied a light essential oil to the scalp					
Massaged oil throughout scalp and hair					
Started by taking two even partings to form a neat row for the cornrow base					
With a tail comb, parted the hair into a panel, using butterfly clips to keep the other hair pinned to either side					
Divided the panel into three even strands					
Placed fingers close to the base					
Crossed the left strand (1) under the center strand (2)					
Crossed the right strand (3) under the center strand (1)					
With each crossing under or revolution, picked up from the base of the panel a new strand of equal size and added it to the outer strand before crossing it under the center strand					
Picked up a strand from the scalp with each revolution, and added it to the outer strand before crossing it under, alternating pick-up sides					
Braided to ends					
Secured ends					
Repeated procedure until all hair was braided					

Essential Review

Using the following words, fill in the blanks below to form a thorough review of Chapter 18, Braiding & Braid Extensions. Words or terms may be used more than once or not at all.

box braids
center strand
challenges
chemicals
coil
coil pattern
cornrows
dampened subsections
diameter
diffuser
double twisting
forehead
invisible
jawline
length
locks
matte finish
maturation
nails
natural curl
network
occupation
oval
ox
palm roll
partial bangs
pomades
rope
rope-like
rotating motion
round
several weeks
shorter
small forehead
softens
spiral configurations
synthetic fiber
temples
visible

1. Braiding styles have been known to distinguish one's tribe, age, economic status, ____________, geographic location, religious standing, and marital status.
2. Hair is referred to as *natural or virgin* if it has had no previous coloring or lightening treatments, ____________, or physical abuse.
3. Natural hairstyling uses no chemicals or tints and does not alter the ____________ or coil pattern of the hair.
4. When referring to braiding and other natural hairstyling, the term *texture* refers to the ____________ of the hair, the wave pattern of the hair, and the feel of the hair.
5. With regard to wave pattern, a ____________ is a very tight curl pattern that is spiral in formation and, when lengthened or stretched, resembles a series of loops.
6. When styling with braids, add height to create the illusion of thinness for the ____________ facial shape.
7. Most braided styles are appropriate for the ____________ facial shape.

Essential Review continued

8. Create styles that are full around the forehead or ____________ to help create a more oval appearance for the diamond facial shape.
9. To create the illusion of length and to soften facial lines for the square facial shape, choose styles that frame the face around the ____________, temples, and jawline.
10. Soft fringes around the forehead will camouflage a ______________ without closing up the triangular-shaped face.
11. Creating full styles can make the oblong face shape appear ____________ or wider.
12. The goal of the inverted-triangle face shape is to minimize the width of the forehead by styling with ____________ or wisps of hair/braids that frame the face.
13. A natural hairbrush, also known as a boar-bristle brush, is best for stimulating the scalp as well as removing dirt and lint from ____________.
14. The tool that dries the hair without disturbing the finished look and without removing moisture is called a ____________.
15. A board made of fine upright ____________ through which human hair extensions are combed is called a *hackle*.
16. A manufactured ________________ of excellent quality that has a texture similar to curly or coiled hair is called *Kanekalon*.
17. A beautiful wool fiber imported from Africa that has a ____________ and comes only in black and brown is known as *lin*.
18. A strong fiber that comes from the domestic ____________ found in the mountains of Tibet and Central Asia is yak.
19. ____________, gels, or lotions can be used to hold the hair in place for a finished look.
20. Textured hair, or hair with a tight ____________, presents certain challenges when styling because it is very fragile when both wet and dry.
21. Blowdrying the hair ____________ it, makes it more manageable, loosens it, and elongates the wave pattern while stretching the hair shaft length.
22. Another term for a/an ____________ braid is inverted.
23. The visible braid is a three-strand braid that employs the underhand technique, in which strands of hair are woven under the ____________.

Essential Review continued

24. A ____________ braid is made with two strands that are twisted around each other.
25. Single braids, ____________, and individual braids are all considered to be free-hanging braids, with or without extensions, that can be extended with either an underhand or overhand stitch.
26. Narrow visible braids that lie close to the scalp are called ____________.
27. There are several ways to cultivate locks such as ______________, wrapping with cord, coiling, braiding, or simply by not combing or brushing.
28. Dreadlocks are natural textured hair intertwined and meshed together to form a single or separate ____________ of hair and are done without the use of chemicals.
29. The method of placing the comb at the base of the scalp and, with a _________________, spiraling the hair into a curl is known as the *comb technique*.
30. The method that involves applying gel to ____________________, placing the portion of hair between the palms of both hands, and rolling in a circular direction is known as *palm roll*.
31. Braids or extensions are an effective way to start locks and involve sectioning the hair for the desired lock and single braiding the hair to the end, with or without adding hair extensions, and waiting for ____________ of growth before employing the palm-roll technique.
32. During the maturation stage of locks, the lock is totally closed at the end and the hair is tightly meshed, giving a ____________ cylinder shape, except where there is new growth at the base.
33. During the prelock stage of locks, the hair is soft and coiled into _________________________ that are smooth and the end is open.

Essential Discoveries and Accomplishments

In the space below, jot some notes about what concepts of this chapter were hardest for you to understand or remember. Imagine finding yourself suddenly in the role of "teacher" and consider what you would tell your "students" about these concepts. Share your Essential Discoveries with some of the other students in your class and ask if they are helpful to them. You may want to revise your discoveries based on good ideas shared by your peers.

Discoveries:

List at least three things you have accomplished since your last entry that relate to your career goals.

Accomplishments:

CHAPTER 19

Wigs & Hair Additions

A Motivating Moment: "A healthy attitude is contagious, but don't wait to catch it from others. Be a carrier!"
—Unknown

Essential Objectives

After studying this chapter and completing the Essential Companion components, you will be able to:

1. **Explain the differences between human hair and synthetic hair.**
2. **Describe the two basic categories of wigs.**
3. **Describe several types of hairpieces and their uses.**
4. **Explain several different methods of attaching hair extensions.**

Essential Aspects of Wigs and Hair Additions

Do people really still wear wigs, and why should I know how to handle them?

Yes, people really do still wear wigs. They wear them for a number of reasons ranging from convenience to need due to hair loss. Celebrities and people in the public eye, both male and female, wear wigs, hairpieces, or toupees regularly to create a different, dramatic look. Like many other cosmetology services you will learn, the use of wigs has been prevalent throughout history from the early Egyptians to the present time. Wigs and hair additions became extremely popular again in the mid-twentieth century and continue to be used extensively in theater, music, and movie productions today.

You will also have clients from time to time who have medical problems or are undergoing chemotherapy treatments. As a result, they may experience partial or total hair loss and will want to use wigs to maintain their personal appearance. You will need to be prepared to provide them the quality service they deserve, especially if they are experiencing a difficult time.

Cosmetologists should study and have a thorough understanding of wigs and hair additions because:

- The market for products and services related to faux hair has expanded to every consumer group, from baby boomers with fine and thinning hair to young trendsetters.
- Hair extensions, additions, and customized wigs can be some of the most lucrative services in the salon.
- Each manufacturer has its own systems, but if you understand the fundamentals, you can easily work with any company on the market.
- The skills you develop will open many doors, from working behind the scenes on Broadway shows to working with celebrities, who today invariably wear faux hair.

Essential Concepts

What can really be so hard about handling wigs, and what do I really need to know?

You need to know about the construction and materials used in wigs and how to care for each type of product, whether it is a human-hair piece or one constructed of synthetic hair. It will be important for you to know how to properly measure a client's head size and properly fit a wig. You will also want to master the special care needed for human-hair and hand-knotted wigs. Wigs that are made of human hair can also be colored to change the client's overall appearance. Hairpieces made of human hair can also be colored to blend with the client's own hair color as necessary. While this may not be the service that you spend the most time on, you will definitely want to be able to offer quality services to meet all of your clients' needs.

Essential Experience 1

The History of Wigs

Conduct research about the history of wigs and write a brief essay on the subject. Be prepared to present the report to the full class if directed by your instructor. There are a number of resources you can refer to including the institution's library or resource center, encyclopedias, the Internet, and the community library. Obtain copies of pictures and prepare drawings to help illustrate your report.

2 Essential Experience

Manufacturer Wig Measurements

Write to at least three different wig manufacturers and obtain their form for measuring wigs. Measure at least three different heads (students or models) and record the required measurements below.

Essential Experience 3

Matching Exercise

Match each of the following essential terms with its definition.

______	**Turned hair**	**1.**	Method of attaching hair extensions in which hair wefts or single strands are attached with an adhesive or bonding agent.
______	**Fusion bonding**	**2.**	Hairpiece on an oblong base with curls or a cluster of curls that offers an endless variety of styling possibilities.
______	**Cascade**	**3.**	Section of hair, machine-wefted on a round base, running across the back of the head.
______	**Capless wig**	**4.**	Also called *Remi hair*; the root end of every single strand is sewn into the base, so that the cuticles of all hair strands move in the same direction: down.
______	**Block**	**5.**	Small wig used to cover the top or crown of the head.
______	**Wig**	**6.**	Hair additions that are secured to the base of the client's natural hair in order to add length, volume, texture, or color.
______	**Full**	**7.**	Artificial covering for the head consisting of a network of interwoven hair.
______	**Hair extensions**	**8.**	Head-shaped form, usually made of canvas-covered cork or Styrofoam, to which the wig is secured for fitting, cleaning, coloring, and styling.
______	**Toupee**	**9.**	Machine-made wig in which rows of wefts are sewn to elastic strips in a circular pattern to fit the head shape.
______	**Bonding**	**10.**	Method of attaching extension in which the extension hair is bonded to the client's own hair with a bonding material that is activated by heat from a special tool.

4 Essential Experience

Crossword Puzzle

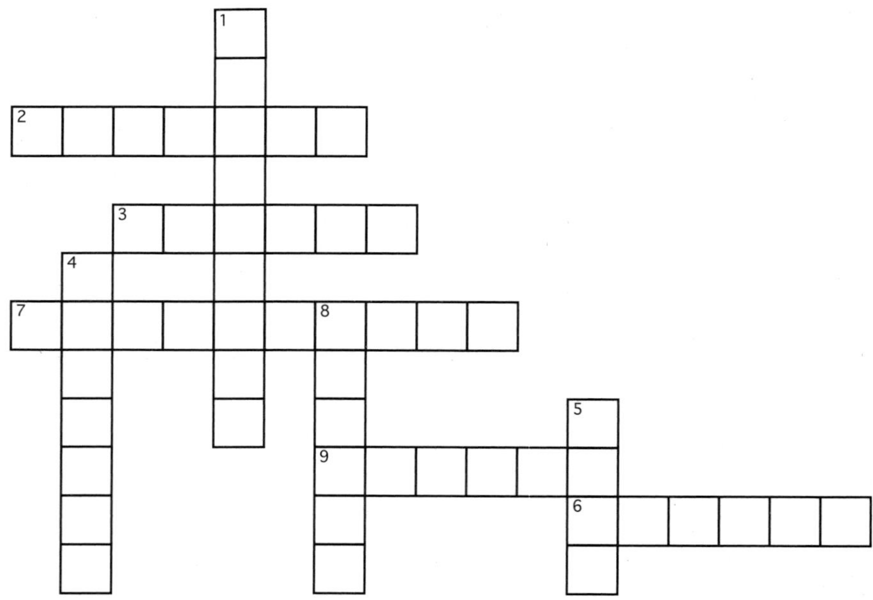

Across

Word	Clue
____________	**2.** Method of attaching hair extensions with adhesive or glue gun
____________	**3.** Wig consisting of elasticized mesh fiber to which hair is attached
____________	**6.** Method of attaching extensions with bonding material activated by heat
____________	**7.** Machine-made wig
____________	**9.** Small wig used to cover top or crown of a man's head

Down

Word	Clue
____________	**1.** Hair addition that sits on top of hair and is usually attached by temporary methods
____________	**4.** Hairpiece with an oblong base and curls or cluster of curls
____________	**5.** Strip of hair woven by hand or machine onto a thread
____________	**8.** Hairpiece consisting of a long length of wefted hair mounted with a loop on the end

Essential Review

Using the following words, fill in the blanks below to form a thorough review of Chapter 19, Wigs & Hair Additions. Words or terms may be used more than once or not at all.

40 percent	**cap**	**fusion**	**split**
60 percent	**cap wigs**	**hand-tied**	**strand test**
70 percent	**capless wigs**	**human hair**	**switch**
angora	**cuticle-intact**	**integration**	**synthetic**
attitudinal	**eight**	**key point checklist**	**ten**
braid-and-sew	**emotional**	**machine-made**	**toupee**
boar bristles	**film**	**oxidizing**	**weft**
bonding	**free-form**	**six**	**wig**
bronze razors			

1. The ancient Egyptians shaved their heads with ____________ and wore heavy wigs to protect them from the sun.
2. A wig service can be a large financial and ____________ investment for a client.
3. Your best tool for achieving good communication during a wig consultation is to follow the ________________.
4. A ____________ can be defined as an artificial covering for the head consisting of a network of interwoven hair.
5. One advantage of ____________ wigs is they have the same styling and maintenance requirements as natural hair.
6. One disadvantage of human hair wigs is that the hair will break and ____________ just like human hair if mistreated by harsh brushing, backcombing, or excessive use of heat.
7. Most ____________ ready-to-wear wigs are cut according to the latest styles, with the cut, color, and texture already set.
8. Well-crafted wigs, such as those used in ____________ work, might be valued at thousands of dollars.
9. Animal hair that may be mixed with human hair to create a wig includes ____________, horse, yak, or sheep hair.
10. Hair that has been "turned" is also known as ____________ hair.
11. ____________ are constructed with an elasticized mesh-fiber base to which the hair is attached.

Essential Review continued

12. ____________ are machine made with the hair woven into long strips called wefts.
13. ____________ wigs are made by inserting individual strands of hair into a mesh foundation and knotting them with a needle.
14. ____________ wigs are divided into three sections: the front edge, the side edge, and the back edge.
15. Canvas wig blocks are available in ____________ sizes.
16. ____________ cutting is usually done on dry hair, which allows you to see more clearly how the hair will fall.
17. Traditionally, brushes made with natural ____________ have been regarded as the best on human hair.
18. Do not use ____________ haircolor or haircolor with peroxide on wig hair that has been treated with metallic hair dye.
19. When coloring wigs or hairpieces, always ____________ the hair prior to full color application.
20. A hairpiece gives 20 percent to ____________ coverage and sits on top of the hair.
21. ____________ hairpieces are very lightweight and natural looking, add length and volume to the client's hair, and allow the client's own hair to be pulled through and blended with the hair of the hairpiece.
22. A ____________ is a small wig used to cover the top and crown of the head.
23. A ____________ is a long length of wefted hair mounted with a loop on the end that covers 10 percent to 20 percent of the head.
24. A wire-based hairpiece combines a hair ____________ with a flexible wire.
25. In the _____________ method, hair extensions are secured at the base of the client's own hair by sewing.

Essential Discoveries and Accomplishments

In the space below, jot some notes about what concepts of this chapter were hardest for you to understand or remember. Imagine finding yourself suddenly in the role of "teacher" and consider what you would tell your "students" about these concepts. Share your Essential Discoveries with some of the other students in your class and ask if they are helpful to them. You may want to revise your discoveries based on good ideas shared by your peers.

Discoveries:

List at least three things you have accomplished since you decided to enroll in school.

Accomplishments:

CHAPTER 20

Chemical Texture Services

A Motivating Moment: "There are two big forces at work, external and internal. We have very little control over external forces such as tornados, earthquakes, floods, disasters, illness and pain. What really matters is the internal force. How do I respond to those disasters? Over that I have complete control."

— Leo F. Buscaglia

Essential Objectives

After studying this chapter and completing the Essential Companion components, you will be able to:

1. Explain the structure and purpose of each of the hair's layers.
2. Explain chemical actions that take place during permanent waving.
3. Explain the difference between an alkaline wave and a true acid wave.
4. Explain the purpose of neutralization in permanent waving.
5. Describe how thio relaxers straighten the hair.
6. Describe how hydroxide relaxers straighten the hair.
7. Describe curl-reforming and what it is best used for.

Essential Chemical Texture Services

What role will permanent waving and hair relaxing have in my career when all I really want to do is style hair?

You will find that being able to provide your client with an appropriate texture service will improve your effectiveness as a hair designer and your ability to earn a higher income. People have been trying to change the texture and curl of their hair since the ancient Roman and Egyptian civilizations. Women wrapped their hair around sticks and men wove their beards around them selves and then applied mud from the river which they allowed to dry in the sun for up to three days to achieve their desired look.

We've come a long way since those primitive methods. We began to make real progress in the first part of the twentieth century when Charles Nessler invented the permanent wave machine. In 1931 the preheat method of perming was introduced. The following year a method using external heat generated by chemical reaction was introduced. By 1941, the cold wave method was discovered, which used chemicals to soften and expand the hair and then reharden it in its newly formed shape. This method does not use heat in any form. Technology continues to improve and new products are introduced regularly that allow the professional cosmetologist to modify the texture of a client's hair and render it more suitable for the desired style.

Our client culture has changed dramatically in the last few decades. Clients today want instant gratification from their salon visit and nearly all want better hair manageability. A texture service can play a huge role in helping the client manage his/her personal style between visits to the salon. Relaxers remove wave or curl from the hair in varying degrees. Many individuals will want the curl in their hair reduced. Hair relaxing services generate significant revenue for you and the salon. As a professional, you will want to be fully prepared to offer a quality service when it is requested.

Cosmetologists should study and have a thorough understanding of chemical texture services because:

- Chemical texture services are problem solvers for stylists and clients in that they change the texture of the hair and can allow a person to wear just about any conceivable hair texture.
- Knowing how to perform these services accurately and professionally will help build a trusting and loyal clientele.

Essential Chemical Texture Services continued

- They are among the most lucrative services in the salon, and many retail products are specific to the hair's condition and the chemical service to which it has been exposed.
- Without a thorough understanding of chemistry, cosmetologists could damage the hair.

Essential Concepts

Exactly what am I going to need to learn about permanent waving and chemical hair relaxing to be considered competent in this particular skill?

Your success in chemical texture services depends on your knowledge of the hair, your understanding of the chemicals used, and your ability to physically perform the service. Other factors relevant to the success of the service are the condition or integrity of the hair. The professional cosmetologist will know how to properly analyze a client's hair and scalp and select the appropriate products to create the desired look. You will also need to know how to select the correct tools and how to properly use them to "set" the perm. In addition, you need to prescribe the proper home care so the service maintains its look for the maximum period of time.

Research and development of relaxer systems continues daily. As a result, we see state-of-the-art formulas and products available for our use in the salon. You will be exposed to these formulas while you are in school as well as in the professional establishment. Many manufacturers provide excellent education in the use of their products, and you will want to take advantage of all that is available to you. In addition to product technology, you will want to learn all about the tools used in relaxing treatments as well as the procedures to follow to ensure success. Finally, you must master all the safety precautions that need to be followed when performing chemical texture services.

1 Essential Experience

Defining Permanent Waving and Identifying Textures

Permanent waving is a chemical and physical process in which the hair is wrapped around a rod, chemically softened and expanded, and finally chemically rehardened into its newly formed shape.

In order to better understand the concept of texture, peruse old magazines (not necessarily beauty-industry related) for examples of different types of textures. You are not looking for texture that involves human hair. Cut out examples of the variety of textures (such as fabrics) and paste them in the space below, creating a texture collage. Beneath the collage, write a brief narrative describing the various textures selected and how they differ from each other. You may choose to create your collage on a poster board rather than in the textbook.

____

____

____

____

Essential Experience

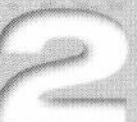

Hair Analysis

Choose three other students and perform a complete consultation and hair analysis on them. Fill out the school's client record card completely. Determine the correct rod size and product choice to create their desired textured look. Ask your instructor to review your record card and make an assessment as to the results you might achieve.

3 Essential Experience

Product Research

Research the various perm products used in your school. Make a chart of the products listing name, pH, key ingredients, and hair type for which they are recommended.

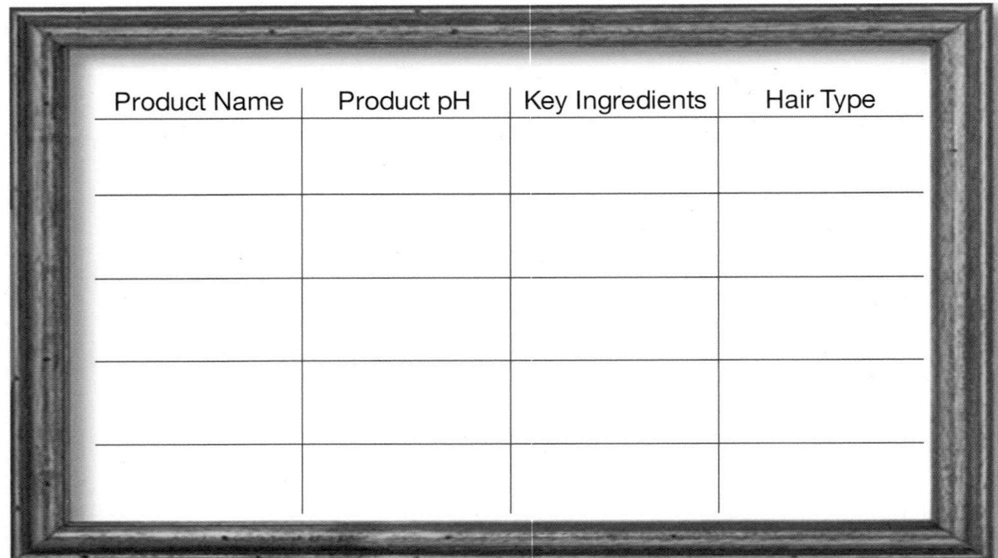

Product Name	Product pH	Key Ingredients	Hair Type

Essential Experience 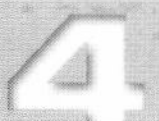

Matching Exercise

Match each of the following essential terms with its identifying phrase or definition.

______	**Coarse texture**	**1.**	Result of overprocessing
______	**Cortex**	**2.**	Processes more quickly than other textures
______	**Cuticle**	**3.**	Usually requires more processing than other textures
______	**Good porosity**	**4.**	Normal hair
______	**Fine texture**	**5.**	Resistant hair
______	**Medium texture**	**6.**	Innermost section of the hair
______	**Medulla**	**7.**	Generally no problems processing
______	**Overporous**	**8.**	Outer covering of the hair
______	**Poor porosity**	**9.**	Major component of the hair structure
______	**Underprocessing**	**10.**	Sulfite permanent
______	**Plastic cap**	**11.**	One end paper folded over hair strand
______	**Elasticity**	**12.**	Hair ends wound from ends toward scalp
______	**Density**	**13.**	The number of hairs per square inch (2.5 square cm)
______	**Body wave**	**14.**	The ability of the hair to stretch and contract
______	**Waving lotion**	**15.**	Porous papers used to cover hair ends
______	**Bookend**	**16.**	Heat is created chemically within the product
______	**Exothermic**	**17.**	Fits over the wrapped rods
______	**Croquignole**	**18.**	Amino acids are bonded together and form these
______	**End papers**	**19.**	Caused by insufficient processing time
______	**Polypeptides**	**20.**	A liquid that softens and swells the hair

5 Essential Experience

Product Research

Research a variety of relaxer products available in your school and found at local supply stores. Use the chart below to track your findings.

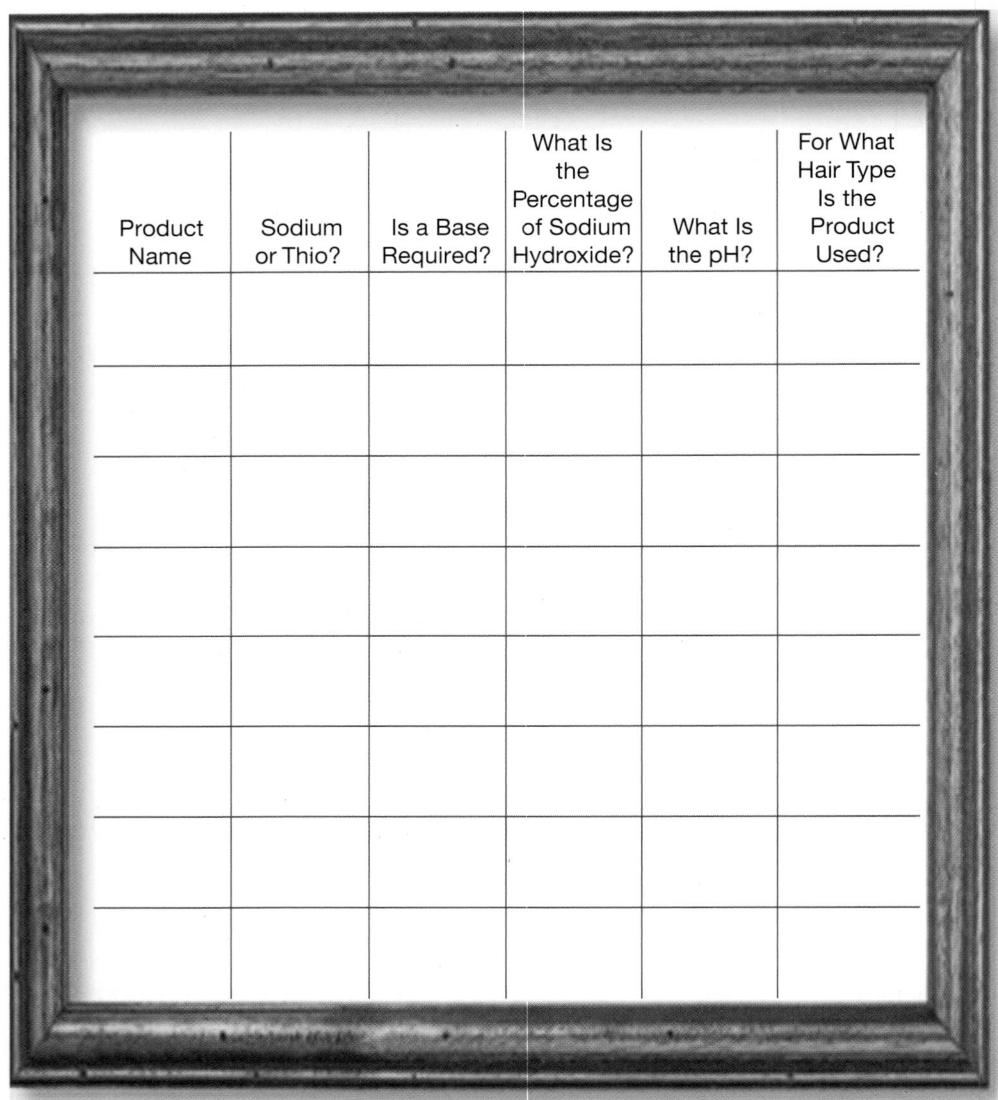

Product Name	Sodium or Thio?	Is a Base Required?	What Is the Percentage of Sodium Hydroxide?	What Is the pH?	For What Hair Type Is the Product Used?

Essential Experience 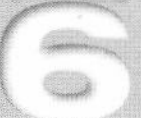

Purpose and Action of Chemical Hair Relaxing

List the products used in sodium hydroxide relaxers.

In your own words, explain the action of hydroxide relaxers on the hair.

What is the common ingredient in a thio-type relaxer and permanent waving solution?

Explain the action of this common ingredient.

What is the purpose of the neutralizer in thio relaxing treatments?

In your own words, explain the difference between *base* and *no-base* formulas, and the purpose of using a base product.

7 Essential Experience

Word Search

After determining the correct word from the clues provided, locate the words in the word search puzzle.

Word	Clue
________________	Perm type having a pH between 7.8 and 8.2
________________	Perm type having a pH between 9.0 and 9.6
________________	Oily cream used to protect the skin and scalp during hair relaxing
________________	Perm wrap in which one end paper is folded in half over hair ends
________________	Rod having a smaller circumference in center than on ends
________________	Hair strands are wrapped from ends to scalp
________________	Partings and bases radiate throughout the panels to follow the curvature of the head
________________	Side bonds between the polypeptide chains in the cortex
________________	Waves activated by an outside heat source
________________	Relatively weak physical side bonds resulting from an attraction between opposite electrical charges
________________	Process by which hydroxide relaxers permanently straighten hair
________________	Process of stopping the action of the permanent wave solution and hardening hair in new form
________________	Also called end bonds
________________	Relaxer having a pH above 10 and a higher concentration of ammonium thioglycolate
________________	Wrapping technique that uses zigzag partings to divide base areas

Essential Experience continued 7

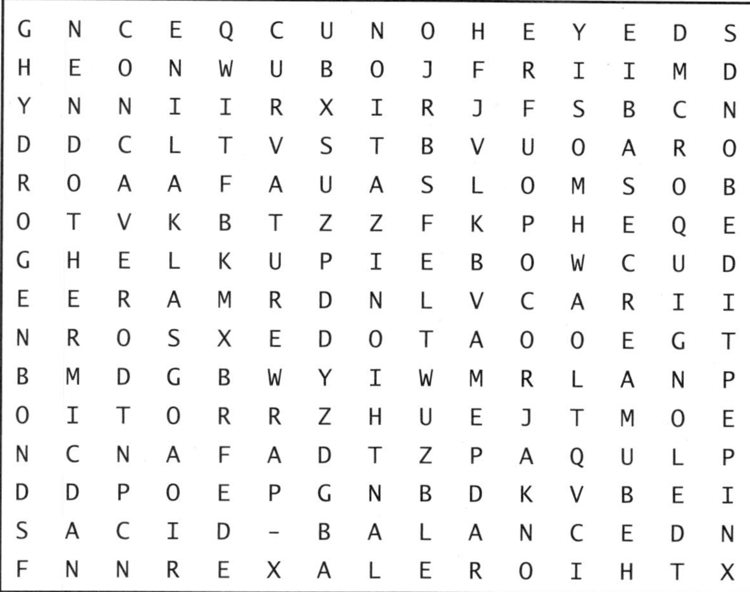

G	N	C	E	Q	C	U	N	O	H	E	Y	E	D	S
H	E	O	N	W	U	B	O	J	F	R	I	I	M	D
Y	N	N	I	I	R	X	I	R	J	F	S	B	C	N
D	D	C	L	T	V	S	T	B	V	U	O	A	R	O
R	O	A	A	F	A	U	A	S	L	O	M	S	O	B
O	T	V	K	B	T	Z	Z	F	K	P	H	E	Q	E
G	H	E	L	K	U	P	I	E	B	O	W	C	U	D
E	E	R	A	M	R	D	N	L	V	C	A	R	I	I
N	R	O	S	X	E	D	O	T	A	O	O	E	G	T
B	M	D	G	B	W	Y	I	W	M	R	L	A	N	P
O	I	T	O	R	R	Z	H	U	E	J	T	M	O	E
N	C	N	A	F	A	D	T	Z	P	A	Q	U	L	P
D	D	P	O	E	P	G	N	B	D	K	V	B	E	I
S	A	C	I	D	-	B	A	L	A	N	C	E	D	N
F	N	N	R	E	X	A	L	E	R	O	I	H	T	X

Essential Rubrics

Rubrics are used in education for organizing and interpreting data gathered from observations of student performance. It is a clearly developed scoring document used to differentiate between levels of development in a specific skill performance or behavior. A rubric is provided in this study guide as a self-assessment tool to aid you in your behavior development.

Rate your performance according to the following scale.

(1) Development Opportunity: There is little or no evidence of competency; assistance is needed; performance includes multiple errors.

(2) Fundamental: There is beginning evidence of competency; task is completed alone; performance includes few errors.

(3) Competent: There is detailed and consistent evidence of competency; task is completed alone; performance includes rare errors.

(4) Strength: There is detailed evidence of highly creative, inventive, mature presence of competency.

Space is provided for comments to assist you in improving your performance and achieving a higher rating.

PERMANENT WAVE AND PROCESSING USING A BASIC PERM WRAP PROCEDURE

Performance Assessed	1	2	3	4	Improvement Plan
Used length of tool to measure width of panels and divided into nine panels					
Kept hair wet during wrapping					
Began wrapping front hairline					
Made a horizontal parting same size as tool					
Held hair at 90-degree angle to head					
Using two end papers, rolled hair down to the scalp					

Essential Rubrics continued

Performance Assessed	1	2	3	4	Improvement Plan
Positioned tool half-off base					
Band was smooth, not twisted, and fastened straight across top of tool					
Inserted picks to stabilize rods and eliminate any tension caused by band as needed					
Continued wrapping remaining eight panels in numerical order, using same technique					
Applied protective barrier cream to hairline and ears					
Applied roll cotton around entire hairline					
Offered client a towel to blot any drips					
Slowly and carefully applied perm solution with a bottle to hair on each tool					
Asked client to lean forward while applying to back area					
Asked client to lean back while applying solution to front and sides.					
Avoided splashing and dripping					
Continued to apply solution until each tool was completely saturated					
If plastic cap was used, punched a few holes in it and covered hair completely					
Did not allow cap to touch skin					

Essential Rubrics continued

Performance Assessed	1	2	3	4	Improvement Plan
Checked cotton and towels					
If saturated with solution, replaced them					
Processed according to manufacturer's directions					
Checked frequently for curl development					
When processing was completed, rinsed hair thoroughly for at least five minutes					
Towel-blotted hair on each tool to remove any excess moisture					
Applied neutralizer slowly and carefully to hair on each tool					
Asked client to lean forward while applying neutralizer to back area					
Asked client to lean back while applying neutralizer to front and sides					
Avoided splashing and dripping					
Continued to apply neutralizer until each tool was completely saturated					
Set timer for according to manufacturer's directions					
After processing, removed tools and worked remaining neutralizer through hair gently					
Rinsed thoroughly					
Styled hair as desired					

CURVATURE PERM WRAP PROCEDURE

Performance Assessed	1	2	3	4	Improvement Plan
Began sectioning at the front hairline on one side of the part					
Combed hair in direction of growth					
Sectioned out individual panels to match length of rod					
Alternated from side to side when sectioning out all curvature panels over entire head					
Began wrapping first panel at front hairline, on one side of part					
Combed out a base section same width as diameter of rod					
Base direction pointed away from face					
Held hair at 90-degree angle to head					
Using two end papers, rolled hair down to scalp					
Positioned rod half-off base					
Remaining base sections in panel were wider on the outside of the panel (the side farthest away from face)					
Continued wrapping rest of rods in panel, alternating rod diameters					

Essential Rubrics continued

Performance Assessed	1	2	3	4	Improvement Plan
When last rod at hairline was reached, combed hair flat at base and directed rod up and toward base, keeping base area flat					
Continued with panel two and repeated the same procedure as on the first panel					
Continued with third panel and repeated same procedure until reaching last two rods at hairline					
Combed hair flat at base and directed last two rods up and toward base, keeping base area flat					
Continued with fourth panel, on the opposite side of head, behind and next to second panel					
Repeated same procedure used with third panel					
Followed same procedure with fifth panel					
The base direction remained consistent with the pattern already established					
The base direction in back flowed around and contoured to the perimeter hairline area					
All panels fit the curvature of the head and blended into surrounding panels					

Essential Rubrics continued

BRICKLAY PERM WRAP PROCEDURE

Performance Assessed	1	2	3	4	Improvement Plan
Began by parting out a base section parallel to front hairline that was the length and width of rod being used					
Base direction was back, away from face					
Held hair at 90-degree angle to head					
Using two end papers, rolled hair down to scalp					
Positioned rod half-off base					
In second row directly behind first rod, parted out two base sections for rods offset from center of first rod					
Held hair at 90-degree angle to head					
Using two ends papers, rolled hair down to scalp					
Positioned rods half-off base					
Began third row by parting out a base section at the point where two rods met in previous row					
Used same pattern throughout entire wrap					
Continued to part out rows that radiated around curve of head through crown area					
Extended rows around and down to side hairline, parting out base sections at center of point where two tools met in previous row					

Performance Assessed	1	2	3	4	Improvement Plan
Stopped the curving rows after wrapping entire crown area					
Parted out horizontal sections throughout the back of head and continued with bricklay pattern					
Length of rods was changed from row to row to maintain pattern as necessary					

SPIRAL PERM WRAP PROCEDURE

Performance Assessed	1	2	3	4	Improvement Plan
Began at nape and worked up toward top of head					
Sectioned out first row along hairline in nape area					
Combed remainder of hair up and secured it out of the way					
Parted out first base section on one side of first row					
Held hair at a 90-degree angle to head					
Using one or two end papers, began wrapping at one end of tool					
Rolled first two full turns at a 90-degree angle to the tool to secure ends of hair					
Then started spiraling the hair on the tool by changing the angle to other than 90-degrees					
Continued to spiral the hair toward the other end of the tool					

Essential Rubrics continued

Performance Assessed	1	2	3	4	Improvement Plan
Rolled hair down to scalp					
Positioned tool half-off base					
Secured it by fastening the ends of the tool together					
Continued wrapping with same technique, in same direction, until first row was completed					
Sectioned out second row above and parallel to first row					
Combed remainder of hair up and secured it to keep it out of the way					
Began wrapping at opposite side from side where first row began					
Moved in the opposite direction established in first row					
Followed same procedure to wrap second row but began wrapping each tool at the opposite end established in first row					
Continued wrapping with same technique, in same direction, until second row was completed					
Sectioned out third row above and parallel to second row					
Followed same wrapping procedure, alternating rows from left to right while moving up the head					

VIRGIN THIO RELAXER PROCEDURE

Performance Assessed	1	2	3	4	Improvement Plan
Parted hair into four sections, from the center of the front hairline to the center of the nape, and from ear to ear					
Clipped the sections up to keep them out of the way					
Applied protective base cream to the hairline and ears					
Wore gloves on both hand					
Began application in the most resistant area, usually at the back of the head					
Made ¼-inch to ½-inch (0.6 to 1.25 cm) horizontal partings and applied relaxer to the top of the strand first, then to the underside					
Applied relaxer ¼-inch to ½-inch (0.6 to 1.25 cm) away from the scalp and up to the porous ends					
Did not allow relaxer to touch scalp until the last few minutes of processing					
Continued applying the relaxer, working down the section toward the hairline					
Continued the same application procedure with the remaining sections; finished the most resistant sections first					
After the relaxer was applied to all sections, used the back of the comb or hands to smooth each section					

Performance Assessed	1	2	3	4	Improvement Plan
Processed according to the manufacturer's directions					
Performed periodic strand tests					
During the last few minutes of processing, worked the relaxer down to the scalp and through the ends of the hair, using additional relaxer as needed					
Carefully combed and smoothed all sections					
Rinsed thoroughly with warm water to remove all traces of the relaxer					
Shampooed with acid-balanced shampoo					
Blotted excess water from hair					
Applied neutralizer in ¼-inch to ½-inch (0.6 to 1.25 cm) sections					
Smoothed with hands or back of comb					
Processed neutralizer according to direction					
Rinsed thoroughly					
Shampooed and conditioned hair					

THIO RELAXER RETOUCH PROCEDURE

Performance Assessed	1	2	3	4	Improvement Plan
Divided hair into four sections, from the center of the front hairline to the center of the nape, and from ear to ear					

Essential Rubrics continued

Performance Assessed	1	2	3	4	Improvement Plan
Clipped sections up to keep them out of the way					
Wore gloves on both hands					
Applied a protective base cream to the hairline and ears					
Began application of the relaxer in the most resistant area, usually at the back of the head					
Made ¼-inch to ½-inch (0.6 to 1.25 cm) horizontal partings and applied the relaxer to the top of the strand					
Applied the relaxer ¼-inch to ½-inch (0.6 to 1.25 cm) away from the scalp and only to new growth					
Did not allow relaxer to touch the scalp until the last few minutes of processing					
Did not overlap the relaxer onto the previously relaxed hair					
Continued applying the relaxer, using the same procedure and working down section toward hairline					
Continued same application procedure with remaining sections, finishing the most resistant sections first					
After the relaxer had been applied to all sections, used the back of the comb or hands to smooth each section					
Processed according to the manufacturer's directions					

Performance Assessed	1	2	3	4	Improvement Plan
Performed periodic strand tests					
During the last few minutes of processing, worked the relaxer down to the scalp					
If the ends of the hair needed additional relaxing, worked the relaxer through to the ends for the last few minutes of processing					
Rinsed thoroughly with warm water					
Shampooed three times with acid-balanced shampoo					
Blotted excess water from hair					
Applied neutralizer in ¼-inch to ½-inch (0.6 to 1.25 cm) sections throughout the hair					
Smoothed with hands or back of comb					
Processed neutralizer according to directions					
Rinsed thoroughly					
Shampooed and conditioned					

SOFT CURL PERMANENT PROCEDURE

Performance Assessed	1	2	3	4	Improvement Plan
NOTE: This assessment begins after the first twelve steps of Procedure 20–10, Applying Hydroxide Relaxer to Virgin Hair.					
Sectioned hair into nine panels using length of rod to measure width of panels					

Performance Assessed	1	2	3	4	Improvement Plan
Rolled hair on the appropriate-sized perm rods					
Wore gloves on both hands					
Began wrapping at the most resistant area					
Applied and distributed thio curl booster to each panel as wrapped					
Make a horizontal parting the same size as the rod					
Held hair at a 90-degree angle to the head					
Using two end papers, rolled hair down to scalp					
Positioned rod half-off base					
Inserted roller picks to stabilize rods and eliminate any tension caused by band					
Continued wrapping first panel using the same technique					
Maintained even dampness as you work					
Continued wrapping the remaining eight panels in numerical order using the same technique					
Placed cotton around the hairline and neck					
Applied thio curl booster to all the curls until they were completely saturated					
Punched a few holes in plastic cap and covered hair completely					

Essential Rubrics continued

Performance Assessed	1	2	3	4	Improvement Plan
Did not allow cap to touch client's skin					
Checked cotton and towels and replaced if saturated					
Processed according to manufacturer's directions					
Checked for proper curl development					
After processing, rinsed the hair thoroughly for at least five minutes					
Towel-blotted hair on each rod to remove excess moisture					
Option: Applied pre-neutralizing conditioner according to the manufacturer's directions					
Applied neutralizer slowly and carefully to the hair on each rod					
Avoided splashing and dripping					
Made sure each rod was completely saturated					
Distributed remaining neutralizer					
Set a timer and neutralized according to the manufacturer's directions					
Removed rods, distributed the remaining neutralizer through the ends of the hair, and rinsed thoroughly					
Option: Shampooed and conditioned					

Essential Review

Complete the following review of Chapter 20, Chemical Texture Services, by circling the correct answer.

1. ____________ rods have a small diameter in the center area and gradually increase to their largest diameter at the ends, resulting in a tighter curl at hair ends, with a loose, wider curl at the scalp.

a) Convex
b) Straight
c) Concave
d) Colored

2. A method of wrapping a permanent wave that is suitable for very long hair is the ____________.

a) double halo method
b) double-rod wrap
c) single halo method
d) straight back method

3. A ____________ is an example of a physical change that results from breaking and re-forming the hydrogen bonds within the hair.

a) blowdry service
b) wet set
c) hair color service
d) comb-out

4. All perm wraps begin by sectioning the hair into panels which are further divided into subsections called ____________.

a) panels
b) base sections
c) base panels
d) base control

5. Always rinse perm solution from the hair for at least ____________ minutes before applying the neutralizer.

a) 2
b) 3
c) 4
d) 5

6. A/an ____________ liquid protein conditioner can be applied to the hair and dried under a warm dryer for five minutes or more prior to neutralization if hair is damaged.

a) alkaline
b) emulsified
c) neutral
d) acidic

7. When hair has been sufficiently straightened, the hair is rinsed rapidly and thoroughly with ____________ water.

a) hot
b) cold
c) cool
d) warm

8. Base control refers to the position of the tool in relation to its ____________ and is determined by the angle at which the hair is wrapped.

   a) panel
   b) base section
   c) base panel
   d) scalp position

9. End wraps are absorbent papers used to ____________ of the hair when wrapping and winding hair on the perm tools.

   a) decrease moisture
   b) control ends
   c) control elasticity
   d) decrease elasticity

10. Hair texture describes the ____________ of a single strand of hair and is classified as fine, medium, or coarse.

    a) length
    b) color
    c) curl
    d) diameter

11. If the hair is not ____________, the hydrogen peroxide in the neutralizer can react with waving lotion and cause the hair color to lighten.

    a) thoroughly shampooed
    b) rinsed properly
    c) lightly shampooed
    d) lightly rinsed

12. If too many ____________ bonds are broken in the perming process, the hair will be too weak to hold a firm curl.

    a) disulfide
    b) hydrogen
    c) salt
    d) polypeptide

13. When processing is complete for a soft curl permanent, what is done after rinsing the hair thoroughly with warm water?

    a) each curl is blotted with towel
    b) conditioner is applied
    c) client is place under dryer
    d) test curl is taken

14. If hair breaks under very slight strain, it has ____________.

    a) excellent elasticity
    b) very good elasticity
    c) average elasticity
    d) little or no elasticity

Essential Review continued

15. In order to make a smooth transition from the rolled section of the head to an unrolled section, use a larger tool for the last tool next to an unrolled section when giving a ____________.

    a) curvature perm b) partial perm
    c) spiral perm d) full perm

16. In neutralization, the bonds in the hair are re-formed ____________.

    a) immediately b) slowly
    c) sporadically d) randomly

17. In permanent waving, most of the processing takes place as soon as the solution penetrates the hair, within the first ____________ minutes.

    a) 1 to 2 b) 2 to 3
    c) 3 to 4 d) 5 to 10

18. Many male clients are looking for added ____________, fullness, style, and low maintenance that only a perm can provide.

    a) color b) shine
    c) texture d) length

19. Metallic salts leave a coating on the hair that may cause ____________, severe discoloration, or hair breakage.

    a) mild odor b) uneven curls
    c) calcification d) smooth curls

20. Neutralization rebuilds the ____________ by removing the extra hydrogen bonds created by the waving solution.

    a) salt bonds b) hydrogen bonds
    c) disulfide bonds d) polypetide chains

21. Perming only a section of a whole head of hair is called ____________.

    a) section perming b) spotmatic perming
    c) partial perming d) limited perming

22. Some manufacturers recommend the application of a ____________ after blotting and before application of the neutralizer.

    a) pre-neutralizing conditioner b) pre-neutralizing shampoo
    c) post-processing moisturizer d) post-processing shampoo

23. The ____________ wrap uses zigzag partings to divide base areas.

a) curvature perm b) weave technique
c) bricklay perm d) straight perm

24. The ____________ wrap creates a movement that curves within sectioned-out panels.

a) curvature perm b) bricklay perm
c) weave technique d) straight perm

25. The basic perm wrap is also called a ____________ wrap.

a) curvature perm b) bricklay perm
c) weave technique d) straight set

26. The chemical action of ____________ breaks the disulfide bonds and softens the hair.

a) ammonia b) hydrogen peroxide
c) waving lotion d) neutralizer

27. The chemical composition of hair consists almost entirely of a protein material called ____________.

a) polypeptides b) keratin
c) cysteine d) melanin

28. Bonds that are formed between two cysteine amino acids located on neighboring polypeptide chains are ____________.

a) salt b) chemical
c) hydrogen d) disulfide

29. The polypeptide chains of this layer of hair are connected by end bonds and cross-linked by side bonds that form the fibers and structure of hair ____________.

a) medulla b) cuticle
c) cortex d) follicle

30. The perm that is activated by heat created chemically within the product is known as ____________.

a) endothermic b) alkaline
c) exothermic d) sodium hydroxide

Essential Review continued

31. The action of waving lotion is to ____________.

a) discolor the hair
b) shrink the hair
c) expand the hair
d) condition the hair

32. The degree to which hair absorbs the waving lotion is related to its ____________.

a) texture
b) length
c) elasticity
d) porosity

33. The length of time required for the hair strands to absorb the waving lotion and for the hair to re-curl is called ____________.

a) application time
b) processing time
c) rinsing time
d) development time

34. The main active ingredient in acid-balanced waving lotions is ____________.

a) glycerol monothioglycolate
b) ammonium thioglycolate
c) hydrogen peroxide
d) sodium hydroxide

35. The main active ingredient or reducing agent in alkaline perms is ____________.

a) glycerol monothioglycolate
b) ammonium thioglycolate
c) hydrogen peroxide
d) sodium hydroxide

36. The ____________ wrap is used to prevent noticeable splits and to blend the flow of the hair.

a) curvature perm
b) bricklay perm
c) spiral perm
d) basic perm

37. The ____________ wrap is done at an angle that causes the hair to spiral along the length of the tool, like the grip on a tennis racquet.

a) spiral
b) croquignole
c) bricklay
d) barber pole

38. The hydrogen atoms in the disulfide bonds are so strongly attracted to the oxygen in the neutralizer that they release their bond with the sulfur atoms and join with the ____________.

a) salt bond
b) nitrogen
c) hydrogen
d) oxygen

39. Underprocessing is caused by ___________ processing time of the waving lotion.

a) excessive
b) increasing
c) insufficient
d) exact

40. Waves that process more quickly and produce firmer curls than true acid waves are considered to be ___________.

a) alkaline
b) acid-balanced
c) ammonium thioglycolate
d) sodium hydroxide

41. What can be used to determine the actual processing time needed to achieve optimum curl results when giving a perm for the first time on a client?

a) patch test
b) strand test
c) porosity test
d) preliminary test curl

42. What type of hair is more fragile, easier to process, and more susceptible to damage from perm services?

a) coarse texture
b) medium texture
c) non-elastic
d) fine texture

43. What type of hair requires more processing than medium or fine hair and may also be more resistant to processing?

a) coarse texture
b) medium texture
c) non-elastic
d) fine texture

44. When the strand of hair is wrapped at an angle 45 degrees beyond perpendicular to its base section, it will result in ___________.

a) half-off base placement
b) off-base placement
c) on-base placement
d) on-stem placement

45. When one end paper is folded in half over the hair ends like an envelope, it is called the ___________.

a) double end paper wrap
b) bookend wrap
c) single end paper wrap
d) top-hand wrap

46. When the strand of hair is wrapped at an angle 90 degrees (perpendicular) to its base section, it will result in ___________.

a) half-off base placement
b) off-base placement
c) on-base placement
d) on-stem placement

47. When performing a procedure for a preliminary test curl, wrap one tool in each different area of the head including the top, the side, and the ____________.

a) bang
b) temple
c) nape
d) occipital

48. When hair has assumed the desired shape, the broken disulfide bonds must be ____________ rebonded.

a) chemically
b) physically
c) temporarily
d) semi-permanently

49. When you place one end wrap on top of the hair strand and hold it flat, it is called the ____________.

a) double flat wrap
b) bookend wrap
c) single flat wrap
d) top-hand wrap

50. A hair relaxing treatment should be avoided when an examination shows the presence of ____________.

a) scalp abrasions
b) strong curl
c) excessive oils
d) pityriasis steadoides

51. After saturating the rods with neutralizer in a soft curl permanent, the next step is to ____________.

a) rinse with hot water
b) remove rods carefully
c) completely dry hair
d) apply protective base

52. After the hair has been processed with a sodium hydroxide relaxer and before the shampoo, the hair should be thoroughly ____________.

a) oiled
b) rinsed
c) dried
d) conditioned

53. Before giving a relaxing treatment to overly curly hair, the cosmetologist must judge its texture, porosity, and ____________.

a) length and elasticity
b) elasticity and silkiness
c) elasticity and extent of damage, if any
d) softness and extent of damage, if any

Essential Review continued

54. If using a *no-base* relaxer, it is recommended that a protective cream be applied ____________.

a) at the nape of the neck
b) over the earlobes
c) the frontal hairline
d) on the hairline and around ears

55. Inspecting the action of the relaxer by stretching the strands to see how fast the natural curls are being removed is called ____________.

a) periodic patch testing
b) periodic relaxer testing
c) periodic strand testing
d) periodic elasticity testing

56. Of the general types of hair relaxers which one does not require pre-shampooing?

a) sodium hydroxide
b) sodium thioglycolate
c) ammonium thioglycolate
d) acid-based relaxers

57. One safety precaution for hair relaxing is to avoid ____________ the scalp with the comb or fingernails.

a) massaging
b) scratching
c) smoothing
d) stimulating

58. Relaxers which are ionic compounds formed by a metal which is combined with oxygen and hydrogen are known as ____________.

a) guanidine hydroxide relaxers
b) metal hydroxide relaxers
c) low-pH relaxers
d) no-base relaxers

59. Sodium hydroxide relaxers are commonly called ____________.

a) guanidine hydroxide relaxers
b) low pH relaxers
c) lithium hydroxide relaxers
d) lye relaxers

60. The action of a sodium hydroxide relaxer causes the hair to ____________.

a) swell
b) shrink
c) harden
d) set

61. The process of breaking the hair's disulfide bonds during processing and converting them to lanthionine bonds when the relaxer is rinsed from the hair is known as ____________.

a) lanolination
b) lanthionization
c) neutralization
d) normalization

62. The scalp and skin are protected from possible burns when using a hair relaxer by applying ___________.

a) cotton
b) stabilizer
c) base
d) shampoo

63. The processing time of a chemical relaxer is affected by ___________.

a) styling products used
b) the client's age
c) the hair's porosity
d) brand of relaxer

64. The relaxer cream is applied near the scalp last because processing is accelerated in this area by ___________.

a) body heat
b) application speed
c) body perspiration
d) sebaceous glands

65. The chemical required to stop the action of the chemical relaxer is a ___________.

a) petroleum cream
b) neutralizer
c) conditioner
d) waving lotion

66. The best type of shampoo to use after the chemical relaxer is ___________.

a) an organic shampoo
b) an antibacterial shampoo
c) a neutralizing shampoo
d) a dry shampoo

67. The strength of relaxer is determined by the strand test. General guidelines suggest that for coarse virgin hair, the following strength is used: ___________.

a) extra mild
b) regular
c) mild
d) strong or super

68. The strength of relaxer is determined by the strand test. General guidelines suggest that for fine, tinted, or lightened hair, the following strength is used: ___________.

a) extra mild
b) regular
c) mild
d) strong or super

69. The process of permanently rearranging the basic structure of overly curly hair into a straight form is called ____________.

a) thermal straightening
b) chemical hair relaxing
c) permanent waving
d) chemical hair softening

70. The combination of a thio relaxer and a thio permanent wrapped on large tools is called a ____________.

a) soft curl permanent
b) thioglycolate reconstructer
c) relaxer curl permanent
d) hard curl permanent

71. The most commonly used methods of hair relaxing are the sodium hydroxide method and the ____________ method.

a) thermal
b) thio
c) ammonia
d) peroxide

72. To check relaxer processing, smooth and press a strand to the scalp using the back of the comb or your finger. If curl returns, ____________.

a) rinse immediately
b) add neutralizer
c) continue processing
d) add conditioner

73. What is used to restore the hair and scalp to their normal acidic pH?

a) cream conditioner
b) medicated shampoo
c) conditioning filler
d) normalizing lotion

74. What stops the action of any chemical relaxer that may remain in the hair after rinsing?

a) softener
b) breakdown cream
c) swelling compound
d) neutralizer

75. What are the two types of formulas for sodium hydroxide chemical hair relaxers?

a) base and no-base
b) lye and no lye
c) stabilizer and no stabilizer
d) cream and no cream

76. What is one safety precaution that must be followed with all chemical hair relaxing services?

a) shampooing the client's hair
b) preconditioning the hair
c) advising the client regarding processing time
d) wearing protective gloves

77. What are the three basic steps used in chemical hair relaxing?

a) wrapping, application, rinsing
b) processing, neutralizing, conditioning
c) shampooing, application, conditioning
d) processing, neutralizing, stabilizing

78. When applying sodium hydroxide relaxer, the processing cream is applied last to the ____________ and ____________.

a) scalp area, middle of hair shaft
b) scalp area, hair ends
c) middle of hair shaft, hair ends
d) nape area, hair ends

79. When performing a sodium hydroxide retouch, where is the product applied first?

a) to the hair ends
b) to the new growth only
c) to middle of the hair shaft
d) to the scalp area only

80. When using the comb method of application, how is the relaxing cream applied?

a) with the back of the comb
b) with the fingers
c) with the applicator brush
d) with the teeth of the comb

Essential Discoveries and Accomplishments

In the space below, jot some notes about what concepts of this chapter were hardest for you to understand or remember. Imagine finding yourself suddenly in the role of "teacher" and consider what you would tell your "students" about these concepts. Share your Essential Discoveries with some of the other students in your class and ask if they are helpful to them. You may want to revise your discoveries based on good ideas shared by your peers.

Discoveries:

____

____

____

____

____

____

____

____

____

____

____

List at least three things you have accomplished since your last entry that relate to your career goals.

Accomplishments:

____

____

____

____

____

CHAPTER 21

Haircoloring

A Motivating Moment: "If you learn to appreciate more of what you already have, you will find yourself having more to appreciate."

—Michael Angier

Essential Objectives

After studying this chapter and completing the Essential Companion components, you will be able to:

1. List the reasons why people color their hair.
2. Explain how the hair's porosity affects haircolor.
3. Understand the types of melanin found in hair.
4. Define and identify levels and their role in formulating haircolor.
5. Identify primary, secondary, and tertiary colors.
6. Know what role tone and intensity play in haircolor.
7. List and describe the categories of haircolor.
8. Explain the role of hydrogen peroxide in a haircolor formula.
9. Explain the action of hair lighteners.
10. List the four key questions to ask when formulating a haircolor.
11. Understand why a patch test is useful in haircoloring.
12. Define what a preliminary strand test is and why it is used.
13. List and describe the procedure for a virgin single-process color service.

Essential Objectives continued

14. Understand the two processes involved in double-process haircoloring.
15. Describe the various forms of hair lightener.
16. Understand the purpose and use of toners.
17. Name and describe the three most commonly used methods for highlighting.
18. Know how to properly cover gray hair.
19. Know the rules of color correction.
20. Know the safety precautions to follow during the haircolor process.

Essential Haircoloring

Will I ever get over my fear of haircolor and be able to formulate and apply it successfully in the salon?

Without a doubt! Haircoloring is an art and you have just begun your training as an artist. This chapter is designed to help you begin to build your confidence with haircoloring in a practical and understandable way. Haircolor is considered to be the "cosmetic for the hair" in today's market. Your clientele are no longer afraid of haircolor and your haircolor clientele will range from teenage boys to grandmothers. By taking the time and effort required to learn haircolor, you will find that it is also a science as well as an art. You will learn that it is fun and easy and all your efforts will be rewarded financially in the salon.

Cosmetologists should study and have a thorough understanding of chemical texture services because:

- Chemical texture services are problem solvers for stylists and clients in that they change the texture of the hair and can allow a person to wear just about any conceivable hair texture.
- Knowing how to perform these services accurately and professionally will help build a trusting and loyal clientele.
- They are among the most lucrative services in the salon and many retail products are specific to the hair's condition and the chemical service to which it has been exposed.
- Without a thorough understanding of chemistry, cosmetologists could damage the hair.

Essential Concepts

What are the key concepts or elements in haircoloring that I need to know to be successful?

You will begin by learning about basic color theory, a refresher from what you learned in elementary school when you studied the colors of the rainbow. You will learn how to lighten dark hair to a light blond as well as how to darken lighter hair. You will learn about the reasons people color their hair and the psychological effects hair color can have on an individual. You will learn about the Level System used by professionals and haircolor manufacturers to analyze the lightness or darkness of a color. As with any professional service, you will gain practice in performing a thorough client consultation prior to providing a haircolor service. Your haircolor training will take you from temporary haircolor through semipermanent, permanent, hair lightening, and special effects haircoloring procedures.

1 Essential Experience

The Color Wheel

In the diagram below, place the colors that correspond with the color found on the wheel. You may use crayons, markers, colored pencils, water-color paint, or cut the various colors out of magazines. Your goal is to depict the primary, secondary, and tertiary colors, and label each accordingly.

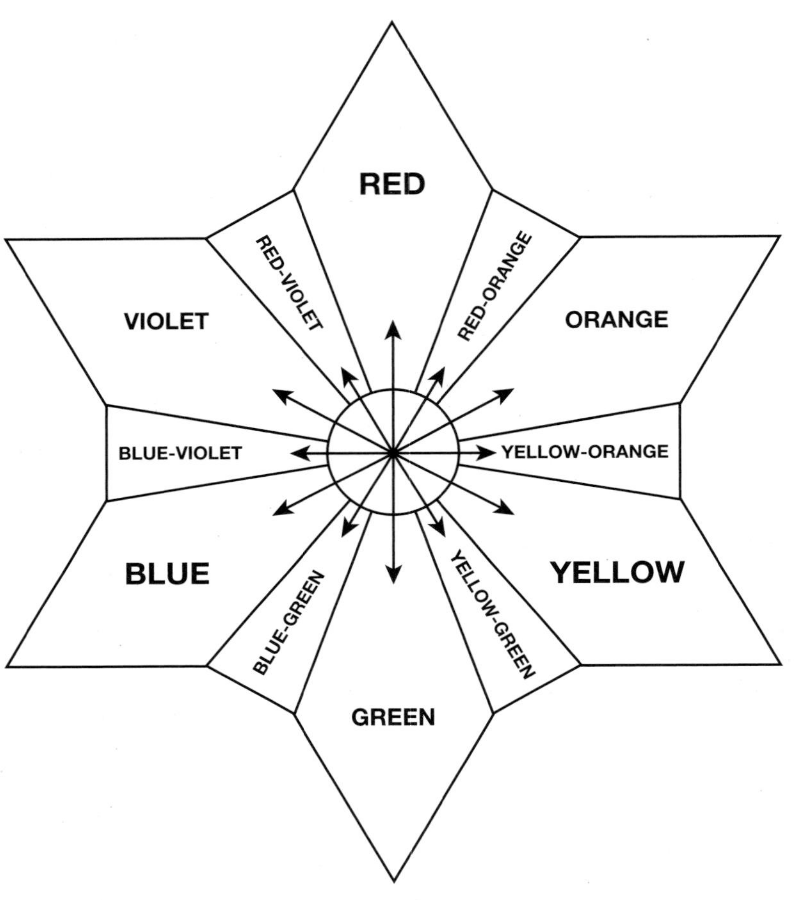

Essential Experience

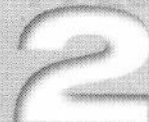

Haircolor Challenges/Corrective Solutions

In the grid below, explain the solutions to the haircoloring challenges listed.

Challenge	Solution
Yellowed Discoloration	
Resistant Gray Hair	
Damaged Hair (due to blowdrying, wind, harsh products, chemical services)	
Damaged, Overly Porous Hair	
Red Hair	
Brunette Hair	

3 Essential Experience

The Level System

Research old magazines with the goal of finding pictures of anything (hair, clothing, etc.) that show the 10 levels of hair or decolorization as stated in the chart below. Cut the colors out and paste them in the appropriate box. Option: Gather actual strands of hair in the various levels. Note: The names for the natural color levels may vary from manufacturer to manufacturer.

Level 1: Black	**Level 2: Very Dark Brown**
Level 3: Dark Brown	**Level 4: Medium Brown**
Level 5: Light Brown	**Level 6: Dark Blond**
Level 7: Medium Blond	**Level 8: Light Blond**
Level 9: Very Light Blond	**Level 10: Lightest Blond**

Essential Experience 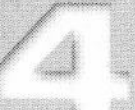

The Four Classifications of Color

Haircolor is divided into four classifications: temporary, traditional semipermanent, demipermanent, and permanent. The classifications indicate color fastness or ability to remain on the hair. They are determined by chemical composition and molecular weight of the pigments and dyes within the products found in each classification. In the chart below, indicate the various characteristics of the three classifications of color. For molecular structure list the size and draw it in as well. Use external research as needed.

Classification	Temporary	Traditional Semipermanent/ Demipermanent	Permanent
Molecular Weight of the Dye Molecule			
Type of pH (acid or alkaline)			
Reaction or Change (physical and/or chemical)			
Color Fastness			
Color Effects (lifts/deposits)			

5 Essential Experience

Windowpane Color Applications

Windowpaning is the process of transferring key elements, points, or steps in a lesson into visual images that are hand sketched into the squares or *panes* of a matrix. Let your mind think in pictures and sketch the essential concepts printed in each of the following windowpanes. Conduct additional research as applicable.

Virgin Tint Going Darker
Darker Retouch
Tint Back to Natural
Virgin Tint Going Lighter
Lighter Tint Retouch
Virgin Lightener
Lightener Retouch
Virgin Toner
Toner Retouch

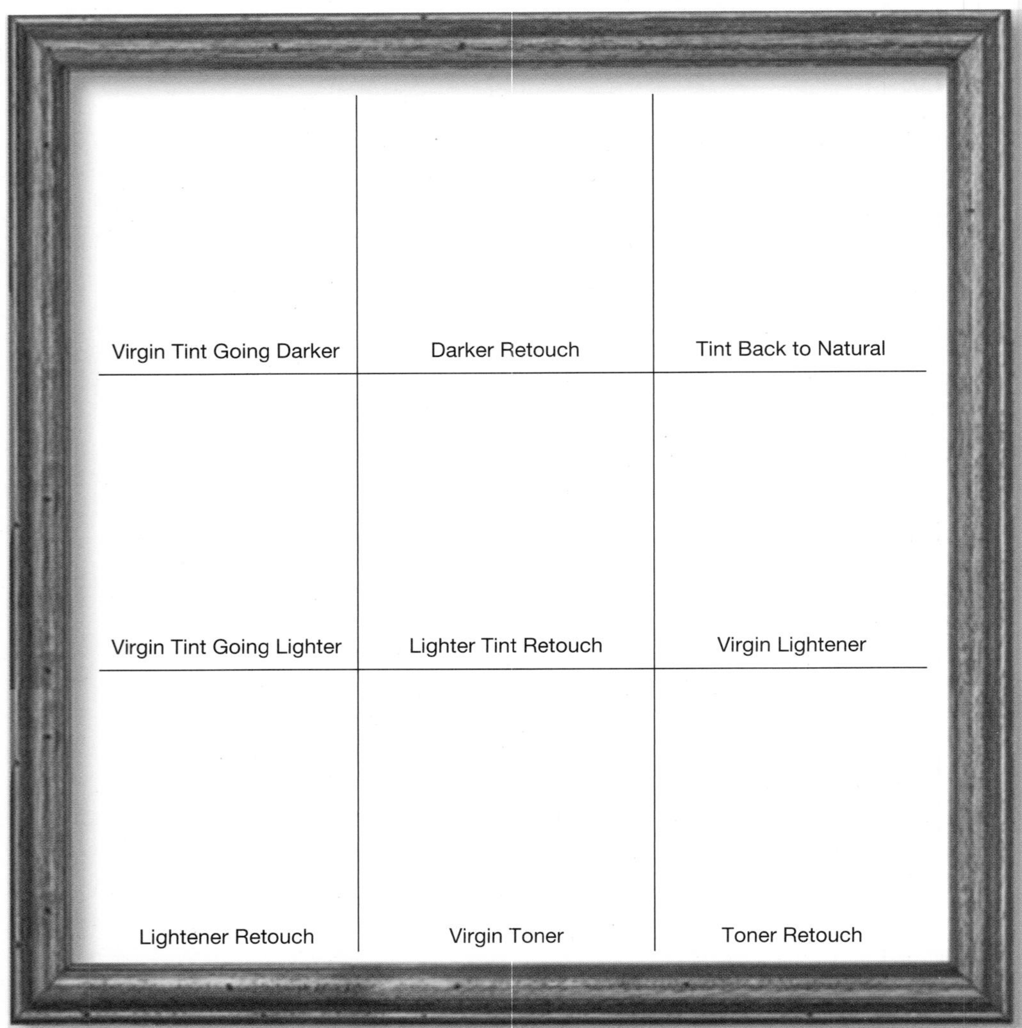

Essential Experience

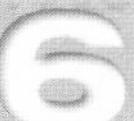

Crossword Puzzle

After identifying the appropriate word from the clues listed below, locate the word in the following crossword puzzle.

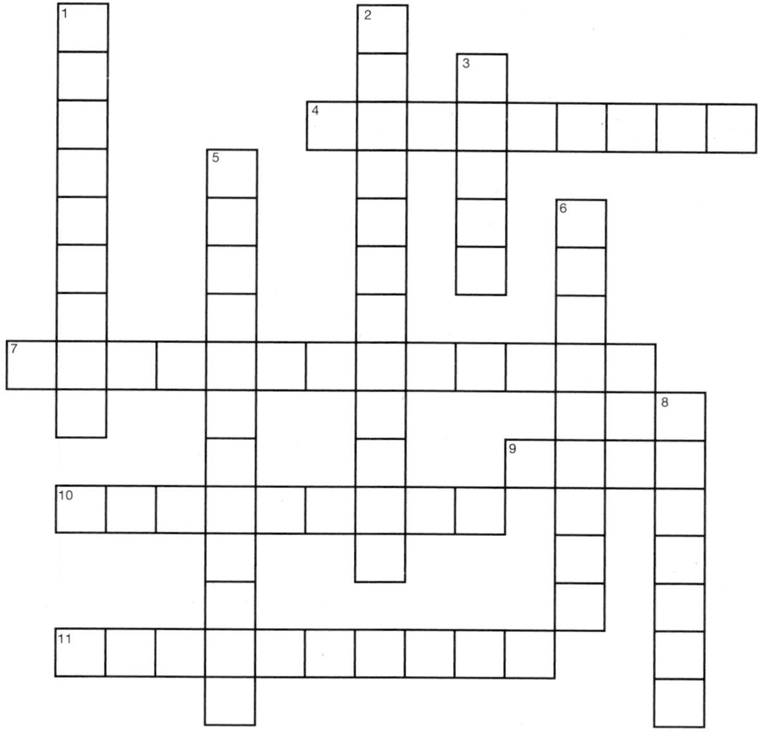

Clues:

Across

4. Oxidizing agent that mixes with an oxidation color and supplies oxygen gas

7. Colors opposite each other on the color wheel

9. Technique involving slicing or weaving out sections

10. Chemical compound for decolorizing hair

11. Color left in hair after it goes through ten stages of lightening

Down

1. Oxidizer added to hydrogen peroxide to increase chemical action

2. Used to treat gray or resistant hair

3. Unit of measurement of lightness or darkness of a color

5. Coloring some strands lighter than natural color

6. Industry term referring to artificial haircolor products

8. ⅛-inch (0.3 cm) section of hair positioned over foil

7 Essential Experience

Word Search

After identifying the correct word from the clues provided, locate the words in the word search puzzle.

Word	Clue
______________	Painting of lightener
______________	Involves pulling hair through a perforated cap
______________	Used to ensure an even shade
______________	Coloring some strands lighter than natural color
______________	Strength of color tone
______________	Haircolor containing metal salts
______________	First step in double-process haircoloring
______________	Process of treating gray or resistant hair to allow better penetration
______________	Pure or fundamental color than cannot be achieved by mixing
______________	Color obtained from mixing equal parts of two primary colors
______________	Involves taking an ⅛-inch (0.3 cm) section of hair and placing it on foil
______________	Intermediate color achieved by mixing a secondary color with its neighboring primary color
______________	Permanent oxidizing color having the ability to lift and deposit in the same process
______________	Used primarily on prelightened hair to achieve pale or delicate colors

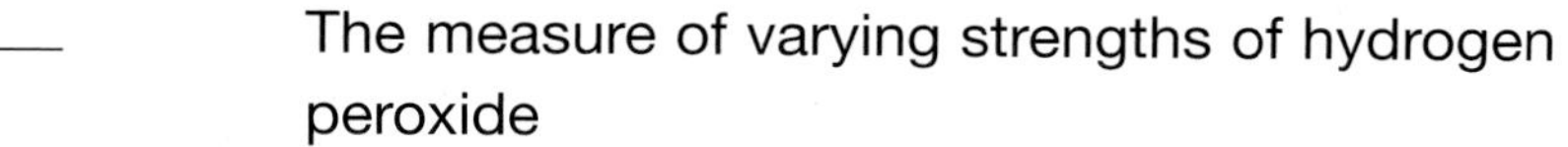

______________ The measure of varying strengths of hydrogen peroxide

______________ Picking up strands with a zigzag motion of the comb

```
C R S F T V W S Y V F J K V H
A C E L G L C N A Y F X I I Y
P R E L I G H T E N I N G N N
T R M C L C Z L Q G F H T J N
E O E P E I I Q O P L Q K J M
C B T S T B F N R I Y H V A B
H M A L O W L I G H T I N G A
N W L G N F M H F Q I R F Y L
I T L P E A T H B R S O U V A
Q N I P R I S E C O N D A R Y
U K C Y N E M G N V E A S R A
E T O G G U Y R A I T R E T G
C H X E L W E A V I N G D Z E
G I V O I A P A U P I G O C E
L L V P N I G N O H T N C D T
```

8 Essential Experience

Matching Exercise

Match each of the following essential terms with its identifying phrase or definition.

_______ **Analysis**	**1.** The predominant color and tone
_______ **Blonding**	**2.** An examination of the hair
_______ **Coating**	**3.** A term applied to lightening the hair
_______ **Degree**	**4.** Pigment that is fundamental and cannot be made
_______ **Base color**	**5.** The cuticle is lifted and the hair is overly porous
_______ **Glaze**	**6.** Residue left on the outside of the hair shaft
_______ **Intensity**	**7.** Strength of color tone
_______ **High porosity**	**8.** Visible line separating colored hair from new growth
_______ **Line of demarcation**	**9.** A no-lift deposit-only color that adds shine and tone
_______ **Primary color**	**10.** Various units of measurement

Essential Experience

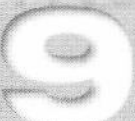

The Client Consultation

In the space provided below, list all the steps required in completing a thorough haircolor consultation. Then choose another student as your partner. Conduct a haircolor client consultation on each other. Record your results on the school's client record card and standard consultation form.

1. ______________________________

____

2. ______________________________

____

3. ______________________________

____

____

4. ______________________________

____

5. ______________________________

____

6. ______________________________

____

7. ______________________________

____

8. ______________________________

____

9 Essential Experience continued

9. ______________________________

____

____

10. ______________________________

____

Essential Rubrics

Rubrics are used in education for organizing and interpreting data gathered from observations of student performance. It is a clearly developed scoring document used to differentiate between levels of development in a specific skill performance or behavior. A rubric is provided in this study guide as a self-assessment tool to aid you in your behavior development.

Rate your performance according to the following scale.

(1) Development Opportunity: There is little or no evidence of competency; assistance is needed; performance includes multiple errors.

(2) Fundamental: There is beginning evidence of competency; task is completed alone; performance includes few errors.

(3) Competent: There is detailed and consistent evidence of competency; task is completed alone; performance includes rare errors.

(4) Strength: There is detailed evidence of highly creative, inventive, mature presence of competency.

Space is provided for comments to assist you in improving your performance and achieving a higher rating.

PATCH TEST PROCEDURE

Performance Assessed	1	2	3	4	Improvement Plan
Selected test area behind ear or on inside of elbow					
Cleaned and dried test area the size of a quarter					
Mixed product					
Applied product to test area					
Left mixture undisturbed for twenty-four to forty-eight hours					
Examined test area					
Recorded results on record card					

Essential Rubrics continued

PRELIMINARY STRAND TEST PROCEDURE

Performance Assessed	1	2	3	4	Improvement Plan
Performed scalp and hair analysis					
Properly draped client					
Parted off a ½-inch (1.25 cm) square section of hair in the lower crown					
Used plastic clips to fasten other hair out of the way					
Placed hair strand over the foil or plastic wrap					
Applied color mixture					
Applied color following proper application method					
Checked development at five minute intervals					
Shampooed hair					
Rinsed hair					
Removed foil or plastic wrap					
Placed towel under strand and misted thoroughly with water					
Added shampoo and massaged through hair					
Rinsed by spraying with water					
Dried strand with towel and observed results					
Made needed adjustments and proceeded with color service					

TEMPORARY HAIRCOLOR APPLICATION PROCEDURE

Performance Assessed	1	2	3	4	Improvement Plan
Draped client for haircoloring service					
Shampooed hair					
Towel-dried hair					
Seated client comfortably at shampoo bowl					
Put on gloves					
Used applicator bottle properly					
Shook product to blend pigments					
Applied color and worked it around entire head					
Blended color with comb, applying more color as necessary					
Did not rinse the hair					
Towel-blotted excess product					

SEMIPERMANENT HAIRCOLOR APPLICATION PROCEDURE

Performance Assessed	1	2	3	4	Improvement Plan
Shampooed client's hair with mild shampoo					
Towel-dried hair					
Put on gloves					
Applied protective cream around hairline and over the ears					
Outlined the hair into four sections, from ear to ear and from front center to center nape					

Performance Assessed	1	2	3	4	Improvement Plan
Used ½-inch (1.25 cm) partings					
Applied color to new growth or scalp area in all four sections					
Worked product through to ends					
Set timer to process					
Massaged color into a lather and rinsed thoroughly					
Removed any stains around hairline with shampoo or stain remover using a towel					
Rinsed thoroughly					
Shampooed and conditioned hair					

SINGLE-PROCESS COLOR ON VIRGIN HAIR APPLICATION PROCEDURE

Performance Assessed	1	2	3	4	Improvement Plan
Draped client for haircolor service					
Put on gloves					
Parted dry hair into four sections					
Applied protective cream to hairline and ears					
Prepared color formula for either bottle or brush application					
Began in most resistant area or where color change was expected to be the greatest					
Parted off ¼-inch (0.6 cm) subsection with the applicator					

Performance Assessed	1	2	3	4	Improvement Plan
Lifted subsection and applied color to the mid-shaft area					
Stayed at least ½ inch (1.25 cm) from the scalp					
Did not go through the porous ends					
Checked color development by following the same steps used in strand testing					
Applied color to the hair at the scalp					
Pulled color through hair ends					
Massaged color into a lather and rinsed thoroughly with warm water					
Removed any stains around hairline with shampoo or stain remover using towel					
Shampooed hair					
Conditioned as needed					

PERMANENT SINGLE-PROCESS RETOUCH WITH GLAZE PROCEDURE

Performance Assessed	1	2	3	4	Improvement Plan
Draped client for haircolor service					
Put on gloves					
Parted dry hair into four sections					
Applied to new growth area using ¼-inch (0.6 cm) partings					

Performance Assessed	1	2	3	4	Improvement Plan
Completed all four sides and set timer for forty-five minutes or according to manufacturer's directions					
Prepared a no-lift deposit-only glaze formula					
Applied no-lift deposit-only glaze to mid-strand and worked through hair					
Checked results before rinsing thoroughly					

LIGHTENING VIRGIN HAIR PROCEDURE

Performance Assessed	1	2	3	4	Improvement Plan
Draped client for haircolor service					
Put on gloves					
Parted hair into four sections					
Applied protective cream around hairline and over ears					
Prepared lightening formula and used immediately					
Placed cotton around and through all four sections to prevent lightener from touching the scalp					
Applied lightener ½ inch (1.25 cm) from scalp, working lightener through the mid-strand, up to the porous ends					
Placed strips of cotton at scalp, between sections throughout head					
Double checked application, adding more lightener as necessary					

Essential Rubrics continued

Performance Assessed	1	2	3	4	Improvement Plan
Did not comb lightener through hair					
Kept lightener moist					
Checked lightening action about fifteen minutes before time indicated by strand test					
Sprayed a hair strand with water and removed lightener with a damp towel					
Examined strand					
Reapplied mixture and continue testing frequently until desired level was reached					
Applied lightener to scalp and ends					
Removed cotton from scalp area					
Applied lightener to hair near scalp with a ⅛-inch (0.3 cm) parting					
Applied lightener to porous ends					
Processed until desired stage is reached					
Rinsed hair thoroughly with warm water					
Shampooed gently and conditioned as needed, keeping hands under hair to avoid tangling					
Applied acid-balanced conditioner					
Reconditioned as necessary					
Towel-dried hair or dried under cool dryer per manufacturer instructions					

Essential Rubrics continued

Performance Assessed	1	2	3	4	Improvement Plan
Examined scalp for abrasions					
Analyzed condition of hair					
Proceeded with toner application if desired					

TONER APPLICATION PROCEDURE

Performance Assessed	1	2	3	4	Improvement Plan
Prelightened hair to desired stage					
Shampooed hair					
Rinsed hair					
Towel-dried hair					
Conditioned as necessary					
Put on gloves					
Selected desired toner shade					
Applied protective cream around hairline and over ears					
Took strand test					
Recorded results on client's service record card					
If using a toner with developer, mixed toner and developer in nonmetallic bowl or bottle, following manufacturer's directions					
Parted hair into four equal sections, using end of tail comb or tint brush					
Avoided scratching scalp					
At crown of back section, parted off ¼-inch (0.6 cm) partings and applied toner from scalp up to, but not including, porous ends					

Performance Assessed	1	2	3	4	Improvement Plan
Took strand test					
Gently worked toner through ends of hair using brush or fingers					
Applied more toner if needed					
Left hair loosely piled to permit air circulation or covered hair with cap if required					
Timed according to strand test					
Removed toner by wetting hair and massaging into a lather					
Rinsed with warm water					
Shampooed gently					
Rinsed thoroughly a second time					
Applied acidic conditioner to close cuticle, lower the pH, and help prevent fading					
Removed toner stains from skin, hairline, and neck					

SPECIAL EFFECTS HAIRCOLORING WITH FOIL PROCEDURE

Performance Assessed	1	2	3	4	Improvement Plan
Draped client for a haircolor service					
Put on gloves					
Parted hair into four sections					
Applied protective cream around hairline and over ears					
Prepared formula and used immediately					

Essential Rubrics continued

Performance Assessed	1	2	3	4	Improvement Plan
Placed cotton around and through all four sections to protect the scalp so the lightener did not contact the scalp					
With a tail comb, took a slice of hair at the lower crown area of the head and placed a piece of foil under the slice of hair					
Held hair taut and brushed on lightener from upper edge of the foil to the hair ends					
Folded foil in half till ends met					
Folded foil in half again					
Used comb to crease foil					
Clipped foil upward					
Took a ¾-inch (1.8 cm) subsection in between foils					
Clipped hair up and out of the way					
Completed back center section					
Continued working down back center of head until section was complete					
Released clipped foils					
Worked to side areas dividing into two smaller sections					
Brought fine slices of hair into foil and applied lightener to hair					
Clipped up foil					

Essential Rubrics continued

Performance Assessed	1	2	3	4	Improvement Plan
Moved to other side of head and completed matching sections					
Took a fine slice of hair off top of a large section, placed on foil, and applied lightener					
Parted out a larger section, and then took a fine slice from top of section, placed it on the foil, and applied lightener					
Continued toward front until last foil is placed					
Checked foils to determine if desired lightness was achieved					
Removed foils one at a time at shampoo area					
Rinsed hair immediately to prevent color from affecting untreated hair					
Applied haircolor glaze to hair from base to ends					
Worked glaze into hair to make sure it was completely saturated					
Processed according to manufacturer's instructions					
Rinsed hair thoroughly					
Shampooed hair					
Conditioned hair					

Essential Review

Complete the following review of Chapter 21, Haircoloring, by circling the correct answer.

1. ____________ are specialized preparations designed to help equalize porosity and deposit a base color in one application.

   a) Presofteners
   b) Color conditioners
   c) Conditioning activators
   d) Fillers

2. A system for understanding color relationships is called ____________.

   a) the law of color
   b) the level system
   c) the color wheel
   d) primary color system

3. A ____________ lightener is strong enough for high-lift blonding, but gentle enough to use on the scalp.

   a) oil
   b) cream
   c) powder
   d) paste

4. A product prepared by combining permanent haircolor, hydrogen peroxide, and shampoo is ____________.

   a) soap cap
   b) highlighting shampoo
   c) color filler
   d) highlighting shampoo tint

5. A mixture of shampoo and hydrogen peroxide creates a ____________.

   a) soap cap
   b) highlighting shampoo
   c) color filler
   d) highlighting shampoo tint

6. A no-lift deposit-only color that adds shine and tone to the hair is called a ____________.

   a) polish
   b) wax
   c) spray
   d) glaze

7. A process that lightens and colors hair in a single application is known as ____________.

   a) double-process haircoloring
   b) temporary rinsing
   c) single-process haircoloring
   d) virgin haircoloring

8. A patch test is generally conducted behind the ear or on the ____________.

   a) inner wrist
   b) inner forearm
   c) temple or forehead
   d) inside of the elbow

9. A combination of equal parts of prepared tint and shampoo that is applied to hair like regular shampoo is called a ____________.

   a) color filler
   b) hair presoftener
   c) soap cap
   d) shampoo tint

10. A/an ____________ contains a powdered oxidizer that is added to hydrogen peroxide to increase its lifting power.

    a) activator
    b) protinator
    c) prohibitor
    d) developer

11. After the hair goes through the 10 stages of decolorizing, the color that is left in the hair is known as its ____________.

    a) foundation
    b) base
    c) vertex
    d) apex

12. An example of a natural or vegetable haircolor obtained from the leaves or bark of plants is ____________.

    a) henna
    b) tint
    c) toner
    d) demipermanent

13. Chemical compounds that lighten hair by dispersing, dissolving, and decolorizing the natural hair pigment are ____________.

    a) dispersers
    b) dissolvers
    c) decolorizers
    d) lighteners

14. Colored mousses and gels are considered to be what haircolor category?

    a) permanent
    b) semipermanent
    c) demipermanent
    d) temporary

15. Colors achieved by mixing equal parts of two primary colors are called ____________ colors.

    a) secondary
    b) tertiary
    c) neutral
    d) protein

Essential Review continued

16. Colors tones that are golden, orange, red, and yellow are considered to be ____________ tones.
    a) warm
    b) cool
    c) neutral
    d) primary

17. Colors tones that are blue, green, and violet are considered to be ____________ tones.
    a) warm
    b) cool
    c) neutral
    d) primary

18. Equal parts of blue and yellow mixed together create ____________.
    a) pink
    b) violet
    c) green
    d) orange

19. Equal parts of red and yellow mixed together create ____________.
    a) pink
    b) violet
    c) green
    d) orange

20. Equal parts of red and blue mixed together create ____________.
    a) pink
    b) violet
    c) green
    d) orange

21. Hair texture is determined by the ____________ of the individual hair strand.
    a) length
    b) strength
    c) diameter
    d) color

22. Haircolor that is able to deposit without lifting because they are less alkaline and are mixed with a low volume developer is ____________.
    a) permanent
    b) semipermanent
    c) demipermanent
    d) temporary

23. Haircolor that is mixed with a developer and remains in the hair shaft until the new growth of hair occurs is called ____________.
    a) permanent
    b) semipermanent
    c) demipermanent
    d) temporary

24. Haircoloring products fall into four classifications including temporary, semipermanent, and ____________.

a) permanent and perpetual
b) permanent and demipermanent
c) demipermanent and perpetual
d) vegetable and demipermanent

25. Metallic haircolors are also called ____________ colors.

a) advancing
b) gradual
c) delayed
d) accelerated

26. One safety precaution in haircoloring is to never apply tint if ____________ are present.

a) parents
b) children
c) abrasions
d) dandruff particles

27. Permanent haircolor is applied by either the bowl-and-brush method or with a/an ____________.

a) spatula and brush
b) applicator bottle
c) bowl-and-bottle
d) brush-and-bottle

28. Porous hair of the same color level will lighten faster than hair that is nonporous, because the bleaching agent can enter the ____________ more rapidly.

a) medulla
b) cortex
c) cuticle
d) follicle

29. Primary and secondary colors that are positioned opposite each other on the color wheel are considered to be ____________.

a) neutral
b) complementary
c) contradictory
d) contrary

30. Products created to remove artificial pigment from the hair are known as ____________.

a) color or tint removers
b) pigment or melanin removers
c) porosity removers
d) highlight removers

31. The predominant tonality of an existing color is referred to as a/an ____________.

a) base color
b) even color
c) neutral color
d) deep color

32. The cortex or middle layer of the hair gives strength and elasticity and contributes about ____________ percent to the overall strength of the hair.

a) 10 b) 20
c) 60 d) 80

33. The strength of a color tone is referred to as ____________.

a) level b) value
c) depth d) intensity

34. The measure of the potential oxidation of varying strengths of hydrogen peroxide is ____________.

a) density b) value
c) volume d) percentage

35. The cuticle of the hair protects the interior and contributes ____________ percent to the overall strength of the hair.

a) 10 b) 20
c) 60 d) 80

36. The U.S. Federal Food, Drug, and Cosmetic Act prescribes that a patch test, also called a/an ____________ test, be given twenty-four to forty-eight hours prior to an application of aniline derivative tint.

a) predisposition b) allergy
c) reaction d) postdisposition

37. The term used to describe the warmth or coolness of a color is ____________.

a) mixed melanin b) contributing pigment
c) tone or tonality d) value or depth

38. The preliminary strand test will tell you how the hair will react to the color formula and indicate ____________.

a) application method b) processing time
c) client satisfaction d) application time

39. The method used to analyze the lightness or darkness of a hair color, whether natural or artificial, is called ____________.

a) the law of color b) the level system
c) the color wheel d) primary color system

40. The tint formula in permanent haircolor contains uncolored dye ____________, which are small compounds that can diffuse into the hair shaft.

a) successors
b) precursors
c) activators
d) protinators

41. The melanin found in red hair is known as ____________.

a) pheomelanin
b) eumelanin
c) neomelanin
d) euromelanin

42. The melanin that gives black and brown color to hair is known as ____________.

a) pheomelanin
b) eumelanin
c) neomelanin
d) euromelanin

43. The ability of the hair to absorb moisture is called ____________.

a) density
b) texture
c) elasticity
d) porosity

44. Haircolor that partially penetrates the hair shaft and stains the cuticle layer, slowly fading with each shampoo, is known as ____________.

a) permanent
b) semipermanent
c) demipermanent
d) temporary

45. The number of hairs per square inch (2.5 square cm) on the head relates to the hair's ____________.

a) density
b) texture
c) elasticity
d) porosity

46. The oxidizer that is added to hydrogen peroxide to increase its chemical action is known as the ____________.

a) generator
b) penetrator
c) activator
d) contributor

47. The two methods of parting hair for a foil technique are ____________.

a) slicing and striping
b) weaving and striping
c) slicing and threading
d) slicing and weaving

Essential Review continued

48. The free-form technique of hair painting is also called ____________.

a) toning
b) baliage
c) brushing
d) swabbing

49. The first important guideline when color services do not turn out as planned or expected is to ____________.

a) call your instructor
b) apply color rinse
c) not panic
d) give money back

50. The system for understanding color relationships is the ____________.

a) Level System
b) Color System
c) Law of Color
d) Law of Hair

51. The process of treating gray or very resistant hair to allow for better penetration of color is known as ____________.

a) presoftening
b) prelightening
c) activating
d) accelerating

52. To some degree, the ____________ is designed to protect the school or salon owner from responsibility for accidents or damages.

a) client record card
b) posted price list
c) release statement
d) indemnity insurance

53. What is added to hydrogen peroxide to increase its chemical action or lifting power?

a) accelerator
b) diffuser
c) dissolver
d) lightener

54. What are the three types of hair lighteners?

a) oil, cream, powder
b) oil, paste, powder
c) cream, powder, paste
d) cream, paste, powder

55. What product is used to open the cuticle of the hair fiber so that tint can penetrate it?

a) hair conditioner
b) color filler
c) alkalizing agent
d) medicated shampoo

Essential Review continued

56. When performing retouches on red hair, the reds will last longer if you create them using a separate formula with a ____________ haircolor product applied to the mid-shaft and ends of the strand.

a) high-lift
b) deposit-only
c) temporary
d) vegetable tint

57. When arranging for a haircolor service consultation, ____________ walls are recommended.

a) pastel-colored
b) white or neutral
c) bright-colored
d) soft, yellow

58. When applying haircoloring products, always follow ____________.

a) manufacturer's directions
b) your instincts
c) client's directions
d) personal preference

59. Which type of lightener is not used directly on the scalp?

a) oil
b) cream
c) powder
d) paste

60. Which type of haircolor product uses the largest pigment molecules?

a) permanent
b) semipermanent
c) demipermanent
d) temporary

Essential Discoveries and Accomplishments

In the space below, jot some notes about what concepts of this chapter were hardest for you to understand or remember. Imagine finding yourself suddenly in the role of "teacher" and consider what you would tell your "students" about these concepts. Share your Essential Discoveries with some of the other students in your class and ask if they are helpful to them. You may want to revise your discoveries based on good ideas shared by your peers.

Discoveries:

List at least three things you have accomplished since your last entry that relate to your career goals.

Accomplishments:

CHAPTER 22

Hair Removal

A Motivating Moment: "You can disagree without being disagreeable."

— Zig Ziglar

Essential Objectives

After studying this chapter and completing the Essential Companion components, you will be able to:

1. **Describe the elements of a client consultation for hair removal.**
2. **Name the conditions that contraindicate hair removal in the salon.**
3. **Identify and describe three methods of permanent hair removal.**
4. **Demonstrate the techniques involved in temporary hair removal.**

Essential Hair Removal

Why do I need to learn about removing unwanted hair when I may never provide such a service?

The technical terms for superfluous hair are *hirsuties* (hur-SUE-shee-eez) and *hypertrichosis* (hy-pur-tri-KOH-sis). Actually, the terms mean nothing more than hair growth occurring in unusual amounts or locations on male and female clients. Often, these clients would like to have the hair removed and this is where the professional cosmetologist comes in. History documents that everything from abrasive pumice stones to sharpened stones and seashells have been used to rub off and pluck out hair. Records also indicate that the Egyptians made a compound of mud and alum for this purpose, and the Turks used a combination of yellow sulfide of arsenic, quicklime, and rose water, which created a primitive depilatory called rusma.

At some point nearly every client will encounter unwanted hair in one area or another. In fact, excessive hair can be extremely embarrassing and unattractive for female clients, especially when the hair is found on the face and chest. It is essential that you master the techniques used for removal of unwanted hair, and also learn to be sensitive when approaching a client about this type of service.

Essential Concepts

What do I need to know about hair removal in order to provide a quality service?

Hair removal falls into two major types: permanent and temporary, with salon techniques generally being limited to temporary methods. Permanent methods of hair removal include electrolysis, which is performed by a licensed electrologist, photoepilation, and laser hair removal. Laws regarding photoepilation and laser hair removal services vary in different states and provinces. However, the licensed cosmetologist should become proficient in all methods of temporary hair removal, including shaving (if allowed in your state or province), tweezing, using depilatories, and a variety of epilation techniques.

Cosmetologists should study and have a thorough understanding of hair removal because:

- Removing unwanted hair is a primary concern for many clients, and being able to advise them on the various types of hair removal will enhance your ability to satisfy your clients.
- Offering clients hair removal services that meet their needs and can be scheduled while they are already in the salon can be a valuable extra service you can offer.
- Learning the proper hair removal techniques and performing them safely makes you an even more important part of a client's beauty regimen.

1 Essential Experience

Temporary and Permanent Methods of Hair Removal

In the space provided, identify the following methods of hair removal as either permanent or temporary.

Hot wax	____________
Shaving	____________
Electrolysis	____________
Tweezing	____________
Electronic tweezing	____________
Epilator	____________
Cold wax	____________
Photoepilation	____________
Laser	____________
Depilatory	____________
Threading	____________
Sugaring	____________

Essential Experience 2

Crossword Puzzle

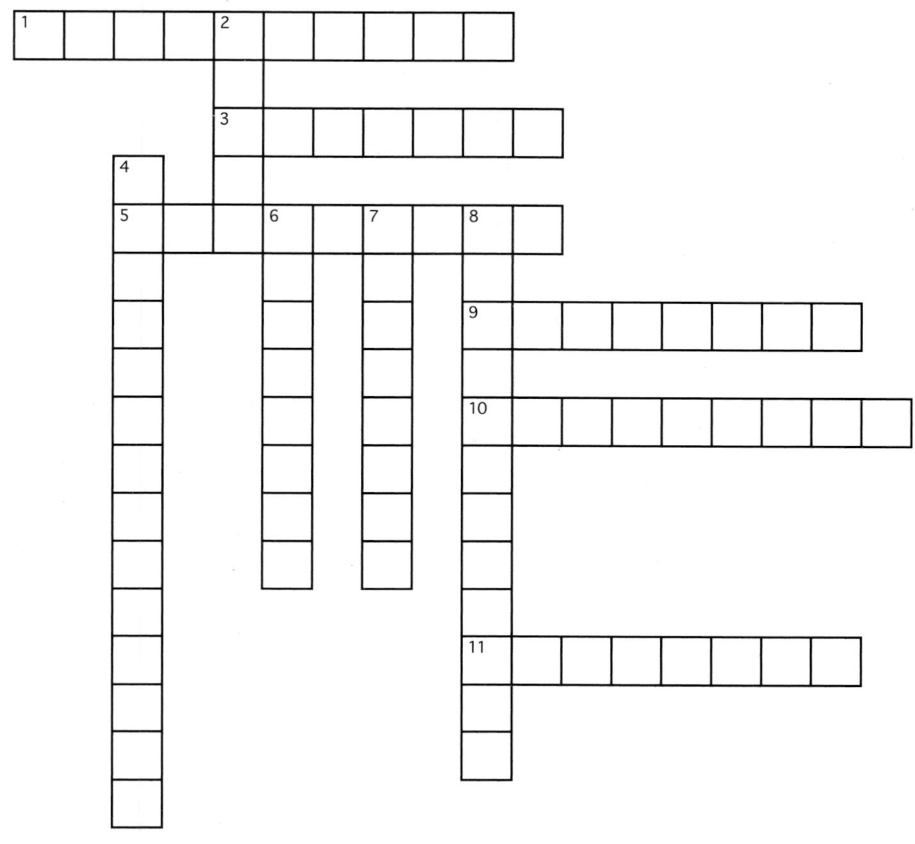

Clues:

Across

Word	Clue
______________	**1.** Substance, usually a caustic alkali preparation, for temporary hair removal
______________	**3.** Recommended when removing unwanted hair in large areas
______________	**5.** Growth of an unusual amount of hair on parts of the body normally bearing only downy hair
______________	**9.** Substance used to remove hair by pulling it out of the follicle

______________ **10.** Temporary hair removal method that involves twisting and rolling cotton thread along the surface of the skin, entwining the hair in the thread, and lifting it from the follicle

______________ **11.** Temporary hair removal that involves the use of a thick, sugar-based paste

Down

Word	Clue
______________	**2.** A beam pulsed on the skin that impairs the hair follicle
______________	**4.** Permanent hair removal treatment that uses intense light to destroy hair follicles
______________	**6.** Advisable to determine whether the individual is sensitive to the action of the depilatory
______________	**7.** Commonly used for shaping eyebrows
______________	**8.** Hair removal by means of an electric current that destroys the hair root

Essential Experience 3

Matching Exercise

Match the following essential terms with their identifying phrases or definition.

______	**Threading**	**1.**	Removes hair in large areas with razor and cream
______	**Cold wax**	**2.**	Depilatory that can be used on the cheeks, chin, upper lip, nape, arms, and legs
______	**Laser hair removal**	**3.**	Radio frequency transmits energy down the hair shaft into the follicle
______	**Tweezing**	**4.**	Does not require fabric strips for removal
______	**Hot wax**	**5.**	A laser beam is pulsed on the skin, impairing the hair follicles
______	**Electronic tweezing**	**6.**	Substance used to remove hair by pulling it out of the follicle
______	**Epilator**	**7.**	The twisting and rolling of cotton thread along the skin surface, entwining the hair in the thread and lifting it from the follicle
______	**Shaving**	**8.**	Commonly used for shaping the eyebrows
______	**Sugaring**	**9.**	Permanent hair removal treatment that uses intense light to destroy the hair follicles
______	**Photoepilation**	**10.**	Temporary method of hair removal that uses a thick, sugar-based paste

4 Essential Experience

Tweezing Eyebrows Procedure

Number the steps for an eyebrow tweezing procedure in the order in which they should occur.

Procedure

_______ Remove the hairs between the brows

_______ Cleanse eyelid area

_______ Brush eyebrows

_______ Brush the eyebrow hair to its normal position

_______ Soften brows

_______ Sponge tweezed area with antiseptic

_______ Apply mild toner

_______ Brush the hair downward

_______ Sponge area with toner to soothe skin

_______ Brush the hairs upward

Essential Experience 5

Eyebrow Waxing Procedure

Number the steps for an eyebrow waxing procedure in the order in which they should occur.

Procedure

______ Lightly massage the treated area

______ Remove remaining wax

______ Cover chair top

______ Put on disposable gloves

______ Place a hair cap or headband on the client's head

______ Spread wax with spatula

______ Apply antiseptic and lotion

______ Apply a fabric strip over the waxed area

______ Melt the wax in the heater

______ Remove fabric strip

______ Remove makeup and cleanse area

______ Test wax on inner wrist

______ Repeat procedure on other eyebrow

Essential Rubrics

Rubrics are used in education for organizing and interpreting data gathered from observations of student performance. It is a clearly developed scoring document used to differentiate between levels of development in a specific skill performance or behavior. A rubric is provided in this study guide as a self-assessment tool to aid you in your behavior development.

Rate your performance according to the following scale:

(1) Development Opportunity: There is little or no evidence of competency; assistance is needed; performance includes multiple errors.

(2) Fundamental: There is beginning evidence of competency; task is completed alone; performance includes few errors.

(3) Competent: There is detailed and consistent evidence of competency; task is completed alone; performance includes rare errors.

(4) Strength: There is detailed evidence of highly creative, inventive, mature presence of competency.

Space is provided for comments to assist you in improving your performance and achieving a higher rating.

TWEEZING PROCEDURE

Performance Assessed	**1**	**2**	**3**	**4**	**Improvement Plan**
Cleansed the eyelid area with cotton balls moistened with gentle eye makeup remover					
Used a small brush to remove any powder or scaliness					
Saturated cotton or towel with warm water and placed over brows for one to two minutes					
Applied a mild toner on a cotton ball prior to tweezing					
Removed hairs between the brows by stretching skin taut					

Essential Rubrics continued

Performance Assessed	1	2	3	4	Improvement Plan
Grasped individual hairs with tweezers and pulled with a quick motion, always in the direction of growth					
Tweezed between the brows and above the brow line first					
Sponged the tweezed area frequently with cotton moistened with an antiseptic lotion					
Brushed hair downward					
Removed excessive hairs from above the eyebrow line without creating a hard line					
Shaped upper section of one eyebrow and then shaped the other					
Frequently sponged the area with toner					
Brushed hairs upward					
Removed hairs from under the eyebrow line					
Shaped lower section of one eyebrow and then shaped the other					
Sponged area with toner or applied emollient cream and massaged the brows					
If applicable, removed cream with cool, wet cotton pads					
After tweezing was completed, sponged eyebrows and surrounding skin with a toner					
Brushed the eyebrow hair to normal position					

Essential Rubrics continued

EYEBROW WAXING PROCEDURE

Performance Assessed	1	2	3	4	Improvement Plan
Melted wax in heater to thickness of a caramel sauce					
Laid a clean towel over the top of the facial chair followed by a layer of disposable paper					
Placed a hair cap or headband on head					
Put on disposable gloves					
Removed client's makeup					
Cleansed area thoroughly with a mild cleanser					
Dried treatment area					
Tested wax temperature and consistency by applying a small drop on your inner wrist					
Using spatula, spread thin coat of wax over area to be treated					
Did not double dip					
Applied a fabric strip over the waxed area					
Ran finger over fabric surface three to five times in direction of hair growth					
Gently applied pressure and quickly removed the fabric strip by pulling it in the direction opposite the hair growth					
Did not pull straight up on the strip					

Essential Rubrics continued

Performance Assessed	1	2	3	4	Improvement Plan
Lightly massaged the treated area					
Removed remaining wax residue from skin with a gentle wax remover					
Repeated procedure on other eyebrow					
Cleansed skin with mild emollient cleanser and applied emollient or antiseptic lotion					

BODY WAXING PROCEDURE

Performance Assessed	1	2	3	4	Improvement Plan
Melted the wax in the heater					
Draped treatment bed with disposable paper or a bed sheet with paper over the top					
If bikini waxing, offered client disposable panties or a small clean towel					
If waxing the underarms, had client remove bra and put on a terry wrap					
Offered terry wrap when waxing legs					
Assisted client onto the treatment bed					
Draped client with towels					
Thoroughly cleansed the area to be waxed with a mild cleanser					
Dried area to be waxed					
Applied a light covering of powder					

Essential Rubrics continued

Performance Assessed	1	2	3	4	Improvement Plan
Tested wax temperature and consistency by applying a small drop to inner wrist					
Using spatula spread a thin coat of wax in direction of hair growth over area to be treated					
Did not double dip					
Applied a fabric strip in the same direction as the hair growth					
Pressed gently, running hand over the surface of the fabric three to five times					
Gently applied pressure and quickly removed wax in the opposite direction of the hair growth					
Did not pull the fabric strip straight upwards					
Applied gentle pressure and lightly massaged the treated area					
Repeated steps, using a fresh fabric strip every time					
If waxing the legs, had client turn over, and repeated procedure on the backs of legs					
Removed remaining residue of powder from skin					
Cleansed area with a mild emollient cleanser					
Applied an emollient or antiseptic lotion					
Undraped client					
Escorted to dressing room					

Essential Review

Using the following words, fill in the blanks below to form a thorough review of Chapter 22, Hair Removal. Words or terms may be used more than once or not at all.

abrasions	**electrolysis**	**needles**
acne	**emollient**	**normal**
adhesives	**epilator**	**opposite**
allergies	**eyebrows**	**patch test**
aloe gel	**fever blisters**	**rosacea**
anagen	**hirsutism**	**sensitive**
beeswax	**hydroquinone**	**shaving**
botox	**hypertrichosis**	**steamed**
client procedure	**hypertrophy**	**strand test**
collagen	**Intense Pulsed Light**	**training and experience**
depilatory	**laser hair removal**	

1. Another technical term for hirsuties is ______________.

2. Both hot and cold wax are made primarily of resins and __________.

3. A client consultation prior to a hair removal service discloses all medications, both topical and oral, along with any known skin disorders or ____________.

4. Facial waxing or tweezing should not be performed on clients who have _____________ or very sensitive skin.

5. Having a history of ____________ or cold sores is considered a contraindication for facial waxing.

6. Use of Retin-A®, Renova®, ______________, or similar products prevent hair removal treatments.

7. Removal of hair by means of an electric current that destroys the root of the hair is known as ____________.

8. Photoepilation uses intense light to destroy hair follicles and has minimal side effects and requires no ___________.

9. A method for the rapid, gentle removal of unwanted hair by means of a beam pulsed on the skin is called _________________.

10. Laser hair removal is most effective when used on follicles in the active growing phase, or ____________.

Essential Review continued

11. ____________ is the most common form of temporary hair removal, particularly of men's facial hair.
12. Correctly shaped ____________ have a strong, positive impact on the overall attractiveness of the face.
13. Washing your hands thoroughly with soap and warm water is critical before and after every ________________ you perform.
14. When tweezing the eyebrows, tweeze between the brows and above the brow line first because the area under the brow line is much more ____________.
15. Threading, sugaring, and specialty waxing, such as Brazilian waxing, are advanced techniques that require additional ________________________.
16. Most manufacturers of electronic tweezers recommend that the area is ____________ first in order to increase efficiency.
17. Depilatories contain detergents to strip the sebum from the hair and ____________ to hold the chemicals to the hair shaft for the five to ten minutes that are necessary to remove the hair.
18. If a client uses a chemical depilatory, you should perform a ____________ to determine whether the individual is sensitive to the action of the product.
19. Wax is a commonly used ____________, applied in either hot or cold form as recommended by the manufacturer.
20. ____________ has a relatively high incidence of allergic reaction.
21. When performing a wax service, the fabric strip and the wax that sticks to it are removed by pulling it in the direction ____________ the hair growth.
22. Do not apply wax over warts, moles, ____________, or irritated or inflamed skin.
23. Apply ____________ to calm and soothe sensitive skin that becomes red or swells due to a waxing procedure.
24. The condition pertaining to an excessive growth or cover of hair is called ____________.
25. ____________________ is also known as photoepilation.

Essential Discoveries and Accomplishments

In the space below, jot some notes about what concepts of this chapter were hardest for you to understand or remember. Imagine finding yourself suddenly in the role of "teacher" and consider what you would tell your "students" about these concepts. Share your Essential Discoveries with some of the other students in your class and ask if they are helpful to them. You may want to revise your discoveries based on good ideas shared by your peers.

Discoveries:

____

____

____

____

____

____

____

____

____

____

____

List at least three things you have accomplished since your last entry that relate to your career goals.

Accomplishments:

____

____

____

____

____

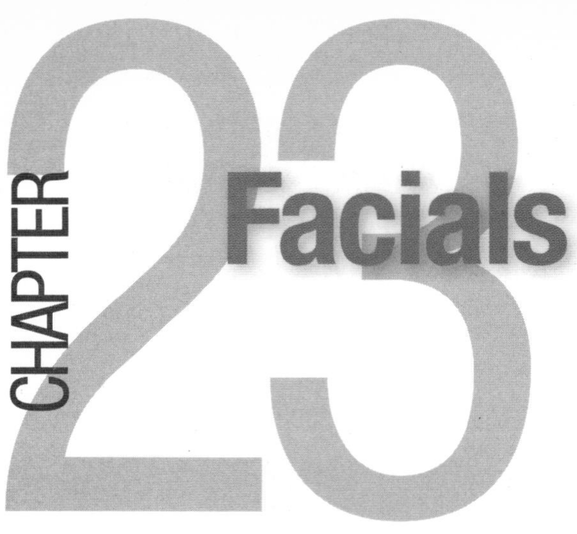

CHAPTER 23 Facials

A Motivating Moment: "Yesterday is but a dream, tomorrow but a vision. But today well lived makes every yesterday a dream of happiness, and every tomorrow a vision of hope. Look well, therefore, to this day."
— Sanskrit Proverb

Essential Objectives

After studying this chapter and completing the Essential Companion components, you will be able to:

1. **Explain the importance of skin analysis and client consultation.**
2. **Understand contraindications and the use of a health screening form to safely perform facial treatments.**
3. **List and describe various skin types and conditions.**
4. **Describe different types of products used in facial treatments.**
5. **Perform a client consultation.**
6. **Identify the various types of massage movements and their physiological effects.**
7. **Describe the basic types of electrical equipment used in facial treatments.**
8. **Identify the basic concepts of electrotherapy and light therapy techniques.**

Essential Theory of Massage

Why do I need to know about the underlying theory of massage, and are facials really that important in my career as a professional cosmetologist?

The term *massage* is of Arabic origin from the word *masa,* meaning to stroke or touch. The therapeutic benefits of massage were used and enjoyed in ancient Greece and are enjoyed more than ever today with the availability of licensed massage therapists. As a professional cosmetologist you will not only be given permission to invade the "comfort zones" of your clients, but you will be asked to actually touch them when you provide various services. For example, a good scalp massage can win the loyalty of your client for years to come. A massage that is both relaxing and stimulating accompanying a facial will inspire client confidence in you and will ensure repeat business. A firm massage given with flexible hands will ensure your clients receive the ultimate benefit from their services.

The generation born between the mid 1940s and the early 1960s is known as the *baby boomer generation*. As we enter the twenty-first century, this generation is growing older, ranging in age from the late 40s to the early 60s. With this aging segment of society, we have grown more interested in the health and beauty of the skin than ever before. Both men and women are buying more skin care products than ever before. The skin care industry is reported to be a multi-million dollar business annually. Professional advice and professional services are essential in ensuring optimum results for those men and women who want to keep their skin looking healthy and youthful. That is where you, the professional cosmetologist, come in. With your knowledge and practiced skills, you can provide the services they desire and increase your yearly income significantly.

Cosmetologists should study and have a thorough understanding of facials because:

- Providing skin care services to clients is extremely rewarding, helps busy clients to relax, improves their appearance, and helps clients feel better about themselves.
- Knowing the basics of skin analysis and basic information about skin care products will enable you to offer your clients help and advice when they ask you for it.
- Although you will not treat a skin disease, you must be able to recognize adverse skin conditions and refer clients to seek medical advice from a physician.

Essential Theory of Massage continued

- Learning the basic techniques of facials and facial massage will give you a good overview of, and an ability to perform, these foundational services.
- You may enjoy this category of services and may consider specializing in skin care services. This study will create a perfect basis for making that decision.

Remember that no matter how the benefits of a service are stressed, unless it is enjoyable to the client the need and demand for the service will decline. A facial service that is accompanied by a good massage will endear you to your clients for years to come. A satisfied client means more clients and more satisfied clients means more income for you!

Essential Concepts

What to do I need to know about the theory of massage and facials in order to provide quality services to my clients?

It is essential that you master the basic manipulations used in massage in order to ensure a satisfactory service as well as to eliminate harm or injury to your client. It will be helpful for you to understand the psychological effects that a good massage will have on your clients. You will master numerous massage manipulations and become familiar with the motor nerve points of the face and the neck.

As a licensed cosmetologist, you will be able to perform many services relating to skin care and makeup. Among those services will be facials, facial massage, packs, and masks. It should be ever present in your mind that you are about to become a professional in the image industry. Therefore, it is essential that you exemplify that role. In addition to learning how to provide the best possible services for your clients, you must be a role model for the industry you represent. You must have the most current hairstyle, the most well-manicured hands and nails, and the best cared for skin. Once you have developed all the applicable skills in this specialty area, you will be in high demand for employment in the high-end, full-service salons in your marketplace.

1 Essential Experience

Motor Nerve Points

On the diagrams below, identify the motor nerve points of the face and neck.

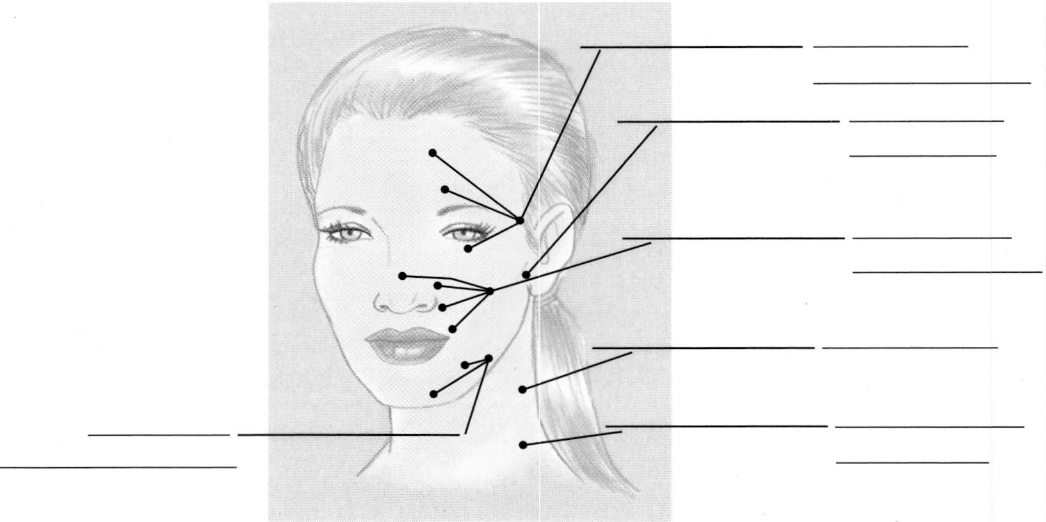

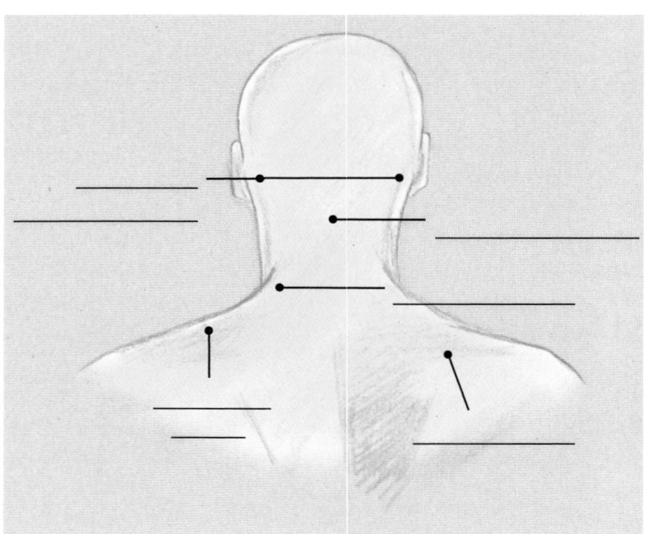

Essential Experience

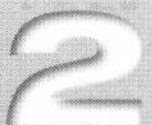

Matching Exercise

Match the following essential terms with their identifying phrases or definition.

______	**Effleurage**	**1.** Tapping, slapping, and hacking movements
______	**Pétrissage**	**2.** Light, continuous, stroking movement
______	**Friction**	**3.** Shaking movement
______	**Percussion**	**4.** Kneading movement
______	**Vibration**	**5.** Deep rubbing movement
______	**Rolling**	**6.** Chopping movement performed with edges of hands
______	**Chucking**	**7.** Another term for percussion
______	**Wringing**	**8.** Pressing and twisting the tissues with a fast back-and-forth movement
______	**Tapotement**	**9.** Grasping flesh firmly in one hand and moving hand up and down along the bone while other hand keeps arm or leg in steady position
______	**Hacking**	**10.** Vigorous movement that applies a twisting motion against the bones in the opposite direction

3 Essential Experience

Massage Manipulations

Label each of the manipulations found below in the space provided.

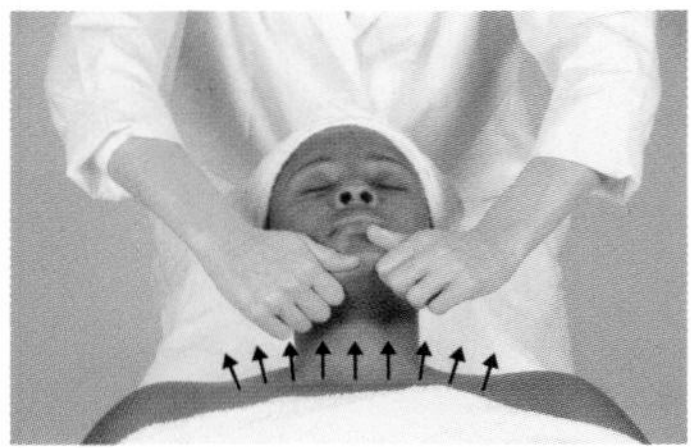

1. ______________________

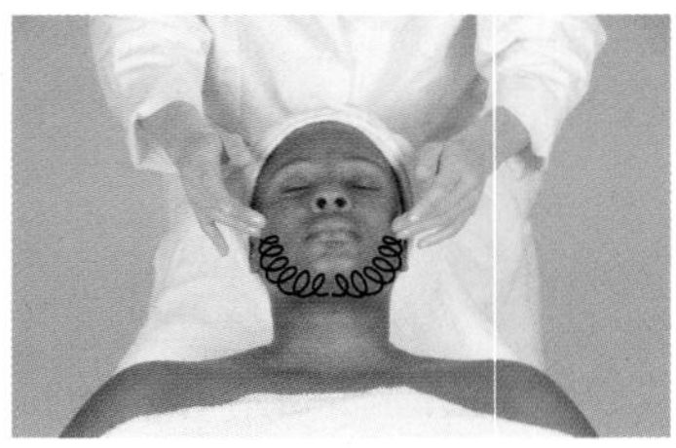

2. ______________________
____

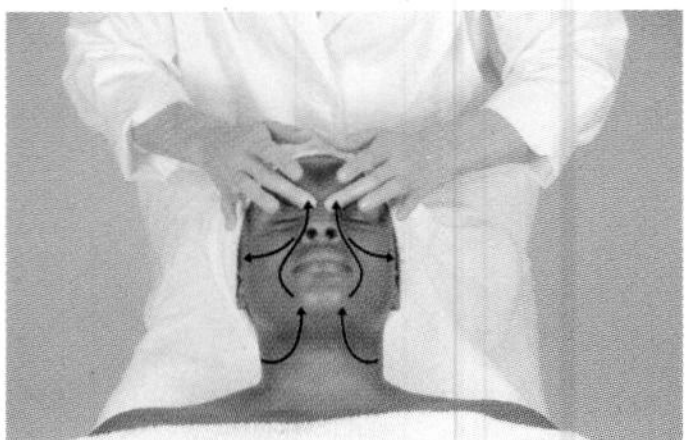

3. ______________________
____

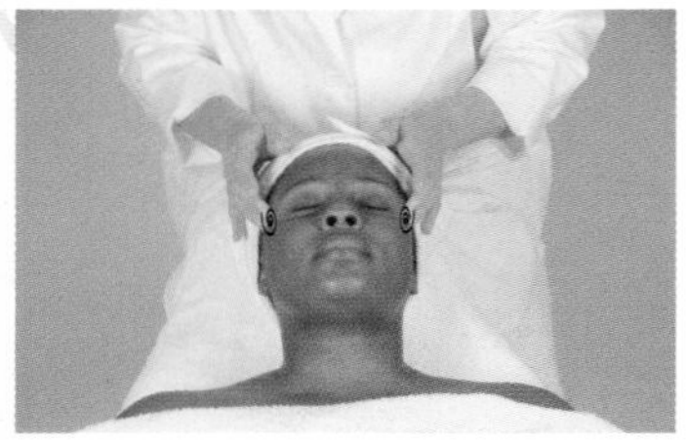

4. ______________________
____
____

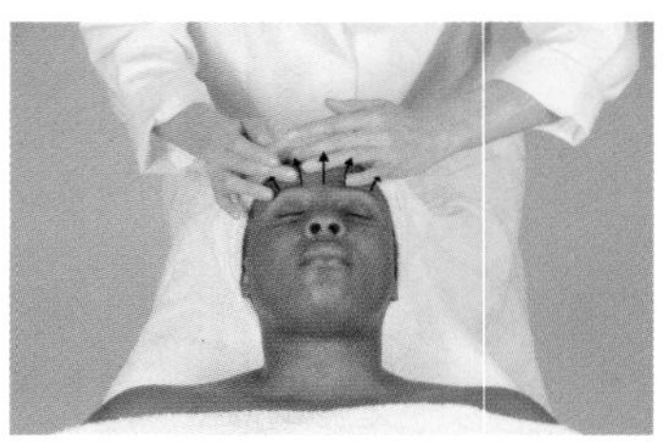

5. ______________________
____

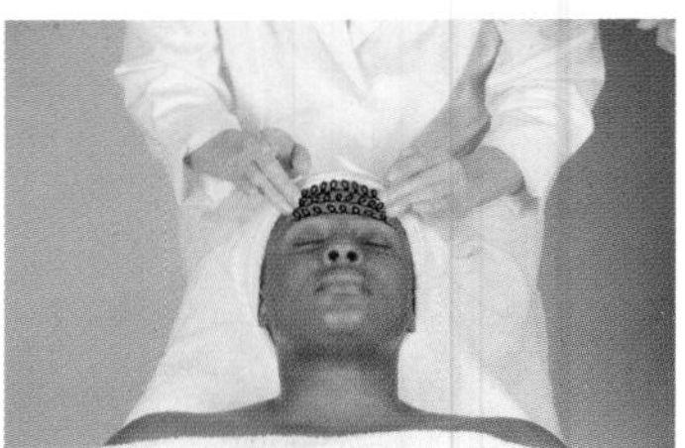

6. ______________________
____

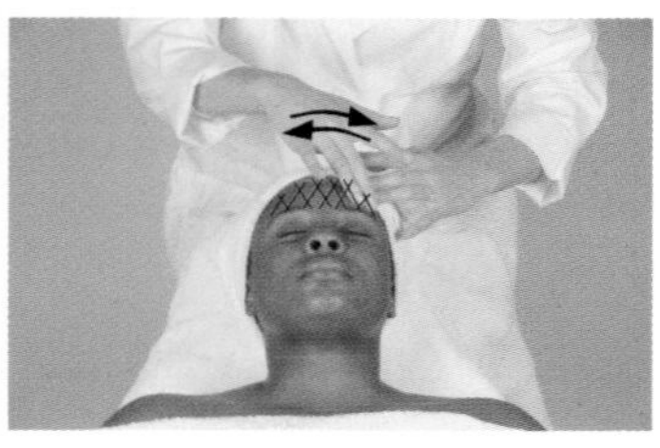

7. ______________________
____

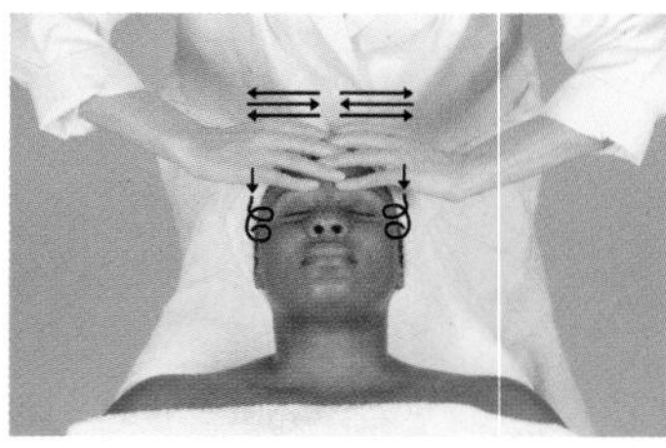

8. ______________________
____

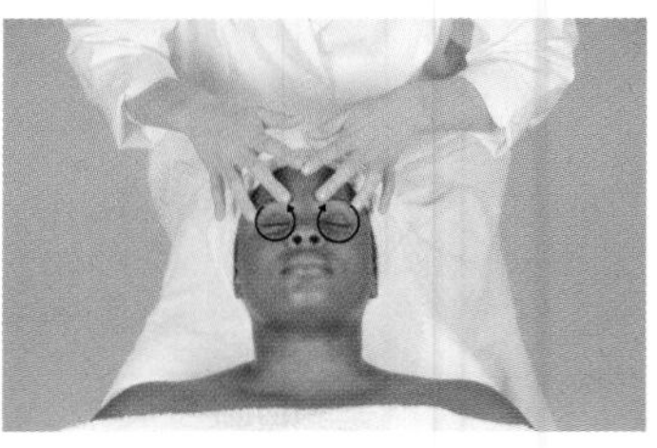

9. ______________________
____

Essential Experience continued 3

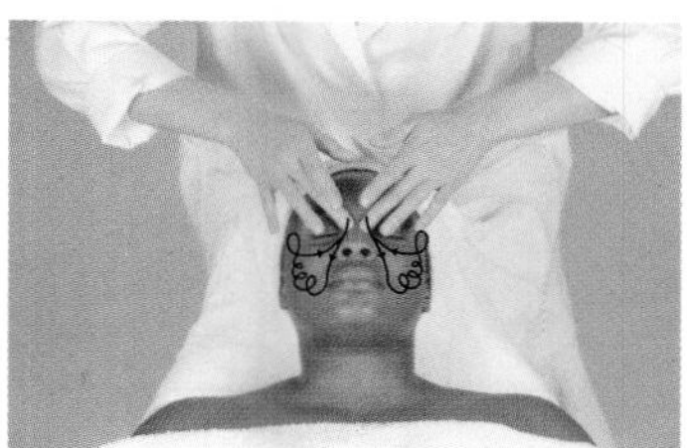

10. ______________________

____

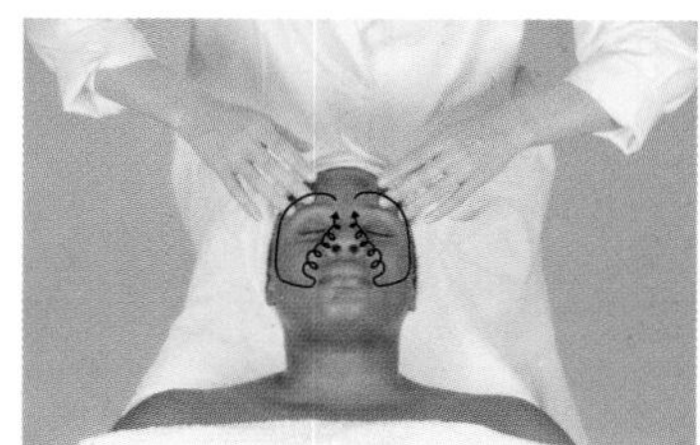

11. ______________________

____

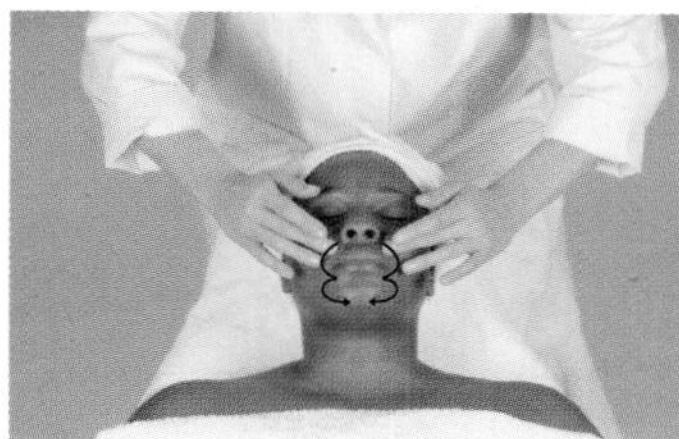

12. ______________________

____

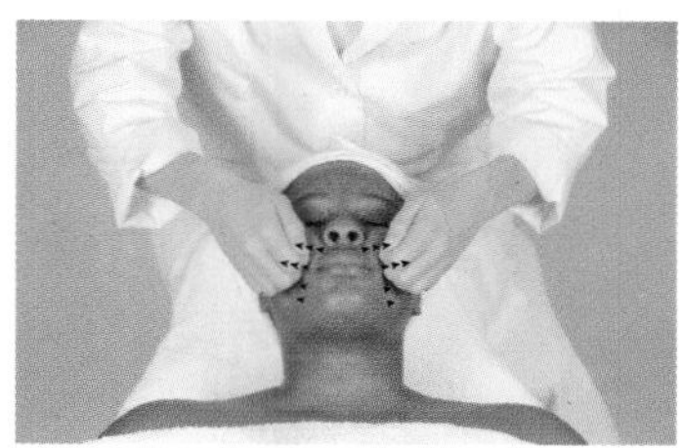

13. ______________________

____

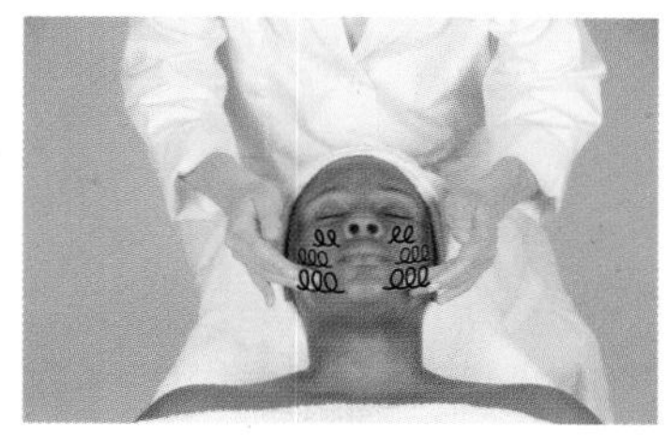

14. ______________________

____

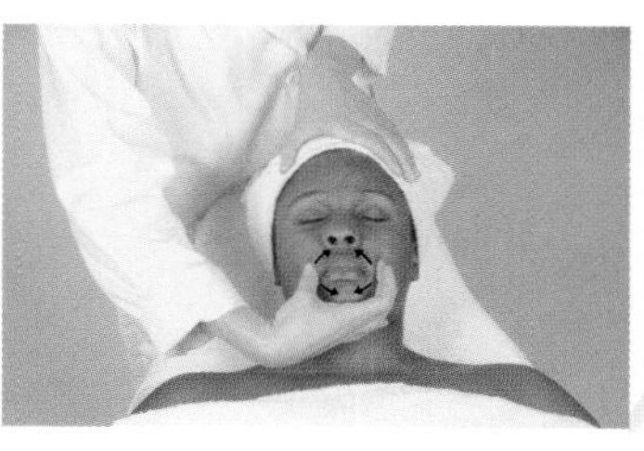

15. ______________________

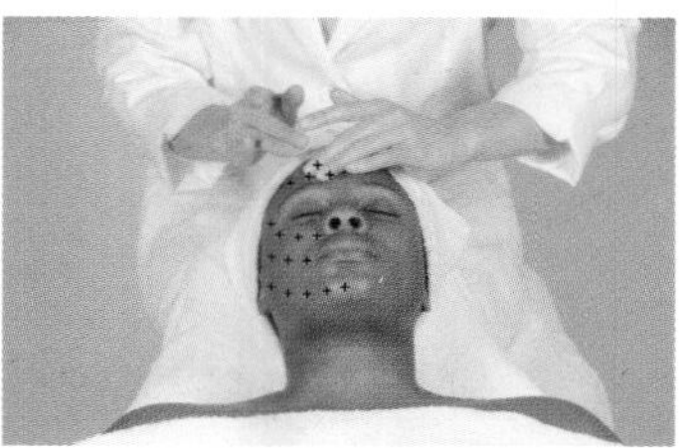

16. ______________________

____

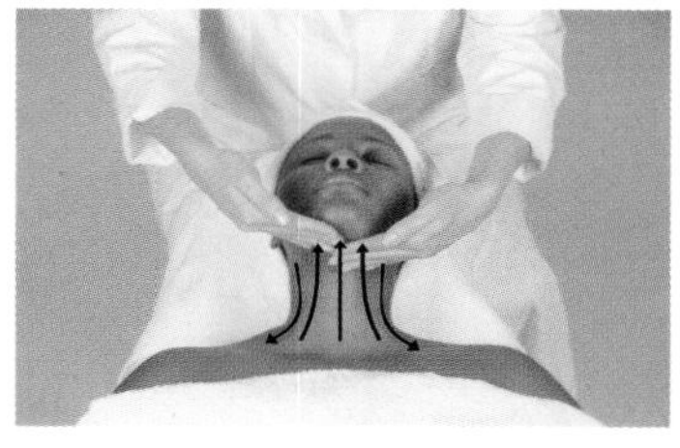

17. ______________________

____

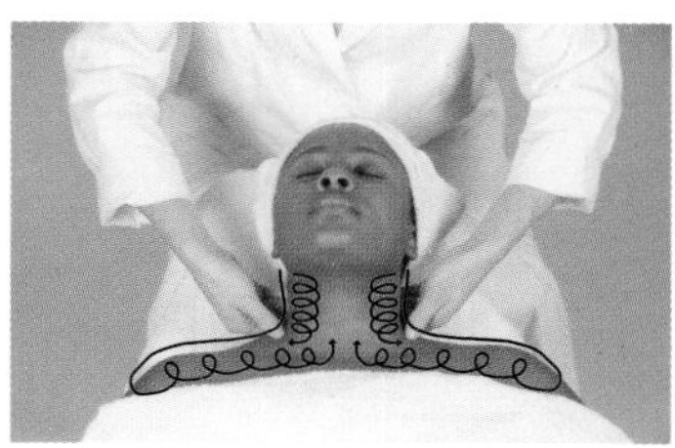

18. ______________________

____

4 Essential Experience

Word Scramble A

Using the clues provided, unscramble the terms below.

Scramble	**Correct Word**
agreleueff	__ __ __ __ __ __ __ __ __ __
	Clue: Light, continuous stroking.
atenotempt	__ __ __ __ __ __ __ __ __ __
	Clue: Tapping, slapping, and hacking.
cepnoirssu	__ __ __ __ __ __ __ __ __ __
	Clue: Tapping, slapping, and hacking.
gilnflu	__ __ __ __ __ __ __
	Clue: Massaging the arms.
njtio	__ __ __ __ __
	Clue: Movable bone.
gmasesa	__ __ __ __ __ __ __
	Clue: Exercises facial muscles.
nbioitarv	__ __ __ __ __ __ __ __ __
	Clue: Shaking movement.
trmoo niopt	__ __ __ __ __ __ __ __ __
	Clue: Each muscle and nerve has one.
rcnfoiti	__ __ __ __ __ __ __ __
	Clue: Deep rubbing movement.
ragtéissep	__ __ __ __ __ __ __ __ __ __
	Clue: Kneading movement.

Essential Experience 5

Crossword Puzzle A

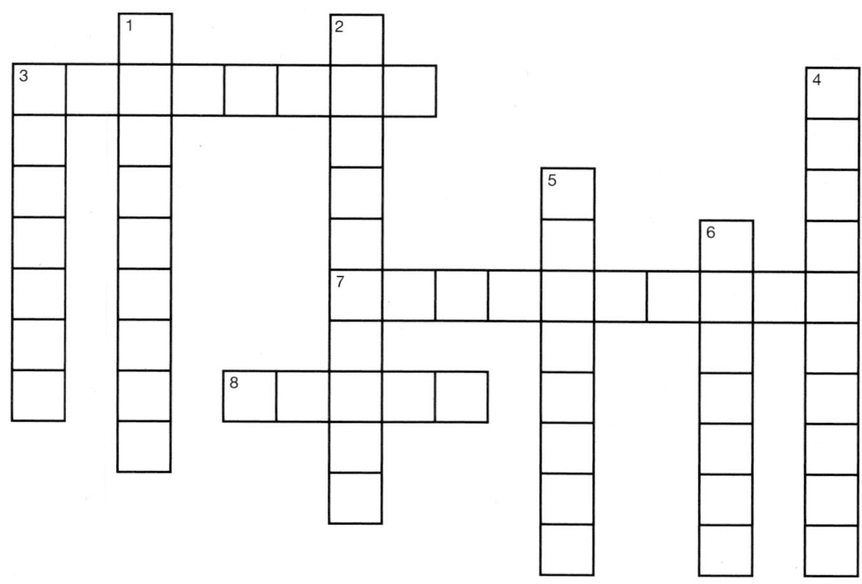

Across

Word	Clue
________________	**3.** A deep rubbing movement
________________	**7.** A kneading movement
________________	**8.** Movable bone

Down

Word	Clue
________________	**1.** A shaking movement accomplished by rapid muscular contractions in your arm
________________	**2.** Every muscle and nerve has one
________________	**3.** A form of pétrissage used mainly for massaging the arms
________________	**4.** Light, continuous stroking movement applied with the fingers
________________	**5.** A vigorous movement in which your hands are placed a short distance apart
________________	**6.** Exercises facial muscles

6 Essential Experience

Massage Movements

In the chart below, describe each massage movement, and list the parts of the body where the movement is used.

Name of Movement	Movement Description	Where Used
Effleurage		
Petrissage		
Friction		
Percussion		
Vibration		

Essential Experience 7

Word Scramble B

Using the clues provided, unscramble the terms below.

Scramble	Correct Word
puekam atyr	_ _ _ _ _ _ _ _ _ _ _ *Clue:* holds cosmetics.
nlaec thsee	_ _ _ _ _ _ _ _ _ _ *Clue:* covering used during basic facial.
laicaf eermtsa	_ _ _ _ _ _ _ _ _ _ _ _ _ *Clue:* moisturizes and softens facial skin.
askm	_ _ _ _ *Clue:* concentrated facial treatment products.
deah vocireng	_ _ _ _ _ _ _ _ _ _ _ _ *Clue:* protects the hair.
eslwot	_ _ _ _ _ _ *Clue:* can replace headbands.
gsespno	_ _ _ _ _ _ _ *Clue:* used for cleansing makeup.
ghhi qcyueerfn	_ _ _ _ _ _ _ _ _ _ _ _ _ *Clue:* uses electrodes for application.
itengtnrsa	_ _ _ _ _ _ _ _ _ _ *Clue:* help rebalance the pH.
fniredar mpal	_ _ _ _ _ _ _ _ _ _ _ _ *Clue:* used to heat skin and increase blood flow.
ngifgniyam amlp	_ _ _ _ _ _ _ _ _ _ _ _ _ _ *Clue:* used in skin analysis.
nolas wong	_ _ _ _ _ _ _ _ _ *Clue:* protects clothing.
pslasuta	_ _ _ _ _ _ _ _ *Clue:* used to remove product from jars.
rireziutsom	_ _ _ _ _ _ _ _ _ _ _ *Clue:* help increase moisture content on skin.

7 Essential Experience continued

scpiitenat	_ _ _ _ _ _ _ _ _ _ _
	Clue: used to clean hands.
irbultacgni ilo	_ _ _ _ _ _ _ _ _ _ _ _ _ _ _ _ _
	Clue: facilitates massage movements.
nottoc awssb	_ _ _ _ _ _ _ _ _ _ _ _
	Clue: used to remove product from skin.
zuega	_ _ _ _ _
	Clue: loosely woven cotton.

Essential Experience

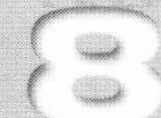

Mind Map Facials

Mind mapping creates a free-flowing outline of material or information. Using the central or key point of preservative and corrective facials, diagram the purpose and benefits of such treatments. Use terms, pictures, and symbols as desired. Using color will increase retention of the material. Keep your mind open and uncluttered and don't worry about where a line or word should go as the organization of the map will usually take care of itself.

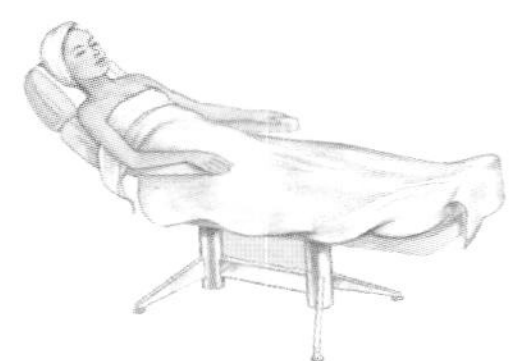

9 Essential Experience

Client Consultation

Choose another student as your partner and conduct a facial treatment consultation on each other. Record your results on the sample record card found below. After the consultations, perform the appropriate facial service on each other. Ask an instructor to evaluate your procedure.

Department of Skin Care

Health Screening Form

Client History

Name____

Address____

City________________State________ Zip Code____________

Home Phone______________ Work Phone________________

Occupation__________Referred by__________Date of Birth________

Is this your first facial treatment? YES___ NO___

Have you ever used:

Retin-A®? YES___ NO___

Accutane® (isotretinoin)? YES___ NO___

Are you using glycolic or alphahydroxy acids? YES___ NO___

Do you smoke? YES___ NO___

Are you pregnant? YES___ NO___

Do you have acne or frequent blemishes? YES___ NO___

Are you nursing? YES___ NO___

Taking birth control pills? YES___ NO___ If so, how long?______________

Have you had skin cancer? YES___ NO___

Do you experience stress? YES___ NO___ If so, how often?______________

Do you wear contact lenses? YES___ NO___

Are you under a physician's care? YES___ NO___

Physician's Name________________________

Do you have any allergies to cosmetics, foods, or drugs? YES___ NO___

Please list____

Are you presently on any medications (oral or topical-dermatological)? YES___ NO___

Please list____

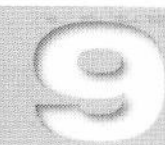

What products do you use presently?______________________________

Please circle: Soap Cleansing Milk Toner Daily Sunscreen Creams

Other____

Please circle if you are affected by or have any of the following:

Have had hysterectomy	Pacemaker/Cardiac Problems	Immune Disorders
Depression or Anxiety	Herpes	Urinary or Kidney Problems
Seborrhea/Psoriasis/Eczema	Chronic Headaches	Hepatitis
Asthma	Fever Blisters	Lupus
High Blood Pressure	Metal Bone Pins or Plates	Epilepsy
Taking Depression/ Mood Altering Medications	Sinus Problems	Other Skin Diseases

Please explain above problems or list any significant others:

____

____

I understand that the services offered are not a substitute for medical care, and any information provided by the therapist is for educational purposes only and not diagnostically prescriptive in nature. I understand that the information herein is to aid the technician in giving better service and is completely confidential.

SALON POLICIES

1. Professional consultation is required before initial dispensing of products.
2. Our active discount rate is only effective for clients visiting every 4 weeks.
3. We do not give cash refunds.

I fully understand and agree to the above salon policies.

______________________________ ______________

Client Signature Date

10 Essential Experience

Crossword Puzzle B

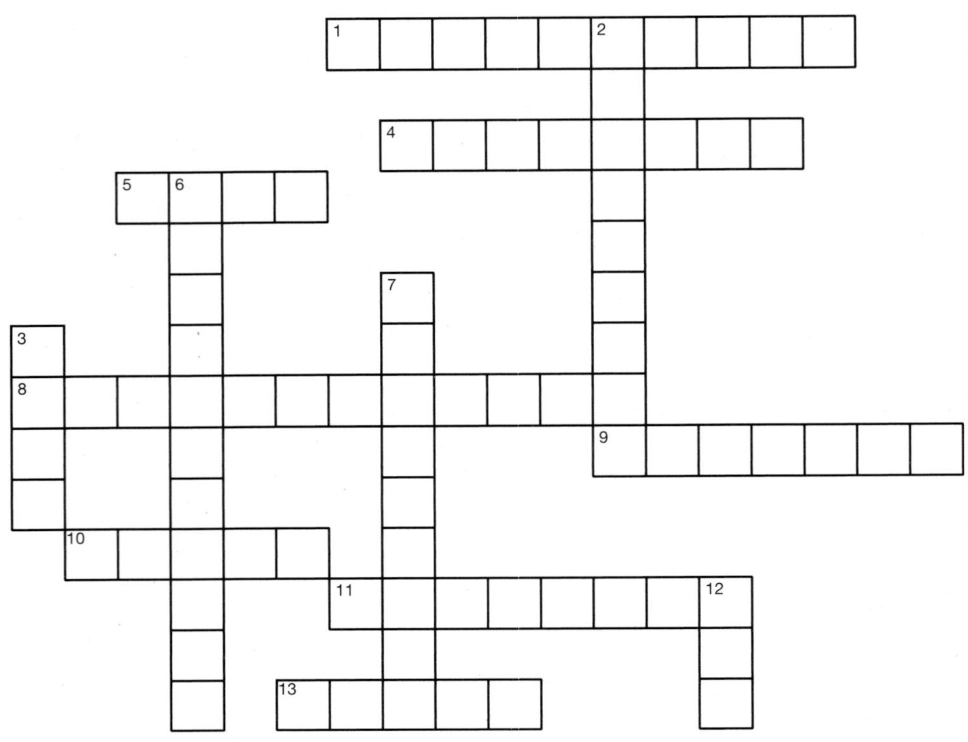

Across

Word	Clue
______________	**1.** Correcting facial skin conditions
______________	**4.** Used to help soften superficial lines and increase blood circulation
______________	**5.** A disorder of the sebaceous glands
______________	**8.** Maintains the health of the skin
______________	**9.** Used to remove the product from containers
______________	**10.** Whiteheads
______________	**11.** Lamp used in facial treatments
______________	**13.** May be made from vegetables, fruits, dairy products, herbs, and/or oils

Down

Word	Clue
________________	**2.** Blackheads
________________	**3.** Used to hold the towel in place
________________	**6.** Gauze used to hold certain mask ingredients on the face
________________	**7.** Covering used to protect the hair
________________	**12.** Skin type caused by insufficient flow of sebum

11 Essential Experience

Skin Care Product Research

Research a variety of skin care products available in your school and found at local supply stores. Include cleansers, toners, moisturizers, astringents, and so on. Use the chart below to track your findings.

Product Name	Pleasant Fragrance (Yes/No) Identify	Texture: How Does Product Feel?	Purpose of the Product	What Skin Type Is Product Used For?

Essential Experience 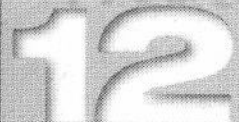

Facial Steaming

Steaming the face can open pores, stimulate circulation, and help masks and creams work more effectively. Steaming should not be done more than once per week and should be accompanied by an appropriate moisturizer to avoid drying out the skin.

Try steaming at home by washing your face thoroughly and pinning or tying back your hair (or wear a shower cap). Boil a large pan of water and put in a handful of herbs based on your ingredient research. For example, chamomile, sage, peppermint, eucalyptus, and lavender disinfect and soothe the skin. They also contain oils that are beneficial to sinus passages. You can also use herbal oils from the health food store. Place the pan on a table or counter of appropriate height that will allow you to sit comfortably and hold your head over the pan. Lower your face over the pan and drape a large towel over your entire head and around the pan so no steam escapes. Now, relax and enjoy a highly rejuvenating experience. Steam for no more than ten minutes. When finished blot your face with a soft cloth. Your skin is now prepared for an effective exfoliation or mask treatment. If not continuing with these treatments, refresh the skin with cool water to close the pores. In the space provided, record the results, your skin's reaction, and how the procedure made you feel.

Essential Rubrics

Rubrics are used in education for organizing and interpreting data gathered from observations of student performance. It is a clearly developed scoring document used to differentiate between levels of development in a specific skill performance or behavior. A rubric is provided in this study guide as a self-assessment tool to aid you in your behavior development.

Rate your performance according to the following scale:

- **Development Opportunity:** There is little or no evidence of competency; assistance is needed; performance includes multiple errors.
- **Fundamental:** There is beginning evidence of competency; task is completed alone; performance includes few errors.
- **Competent:** There is detailed and consistent evidence of competency; task is completed alone; performance includes rare errors.
- **Strength:** There is detailed evidence of highly creative, inventive, mature presence of competency.

Space is provided for comments to assist you in improving your performance and achieving a higher rating.

BASIC FACIAL PROCEDURE

Performance Assessed	1	2	3	4	Improvement Plan
Removed jewelry					
Escorted client to dressing room					
Offered assistance					
Placed clean towel across back of facial table or chair					
Helped client onto facial bed					
Placed towel across chest and sheet over body, folding top of towel over it					
Removed client's shoes and tucked cover around feet					
Used disposable slippers if available					

Essential Rubrics continued

Performance Assessed	1	2	3	4	Improvement Plan
Fastened headband or towel around head to protect hair					
Removed lingerie straps from shoulders or tucked into topless gown					
Removed makeup					
Applied cleanser					
Removed cleanser with facial sponges, tissues, moist cotton pads, or warm, moist towels					
Started at forehead and followed contours of face					
Removed all cleanser from one area of face before proceeding to the next					
Finished with neck, chest, and back					
Analyzed skin					
Steamed the face using warm, moist towels, or a facial steamer					
Covered client's eyes with cotton pads moistened with distilled water or alcohol-free freshener					
For nonsensitive skin, applied a granular scrub to face					
Gently massaged the scrub in small circular movements					
Did not use near eye area					
Massaged the face using basic facial manipulations					

Essential Rubrics continued

Performance Assessed	1	2	3	4	Improvement Plan
Removed massage cream using warm, moist towels, moist cleansing pads, or sponges					
Sponged face using cotton pledgets moistened with toner or freshener					
Applied a treatment mask using product formulated for the client's skin condition					
Removed mask using wet cotton pledgets, sponges, or towels					
Applied toner, astringent, or freshener					
Applied a moisturizer or sunscreen					

FACIAL FOR DRY SKIN PROCEDURE

Performance Assessed	1	2	3	4	Improvement Plan
Properly draped chair and client					
Removed eye makeup					
Applied cleanser					
Removed cleanser residue					
Steamed face					
Exfoliated face					
Applied eye cream under eyes					
Applied moisturizer or massage cream					
Performed basic facial manipulations					

Essential Rubrics continued

Performance Assessed	1	2	3	4	Improvement Plan
Removed massage cream					
Option #1: Performed galvanic treatment					
Option #2: Performed high-frequency treatment					
Applied additional moisturizer					
Applied mask					
Applied cold cotton eye pads					
Removed mask					
Applied toner					
Applied moisturizer or sunscreen					
Proceed with additional desired service					
Post-service cleanup and appointment scheduling completed					

FACIAL FOR OILY SKIN WITH OPEN COMEDONES PROCEDURE

Performance Assessed	1	2	3	4	Improvement Plan
Properly draped chair and client					
Removed eye makeup					
Applied cleanser					
Removed cleanser residue					
Steamed face					
Exfoliated face					
Applied desincrustation lotion or gel					
Extracted comedones					
Applied astringent					

Essential Rubrics continued

Performance Assessed	1	2	3	4	Improvement Plan
Applied high-frequency current					
If skin clogged, proceeded to mask step					
If not clogged, applied hydration fluid and performed massage manipulations					
Applied mask					
Removed mask					
Applied toner					
Applied moisturizer or sunscreen					
Proceeded with additional desired service					
Post-service cleanup and appointment scheduling completed					

FACIAL FOR ACNE-PRONE AND PROBLEM SKIN PROCEDURE

Performance Assessed	1	2	3	4	Improvement Plan
Properly draped chair and client					
Removed eye makeup					
Applied cleanser					
Removed cleanser residue					
Steamed face					
Applied desincrustation lotion or gel and removed					
Extracted comedones					
Applied high-frequency treatment					
Applied positive galvanic current					

Essential Rubrics continued

Performance Assessed	1	2	3	4	Improvement Plan
Performed facial massage manipulations					
Applied mask					
Removed mask					
Applied toner					
Applied moisturizer or sunscreen					
Proceeded with additional desired service					
Post-service cleanup and appointment scheduling completed					

Essential Review

Using the following words, fill in the blanks below to form a thorough review of Chapter 23, Facials. Words or terms may be used more than once or not at all.

5 to 7
7 to 10
astringents
clay masks
cleansing lotion
cleansing milk
client consultation
combination
dehydration
dry
effleurage
emollients
enzyme peels
essential oils
exfoliation
fresheners
from insertion to origin
fulling
gauze
gommage
hacking movement
hands and arms
massage
massage cream
microdermabrasion
modelage
moisturizers
motor
normal
oily
open skin pores
origin
paraffin
percussion
pétrissage
preservative
relaxation
rolling
soft hands
tonic lotions
treatment
vibration
warm, moist towels
wringing

1. ____________ creams are used to hydrate and condition the skin during the night when normal tissue repair is taking place.
2. ____________ can be used to hold in place certain mask ingredients that tend to run.
3. ____________ is a vigorous movement in which your hands are placed a little distance apart on both sides of the client's arm or leg. While working downward, a twisting motion is applied against the bones in the opposite direction.
4. ________________ is used to achieve good slip during a massage.
5. A water-based emulsion that can be used twice daily on normal and combination skin for the purpose of removing makeup and soil is known as ________________.
6. A non-foaming lotion cleanser for the face is called ________________.
7. A light, continuous movement applied with fingers and palms in a slow, rhythmic manner without pressure is called ________________.

Essential Review continued

8. A form of pétrissage in which the tissue is grasped, gently lifted, and spread out and used mainly on the arms is called ________________.

9. A shaking movement accomplished by rapid muscular contractions in the cosmetologist's arms, while the balls of the fingertips are pressed firmly on the point of application is known as ________________.

10. Oily or fatty ingredients that block moisture from leaving the skin are called ________________.

11. An enzyme peel in which a cream is applied to the skin before steaming and forms a hardened crust that is then massaged or "rolled" off the skin is called ________________.

12. Another name for chemical exfoliation procedures is ________________.

13. Aromatherapy refers to the therapeutic use of ________________.

14. Clay preparations used to stimulate circulation and temporarily contract the pores of the skin are ________________.

15. Cleansing cream is removed from the skin with tissues, moist cotton pads, facial sponges, or ________________.

16. Cosmetology services are generally limited to the scalp, face, neck, shoulders, upper chest, back, feet, lower legs, and ________________.

17. Every muscle and nerve has a ________________ point which is the point over the muscle where pressure or stimulation will cause contraction of the muscle.

18. Fresheners, tonics, and astringents are all used to remove excess cleansers and residue left behind by face wash cleansers and are called ________________.

19. In addition to a firm sure touch and strong flexible hands, quality massage requires self-control and ________________.

20. Maintaining the health of the facial skin by using correct cleansing methods, increasing circulation, relaxing the nerves, and activating the skin glands and metabolism through massage is known as ________________ facial treatment.

21. Masks that are melted at a little more than body temperature before application are ________________ masks.

22. Masks that contain special crystals of gypsum that harden when mixed with cold water immediately before application are ________________ masks.

Essential Review continued

23. Examples of mechanical exfoliants that work physically by bumping off dead cell buildup are granular scrubs, roll-off masks, and the use of ________________.

24. Skin that may have either oily and normal areas or normal and dry areas is known as ________________.

25. Skin that is lacking in oil and often dehydrated is considered to be ________________.

26. Skin that has an overabundance of sebum is considered to be ________________.

27. Skin that is usually in good condition and has an adequate supply of sebum and moisture is considered to be ________________.

28. Steam the face mildly with warm, moist towels or with a facial steamer in order to ________________.

29. The fixed attachment of one end of the muscle to a bone or tissue is called the ________________ of the muscle.

30. The most stimulating form of massage that is performed by tapping, slapping, or hacking movements is called ________________ or tapotement.

31. ________________ and astringents are usually stronger products, often with higher alcohol content, and are used to treat oilier skin types.

32. The manual or mechanical manipulation of the body by various movements to increase metabolism and circulation, promote absorption, and relieve pain is ________________.

33. The direction of massage movements should always be ____________________.

34. The result achieved through light but firm, slow rhythmic movements, or very slow, light hand vibrations over the motor points for a short time is ________________.

35. The ________________ movement involves pressing and twisting the tissues with a fast back-and-forth movement.

36. The condition that causes skin to feel dry and flaky because of an insufficient amount of water in the body is ________________.

37. The first step of all facial treatments is the ________________.

38. Use of the wrists and outer edges of hands in fast, light, firm, flexible motions against the skin in alternate succession is called ________________.

Essential Review continued

39. Water-based emulsions that are absorbed quickly without leaving any residue on the skin surface are called ________________.

40. When the skin is grasped between the fingers and palms and tissues are lifted from the underlying structures and squeezed, rolled, or pinched with light, firm pressure, it is called ________________.

Essential Discoveries and Accomplishments

In the space below, jot some notes about what concepts of this chapter were hardest for you to understand or remember. Imagine finding yourself suddenly in the role of "teacher" and consider what you would tell your "students" about these concepts. Share your Essential Discoveries with some of the other students in your class and ask if they are helpful to them. You may want to revise your discoveries based on good ideas shared by your peers.

Discoveries:

____

____

____

____

____

____

____

____

____

____

____

List at least three things you have accomplished since your last entry that relate to your career goals.

Accomplishments:

____

____

____

____

____

CHAPTER 24 Facial Makeup

A Motivating Moment: "Keep your face to the sunshine and you cannot see the shadow."
— Helen Adams Keller

Essential Objectives

After studying this chapter and completing the Essential Companion components, you will be able to:

1. **Describe the various types of cosmetics and their uses.**
2. **Demonstrate an understanding of cosmetic color theory.**
3. **Perform a consultation for the basic makeup procedure for any occasion.**
4. **Understand the use of special-occasion makeup.**
5. **Identify different facial types and demonstrate procedures for basic corrective makeup.**
6. **Demonstrate the application and removal of artificial lashes.**

Essential Facial Makeup

What makes applying makeup such a critical part of my career as a cosmetologist?

We have already discussed the fact that today's society is aging. As people age, they will do almost anything to feel and look younger. Women have the opportunity to apply makeup, which can do a great deal to emphasize their most attractive facial features and minimize those features that are not so attractive or are out of balance. Even though today's society places so much emphasis on this particular aspect of life, it is not a new concept. History shows that both men and women as far back as the New Stone Age used tattooing and body paint for ornamentation. Makeup has been used for tribal identification, religious ceremonies, preparation for war (remember Mel Gibson in the movie *Braveheart*), and a number of other occasions or events. The Egyptians were quite innovative and used a combination of ground alabaster or starch mixed with vegetable dyes and mineral salts.

We have Elizabeth Arden and Max Factor to thank for turning cosmetic makeup into an industry all its own back in the 1930s. Without a doubt cosmetic makeup is here to stay. For a cosmetologist, that means more opportunity and more money!

Cosmetologists should study and have a thorough understanding of facial makeup because:

- Clients will rely on you to advise them on tips and techniques that will help them look their best.
- You will want to use basic makeup techniques to enhance the hair and chemical services you provide for clients, offering them a total look that is harmonious and balanced.
- You will need to understand the various categories of facial makeup products available so that you know when and on whom they should be used.
- You will also learn about highlighting and contouring and will use these methods to help clients accent attractive features, hide not-so-attractive features, and change the appearance of their face shape.

Essential Concepts

What to do I need to know about facial makeup in order to provide a quality service?

You need to consider the structure of the client's face, the color of the eyes, skin, and hair. You will need to consider how the client wants to look, keeping in mind the reasonable results you will be able to achieve. For example, you can't change a huge nose into a petite nose. You can, however, artistically and scientifically apply makeup and arrange hair so as to minimize the size of the nose. You will truly become an artist when you can apply color, shading, and highlighting to create illusions that present the client in the most attractive manner. You will need to know all the techniques used for face shapes and features, and, as a professional cosmetologist, you will be able to apply all those techniques combined with the appropriate hair color and design to create the best possible image for your client.

1 Essential Experience

Commercial Cosmetics

Choose a partner and conduct a joint research project. Your goal is to create a collage of commercial cosmetics in at least two categories, such as daytime makeup, evening makeup, normal skin, dry skin, or oily skin.

Look through industry and fashion magazines and choose ads that depict various types of cosmetics, such as lipstick, eye cream, moisturizer, foundation, mascara, etc. Cut out the ads, use colored markers, and any other implements to create an artistic representation for your chosen category.

Your collage, built on a large poster board or other suitable background, should depict a complete cosmetic and skin care regimen for the category you have chosen.

Be prepared to do an oral presentation to your classmates about your project, explaining each product's purpose and how it is used.

Essential Experience 2

Windowpane Face Shapes

Windowpaning is the process of transferring key elements, points, or steps in a lesson into visual images that are hand sketched into the squares or *panes* of a matrix. Let your mind think in pictures and sketch the essential concepts printed in each of the following windowpanes. Don't be concerned with your artistic ability. Use lines and stick figures to depict the concepts requested.

Oval Face Shape
Round Face Shape
Square Face Shape
Triangle Face Shape
Inverted Triangle Face Shape
Diamond Face Shape
Oblong Face Shape

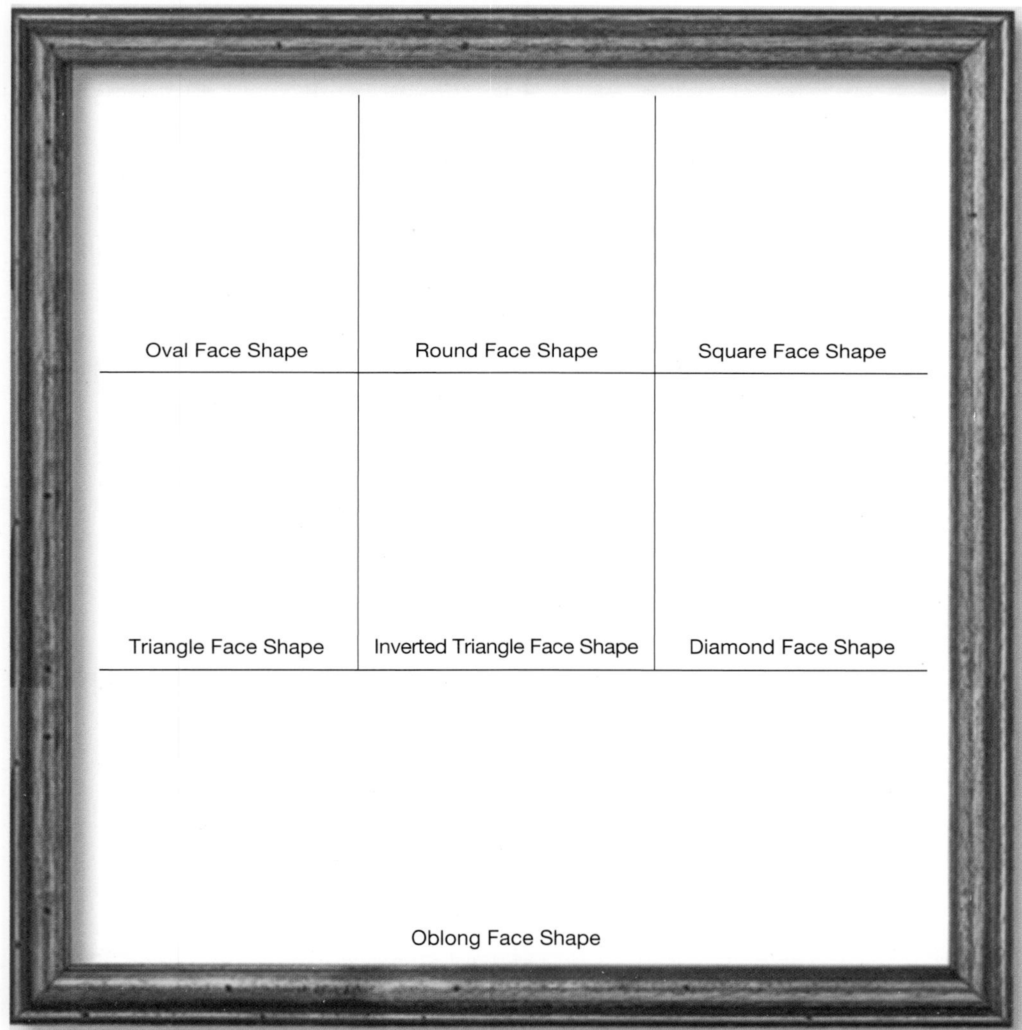

3

Essential Experience

Word Scramble

Using the clues provided, unscramble the terms below.

Scramble	**Correct Word**
ragel sone	_ _ _ _ _ _ _ _ _ *Clue:* Apply a darker foundation on the nose and a lighter foundation on the cheeks at the sides of the nose.
talf seon	_ _ _ _ _ _ _ _ *Clue:* Apply a lighter foundation down the center of the nose, stopping at the tip.
esolc tes seye	_ _ _ _ _ _ _ _ _ _ _ _ *Clue:* Apply shadow lightly up from the outer edge of the eyes.
wanorr enaliwj	_ _ _ _ _ _ _ _ _ _ _ _ _ *Clue:* Highlight by using a lighter shade foundation over the prominent area of the jawline.
ayveh dilded	_ _ _ _ _ _ _ _ _ _ _ *Clue:* Shadow evenly and lightly across the lid from the edge of the eyelash line to the small crease in the eye socket.
tsorh chtik nekc	_ _ _ _ _ _ _ _ _ _ _ _ _ _ *Clue:* Use a darker foundation on the neck than the one used on the face.
doarb osen	_ _ _ _ _ _ _ _ _ *Clue:* Use a darker foundation on the side of the nose and nostrils.
wedi tes	_ _ _ _ _ _ _ *Clue:* Extend brow lines to inside corners of the eye.
doabr wajenil	_ _ _ _ _ _ _ _ _ _ _ _ *Clue:* Apply a darker shade of foundation over the heavy area of the jaw, starting at the temples.
ugnibgl yees	_ _ _ _ _ _ _ _ _ _ _ *Clue:* Minimize by blending the shadow carefully over the prominent part of the upper lid.

Essential Experience continued 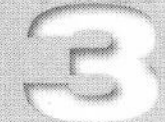

gnol niht kcne — — — — — — — — — — — —

Clue: Apply a lighter shade foundation on the neck than the one used on the face.

dnuor seye — — — — — — — — — —

Clue: Lengthen by extending the shadow beyond the outer corner of the eyes.

4 Essential Experience

Corrective Lip Treatment

On the diagrams below, use colored pencils to illustrate how lipstick can be applied to create the illusion of more balanced and proportioned lips.

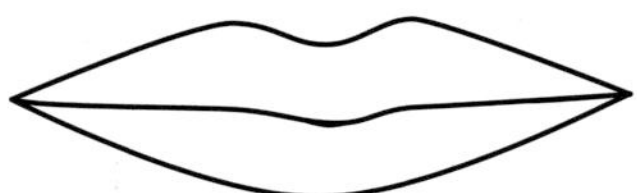

Thin lower lip

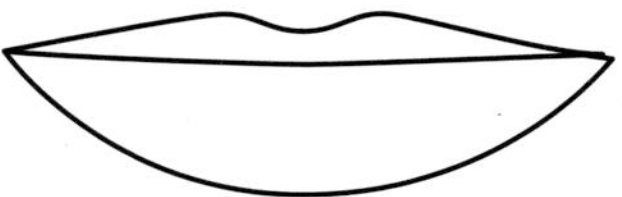

Thin upper lip

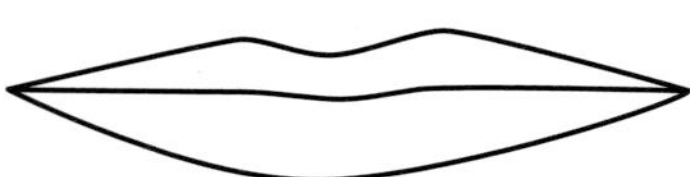

Thin lips

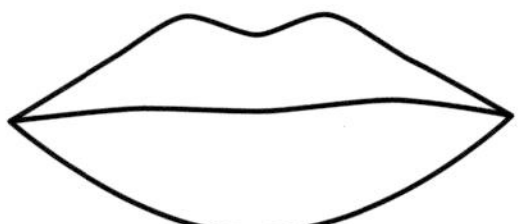

Small mouth

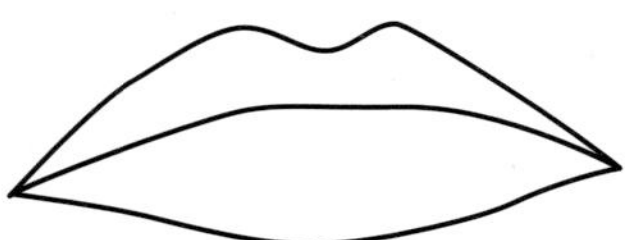

Drooping corners

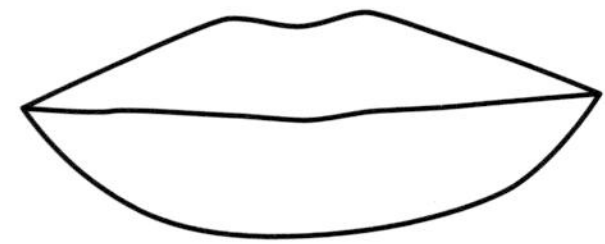

Oval lips

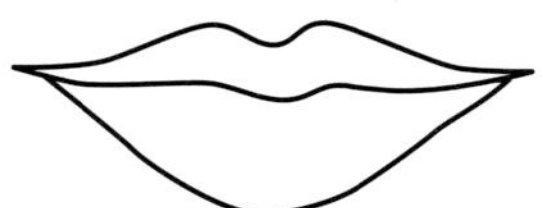

Sharp peaks

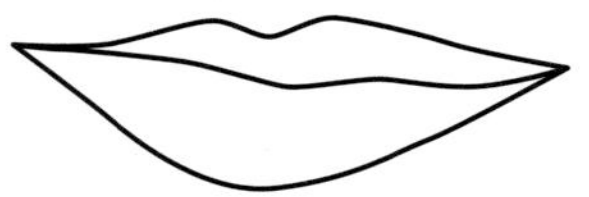

Uneven lips

Essential Experience 5

Crossword Puzzle

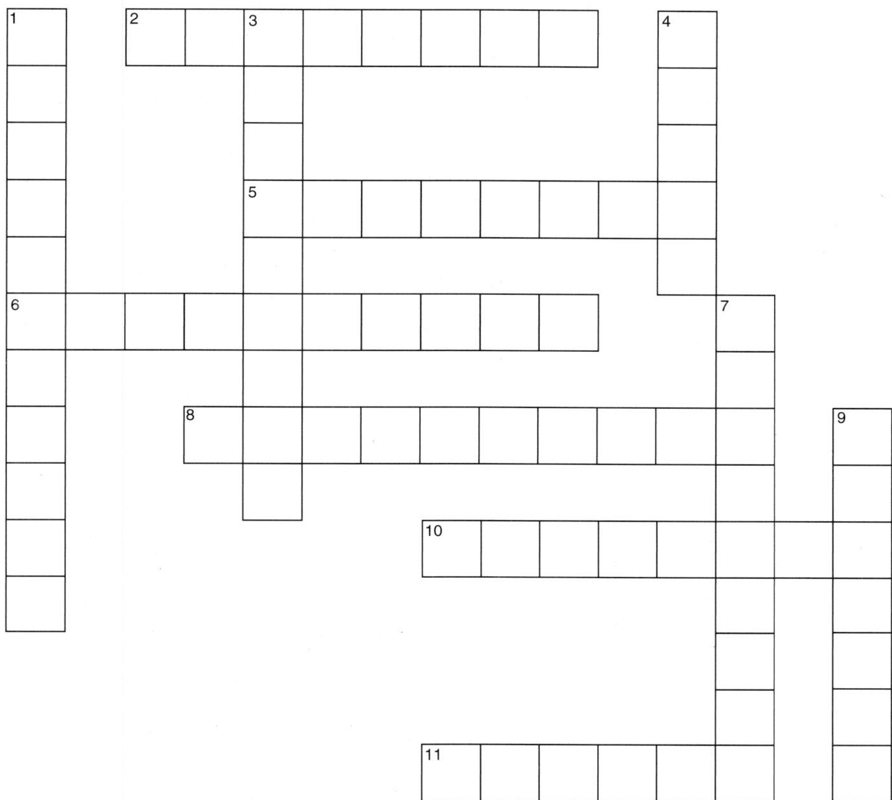

Across

Word	Clue
________________	**2.** Part of a complete and effective makeup application if well groomed
________________	**5.** Used to remove makeup from containers
________________	**6.** Individual artificial eyelashes
________________	**8.** Base or protective film
________________	**10.** Used to remove excess facial hair
________________	**11.** Used to add matte finish to face

5 Essential Experience continued

Down

Word	**Clue**
______________	**1.** Used for theatrical purposes
______________	**3.** Used to accentuate eyelids
______________	**4.** Used to color cheeks
______________	**7.** Used to cover blemishes
______________	**9.** Used to darken, define, and thicken lashes

Essential Experience 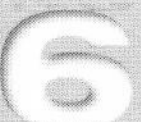

Band Lash Procedure

Number the following steps in the preparation, procedure, and cleanup activities for applying artificial band eyelashes in the order they should occur.

Procedure

______ Apply adhesive. Apply a thin strip of lash adhesive to the base of the lash and allow a few seconds for it to set.

______ Prepare lashes. Brush the client's eyelashes to make sure they are clean and free of foreign matter, such as mascara particles. If the client's lashes are straight, they can be curled with an eyelash curler before you apply the artificial lashes.

______ Carefully remove the eyelash band from the package.

______ Feather lash. Feather the lash by nipping into it with the points of your scissors. This creates a more natural look.

______ Apply the lower lash. Lower lash application is optional, as it tends to look more unnatural. Trim the lash as necessary and apply adhesive in the same way you did for the upper lash. Place the lash on top of the client's lower lash. Place the shorter lash toward the center of the eye and the longer lash toward the outer part of the lid.

______ Shape eyelash. Start with the upper lash. If it is too long to fit the curve of the upper eyelid, trim the outside edge. Use your fingers to bend the lash into a horseshoe shape to make it more flexible so it fits the contour of the eyelid.

______ Apply the lash. Start with the shorter part of the lash and place it on the inner corner of the eye, toward the nose. Position the rest of the artificial lash as close to the client's own lash as possible. Use the rounded end of a lash liner brush or tweezers to press the lash on. Be very careful and gentle when applying the lashes. If eyeliner is to be used, the line is usually drawn on the eyelid before the lash is applied and retouched when the artificial lash is in place.

Essential Rubrics

Rubrics are used in education for organizing and interpreting data gathered from observations of student performance. It is a clearly developed scoring document used to differentiate between levels of development in a specific skill performance or behavior. A rubric is provided in this study guide as a self-assessment tool to aid you in your behavior development.

Rate your performance according to the following scale:

(1) Development Opportunity: There is little or no evidence of competency; assistance is needed; performance includes multiple errors.

(2) Fundamental: There is beginning evidence of competency; task is completed alone; performance includes few errors.

(3) Competent: There is detailed and consistent evidence of competency; task is completed alone; performance includes rare errors.

(4) Strength: There is detailed evidence of highly creative, inventive, mature presence of competency.

Space is provided for comments to assist you in improving your performance and achieving a higher rating.

PROFESSIONAL MAKEUP APPLICATION PROCEDURE

Performance Assessed	1	2	3	4	Improvement Plan
Draped client					
Cleansed face and removed cleanser					
Applied astringent or toner					
Applied moisturizer					
Groomed eyebrows, if needed					
Applied foundation					
Blended foundation					
Applied concealer					
Applied powder					
Applied eye color					
Applied eyeliner					

Performance Assessed	1	2	3	4	Improvement Plan
Applied eyebrow color					
Applied mascara					
Applied cheek color					
Applied lip color					

BAND LASH APPLICATION PROCEDURE

Performance Assessed	1	2	3	4	Improvement Plan
Draped client					
Removed contact lenses, if applicable					
Removed makeup					
Brushed eyelashes					
Removed eyelash back from package					
Trimmed eyelash band to fit eye					
Feathered lash if needed					
Applied thin strip of adhesive					
Applied upper band lashes					
Applied lower band lashes if desired					

Essential Review

Using the following words, fill in the blanks below to form a thorough review of Chapter 24, Facial Makeup. Words or terms may be used more than once or not at all.

antiseptic	**eye tabbing**	**paste-like**
bleeding	**eyeliner**	**pink**
blend	**face powder**	**powder foundation**
blues	**foundation**	**shape**
cheek color	**frame**	**smooth**
complementary	**high arch**	**straight**
concealers	**inner rim**	**strip**
contour	**lighter**	**thicker**
cream	**lip**	**widening**
discolorations	**matte**	**yellow**
double-dip	**paraffin**	**yellow or gold**

1. Affixing individual eyelashes to a client is referred to as ______________.
2. A cosmetic, usually tinted, that is used as a base or as a protective film applied before powder is known as ______________.
3. ______________ foundation, also known as oil-based, is a considerably thicker product, often sold in a jar or a tin and may or may not contain water.
4. Mineral __________________ is applied with a large fluffy brush and contains a lot of pigment for coverage.
5. ______________ are available in tins, jars, and tubes with wands in a range of colors to coordinate with or match natural skin tones.
6. ______________ is a cosmetic powder, sometimes tinted or scented, that is used to add a matte or nonshiny finish to the face.
7. ______________ gives a natural-looking glow to the cheeks, but can also be used to add a little color to the face.
8. When applying cheek color, ______________ outward and upward toward the temples.
9. Lip color is a cosmetic in a ______________ form, usually in a metal or plastic tube, manufactured in a wide range of colors.

Essential Review continued

10. In addition to outlining the lips, lip liner helps to keep lip color from ______________ into the small lines around the mouth.

11. Eye shadows are applied on the eyelids to accentuate or contour them and come in a variety of finishes, including metallic, ______________, frost, shimmer, and dewy.

12. A highlight color is ______________ than the client's skin tone and may have any finish, including matte or iridescent.

13. A ______________ color is deeper and darker than the client's skin tone and is applied to minimize a specific area to create contour.

14. The cosmetic used to outline and emphasize the eyes is called ______________.

15. Eyeliner pencils consist of a ______________ wax or hardened oil base with a variety of additives to create color.

16. According to the American Medical Association, eye pencils should not be used to color the ______________ of the eyes.

17. Eyebrow pencils or shadows are used to darken eyebrows, to fill in sparse areas, or to ______________ the eyebrows.

18. Mascara is used to enhance the natural lashes making them appear ______________ and longer.

19. Warm colors are dominated by ______________ tones.

20. Cool colors suggest coolness and are dominated by ______________.

21. When choosing eye makeup colors, consider contrasting eye color with ______________ colors to emphasize the eye color most effectively.

22. When choosing makeup colors, take care to coordinate cheek and ______________ colors within the same color family.

23. When applying mascara to a client, use a disposable mascara wand and dip into a clean tube of mascara, taking care to never ______________.

24. If eyes are close-set, they can be made to appear farther apart by ______________ the distance between the eyebrows and extending them outward slightly.

25. When arching brows for a long face, making them almost ______________ can create the illusion of a shorter face.

26. A square face will appear more oval if there is a ______________ on the ends of the eyebrows.

27. For ruddy skin, apply a ______________ or green foundation to affected areas, blending carefully.

28. For sallow skin, apply a ______________ or violet-based foundation on the affected areas and blend carefully into the jaw and neck.

29. Band lashes are also called ______________ lashes.

30. As a safety precaution when giving a facial, keep fingernails ______________ and avoid scratching the client's skin.

Essential Discoveries and Accomplishments

In the space below, jot some notes about what concepts of this chapter were hardest for you to understand or remember. Imagine finding yourself suddenly in the role of "teacher" and consider what you would tell your "students" about these concepts. Share your Essential Discoveries with some of the other students in your class and ask if they are helpful to them. You may want to revise your discoveries based on good ideas shared by your peers.

Discoveries:

____

____

____

____

____

____

____

____

____

____

____

List at least three things you have accomplished since your last entry that relate to your career goals.

Accomplishments:

____

____

____

____

____

CHAPTER 25–26

Manicuring & Pedicuring

This chapter contains information and activities related to both Chapter 25, Manicuring, and Chapter 26, Pedicuring, of *Milady Standard Cosmetology*, 2012 edition.

A Motivating Moment: "An optimist is a person who sees a green light everywhere. The pessimist sees only the red light. But the truly wise person is color blind."

— Dr. Albert Schweitzer

Essential Objectives

After studying this chapter and completing the Essential Companion components, you will be able to:

1. **Identify the four types of nail implements and/or tools required to perform a manicure or pedicure.**
2. **Explain the difference between reuseable and disposable implements.**
3. **Describe the importance of hand washing in nail services.**
4. **Explain why a consultation is necessary each time a client has a service in the salon.**
5. **Name the five basic nail shapes for women and the most popular nail shape for men.**
6. **List the types of massage movements most appropriate for a hand and arm massage.**
7. **Explain the difference between a basic manicure and a spa manicure.**
8. **Describe how aromatherapy is used in manicuring services.**

Essential Objectives continued

9. Explain the use and benefits of paraffin wax in manicuring.
10. Name the correct cleaning and disinfection procedure for nail implements, tools, and pedicure baths.
11. Describe a proper setup for the manicuring/pedicuring table.
12. List the steps in the post-service procedure.
13. List the steps taken if there is an exposure incident in the salon.
14. List the steps in the basic manicure.
15. Describe the proper technique for the application of nail polish.
16. Describe the procedure for a paraffin wax hand treatment before a manicure.
17. Describe a callus softener and how it is best used.
18. Explain the differences between a basic and a spa pedicure.
19. Describe reflexology and its use in pedicuring.
20. Describe the proper tool and technique to reduce the instance of an ingrown toenail.
21. Demonstrate the proper procedures for a basic pedicure and foot and leg massage.

Essential Manicuring and Pedicuring

Why are manicuring and pedicuring so important in my career as a cosmetologist?

It may help to understand a little of the history of manicuring in order to understand its relevance in today's society. The word manicure comes from the Latin word *manus* (which means hand) and the word *cura* (which means care). So, manicuring means just that, to improve the appearance of the hands and nails. You need to be able to provide this important service to your clients, but you also must maintain your own hands and nails in the best possible condition. After all, you will be touching your clients with your hands during every service you offer. It is important that your nails are smooth and do not scratch the client's skin or scalp.

The early societies of Egypt and China considered long, polished, and colored fingernails as a mark of distinction between the aristocrats and the commoners. Nails were shaped with pumice stones and colored with vegetable dyes. In the late 1800s, painted fingernails became a trend among the elite in Paris. Manicuring as a service and wearing nail polish became so popular in the 1920s that barber shops began to offer services for nails to both men and women. By the late 1950s, most states began to require licensure for this special service.

Cosmetologists should study and have a thorough understanding of manicuring and pedicuring because:

- It will enable you to offer your clientele a variety of services they want and enjoy.
- As a professional you should be able to easily recognize manicuring and pedicuring tools and how they are properly used.
- You will be able to perform a manicure or pedicure safely and correctly.

Essential Concepts

What do I need to know about manicuring and pedicuring in order to provide a quality service?

As with other services you provide, you will need to thoroughly consult with each client to learn what his or her specific desires are with the nail service. You will need to be able to file and shape the nails to the desired shape. You must be able to gather and properly use all the implements and equipment required in the various nail procedures. You will learn the importance of being able to provide an effective hand and arm or foot massage in manicuring and pedicuring.

1

Essential Experience

Windowpane Nail Shapes

Windowpaning is the process of transferring key elements, points, or steps in a lesson into visual images that are hand sketched into the squares or *panes* of a matrix. Let your mind think in pictures and sketch the essential concepts printed in each of the following windowpanes. Don't be concerned with your artistic ability. Use lines and stick figures to depict the concepts requested.

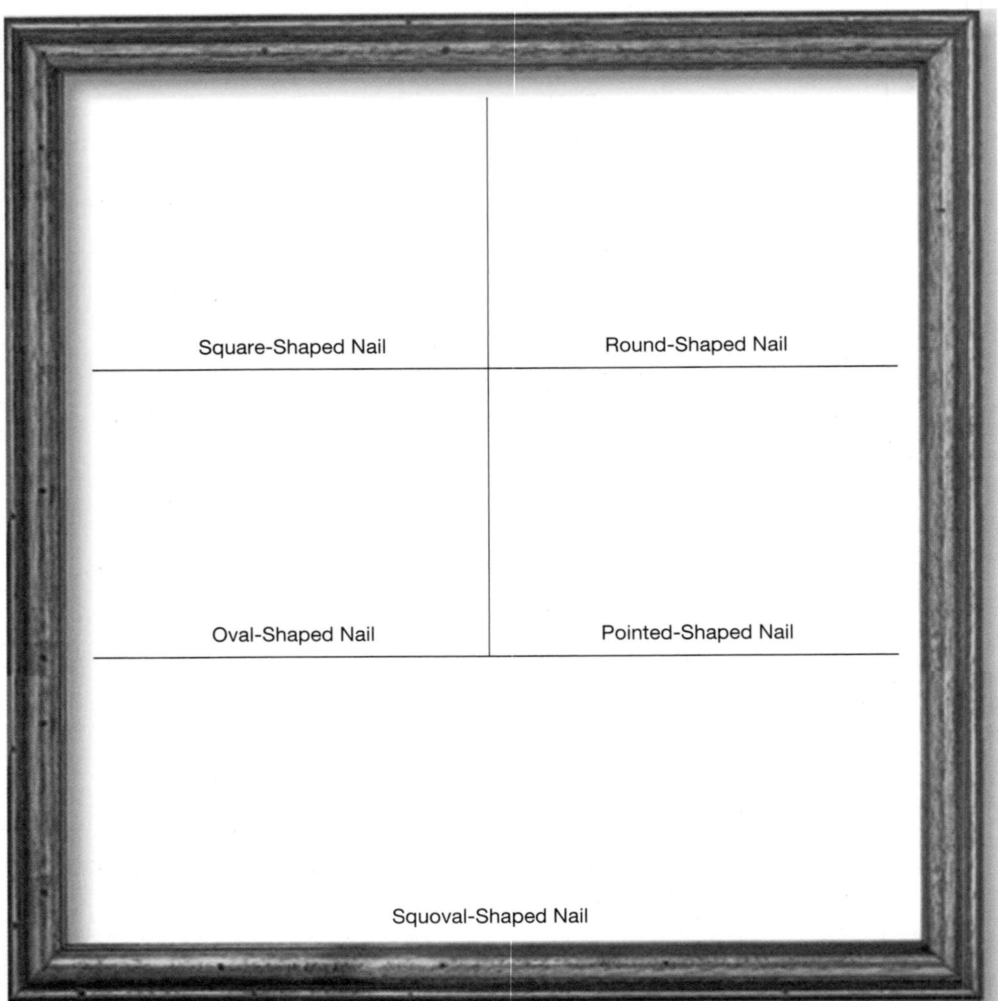

Essential Experience 2

Implements

Identify each of the manicuring implements depicted below.

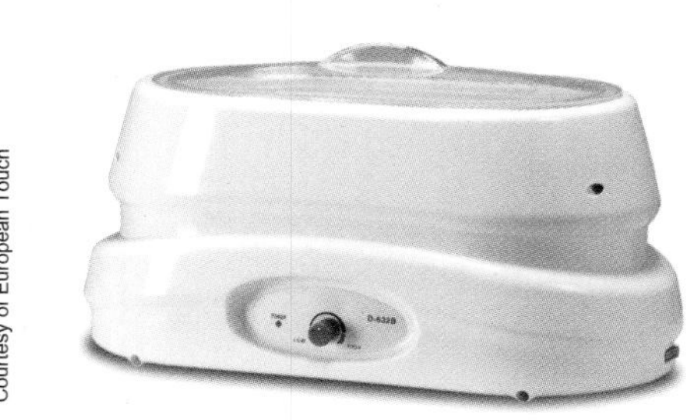

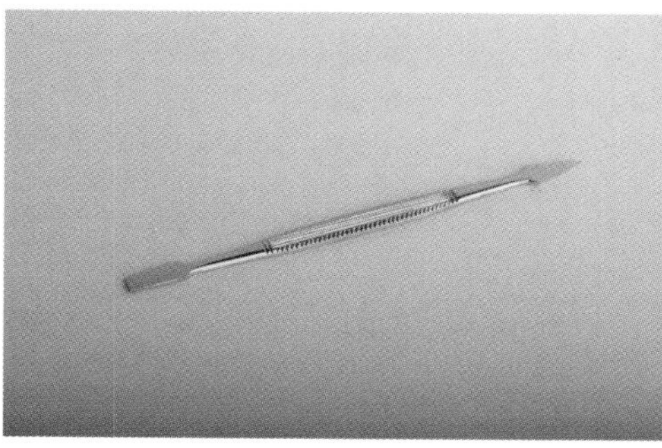

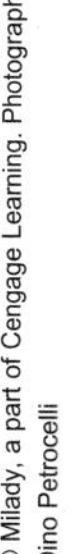

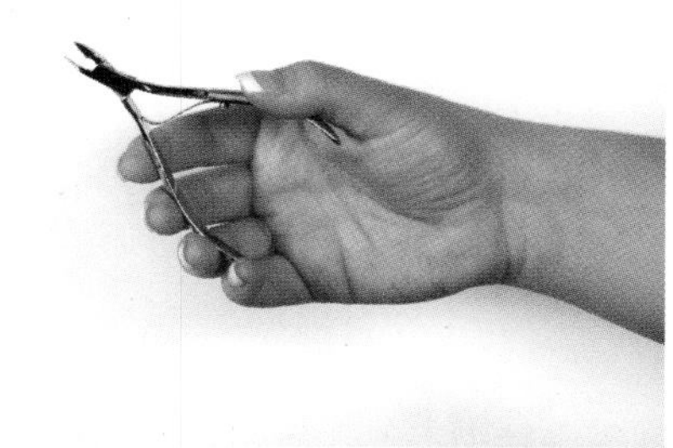

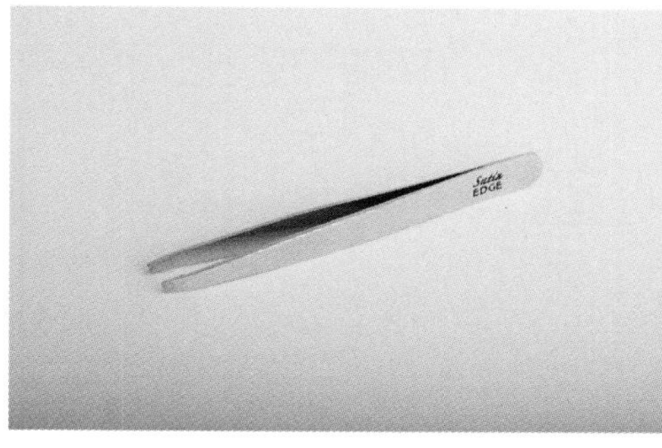

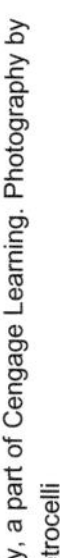

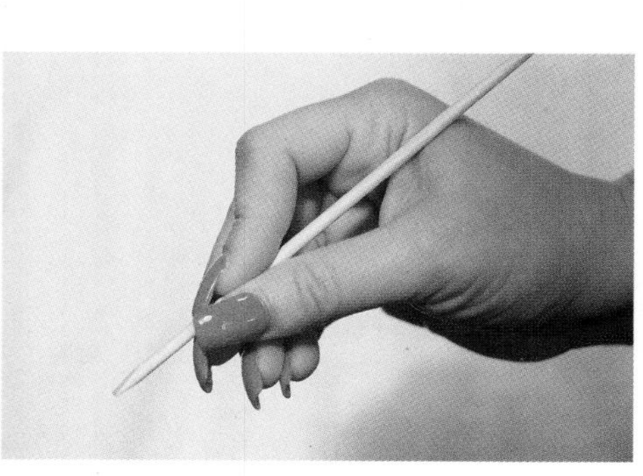

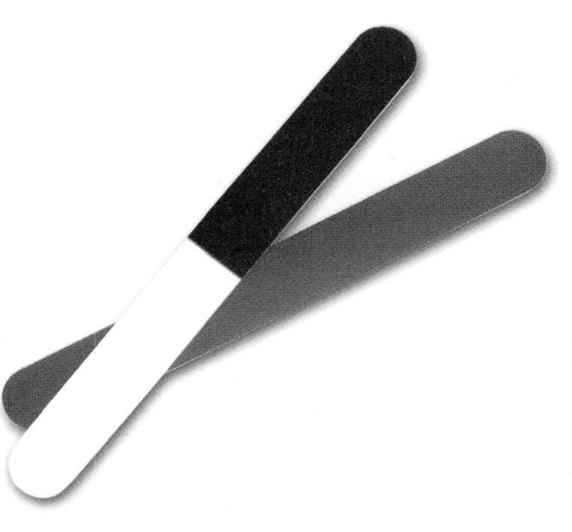

3 Essential Experience

Matching Exercise

Match the following essential terms with their identifying phrases or definition.

______ **Essential oil**	**1.** Used to add shine to the nail and smooth wavy ridges
______ **Chamois buffer**	**2.** Holds cosmetics
______ **Mild abrasives**	**3.** Used to lift small bits of debris from nail plate
______ **Cotton balls**	**4.** Used to clean fingernails
______ **Pumice powder**	**5.** Used to shorten the nail plate
______ **Supply tray**	**6.** Used to remove cuticle tissue from nail plate
______ **Wooden pusher**	**7.** Oils extracted using distillation from the seeds, bark, roots, leaves, wood, and/or resin of plants
______ **Tweezers**	**8.** Used to smooth nails and skin
______ **Nail brush**	**9.** Used to remove polish
______ **Nail clippers**	**10.** Abrasive derived from volcanic rock

Essential Experience

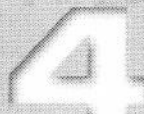

Word Scramble

Using the clues provided, unscramble the terms below.

Scramble	**Correct Word**
alin life	_ _ _ _ _ _ _ _ *Clue:* Used for shaping and smoothing the free edge.
litucce presinp	_ _ _ _ _ _ _ _ _ _ _ _ _ _ *Clue:* Used for trimming the cuticle.
lian fubref	_ _ _ _ _ _ _ _ _ _ *Clue:* Used for buffing and polishing the nail.
rengfi wblo	_ _ _ _ _ _ _ _ _ _ *Clue:* Holds warm, soapy water.
tuclice hspure	_ _ _ _ _ _ _ _ _ _ _ _ _ *Clue:* Loosens and pushes back the cuticle.
cirtleec retahe	_ _ _ _ _ _ _ _ _ _ _ _ _ _ *Clue:* Heats oil.
ailn sbruh	_ _ _ _ _ _ _ _ _ *Clue:* Used for cleansing nails and fingertips.
yulpps ytar	_ _ _ _ _ _ _ _ _ _ *Clue:* Holds cosmetics for the nails.
ezsewret	_ _ _ _ _ _ _ _ *Clue:* Used for lifting small bits of cuticle.
rnienaotc	_ _ _ _ _ _ _ _ _ *Clue:* Holds clean absorbent cotton.

5 Essential Experience

Table Setup Procedure

Put the following steps for a pre-service table setup procedure in the proper order.

______ Place polishes

______ Place finger bowl

______ Prepare for waste disposal

______ Prepare arm cushion

______ Prepare drawer

______ Fill disinfectant container

______ Clean table and drawer

______ Place abrasives and buffers

Essential Experience

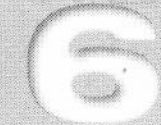

Pre-Service Procedure

Put the following steps for the pre-service procedure in the proper order.

_______ Wash hands

_______ Remove implements

_______ Store implements

_______ Clean implements

_______ Rinse implements

_______ Immerse implements

_______ Wear gloves

7 Essential Experience

Manicure Procedure

Put the following steps for a basic manicure in the appropriate order.

_______ Choose polish color

_______ Dry hands

_______ Repeat steps 5 through 10 on opposite hand

_______ Remove debris

_______ Loosen and remove cuticles

_______ Buff with high shine buffer

_______ Apply nail oil

_______ Brush nails

_______ Remove traces of oil

_______ Clean under free edge

_______ Apply cuticle remover

_______ Apply bleach

_______ Bevel nails

_______ Remove polish

_______ Apply lotion and massage

_______ Shape nails

_______ Soften eponychium

_______ Nip dead tags of skin

_______ Apply polish

Essential Experience 8

Partners for Pedicure

Choose a partner and provide a pedicure service to each other. Rate each other's procedure according to the following evaluation form. Circle the numeric score you would assign the service you just received, using the following rating scale.

1 = Poor; 2 = Below Average; 3 = Average; 4 = Good; 5 = Excellent

1 2 3 4 5 **1.** You were seated comfortably and asked to remove shoes and socks or stockings.

1 2 3 4 5 **2.** All required equipment, implements, and materials were arranged.

1 2 3 4 5 **3.** Your feet were placed on clean paper towels on a footrest.

1 2 3 4 5 **4.** Technician's hands were washed and sanitized.

1 2 3 4 5 **5.** Two basins were filled with warm water to cover ankles.

1 2 3 4 5 **6.** Antiseptic or antibacterial soap was added to one basin; both feet were placed in bath for three to five minutes.

1 2 3 4 5 **7.** Feet were removed, rinsed, and wiped dry.

1 2 3 4 5 **8.** Old polish was thoroughly removed from nails of both feet.

1 2 3 4 5 **9.** Toenails of left foot were clipped.

1 2 3 4 5 **10.** Toe separators were inserted.

1 2 3 4 5 **11.** Toenails were filed straight across, rounding them slightly at the corners to conform to the shape of the toes.

1 2 3 4 5 **12.** Foot file was used on ball and heel of left foot to remove dry skin and smooth down callus growth.

1 2 3 4 5 **13.** Toe separators were removed and left foot was placed in warm, soapy water.

1 2 3 4 5 **14.** Steps were completed on the right foot.

1 2 3 4 5 **15.** Left foot was removed from basin, rinsed, dried, and toe separators were inserted.

8 Essential Experience continued

1 2 3 4 5 **16.** Cuticle solvent was applied under free edge of each toenail of left foot with cotton-tipped orangewood stick.

1 2 3 4 5 **17.** Cuticle was gently loosened with the cotton-tipped orangewood stick. Cuticle was kept moist with additional lotion or water. Excessive pressure was not used. Cuticle was not cut.

1 2 3 4 5 **18.** Left foot was rinsed and dried.

1 2 3 4 5 **19.** Cream or lotions were applied.

1 2 3 4 5 **20.** Left foot was massaged and placed on a clean towel on floor.

1 2 3 4 5 **21.** Steps were repeated on the right foot.

1 2 3 4 5 **22.** Lotion or cream was removed from toenails.

1 2 3 4 5 **23.** Base coat, two color coats, and top coat were applied.

1 2 3 4 5 **24.** Post-service steps were completed.

Essential Experience 9

Select a partner and fill in the blanks below on the reflexology foot chart below. You may need to conduct research through the internet or other sources to find accurate information.

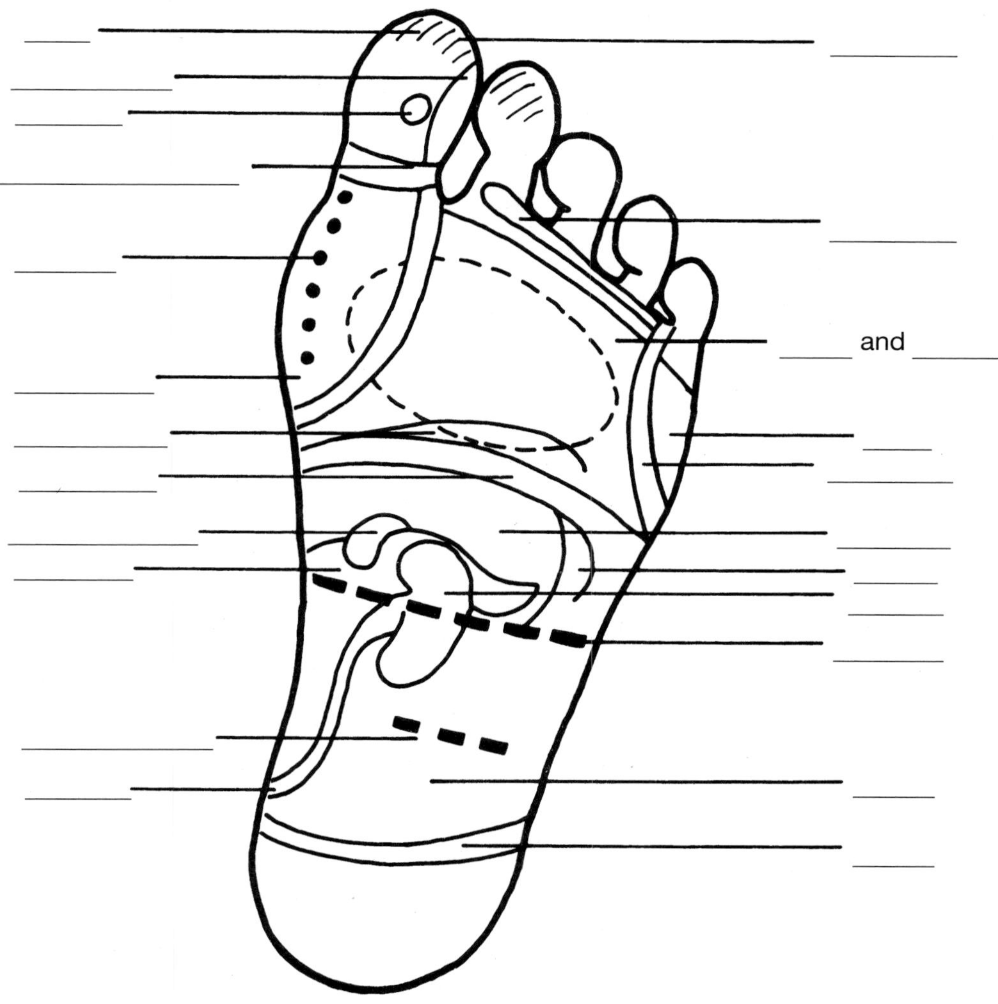

Essential Rubrics

Rubrics are used in education for organizing and interpreting data gathered from observations of student performance. It is a clearly developed scoring document used to differentiate between levels of development in a specific skill performance or behavior. A rubric is provided in this study guide as a self-assessment tool to aid you in your behavior development.

Rate your performance according to the following scale:

(1) Development Opportunity: There is little or no evidence of competency; assistance is needed; performance includes multiple errors.

(2) Fundamental: There is beginning evidence of competency; task is completed alone; performance includes few errors.

(3) Competent: There is detailed and consistent evidence of competency; task is completed alone; performance includes rare errors.

(4) Strength: There is detailed evidence of highly creative, inventive, mature presence of competency.

Space is provided for comments to assist you in improving your performance and achieving a higher rating.

MANICURE TABLE PREPARATION PROCEDURE

Performance Assessed	1	2	3	4	Improvement Plan
Cleaned table with disinfectant solution					
Prepared arm cushion					
Filled disinfectant container					
Placed abrasives					
Placed finger bowl and brush					
Prepared for waste disposal					
Placed polishes					
Prepared drawer					

PRE-SERVICE PROCEDURE

Performance Assessed	1	2	3	4	Improvement Plan
Wore gloves					
Cleaned implements					
Rinsed implements					
Immersed implements					
Removed implements					
Stored implements					
Washed hands					
Greeted client					
Client washed hands					
Used clean towels					
Made client comfortable					
Performed consultation					

POST-SERVICE PROCEDURE

Performance Assessed	1	2	3	4	Improvement Plan
Advised client on home maintenance					
Suggested needed retail products					
Scheduled next appointment					
Thanked client					
Recorded information					
Prepared work area					
Followed pre-service procedures					
Reset work area					

Essential Rubrics continued

HAND MASSAGE PROCEDURE

Performance Assessed	1	2	3	4	Improvement Plan
Applied massage lotion					
Performed relaxer movement					
Performed joint movement on fingers					
Performed circular movement in palm					
Performed circular movement on wrist					
Performed transition movement and finger massage					
Performed arm massage					
Performed under arm massage					
Performed elbow movement					
Pulled and pressed fingers and feathered off					
Covered client's hands					

BASIC MANICURE PROCEDURE

Performance Assessed	1	2	3	4	Improvement Plan
Removed polish					
Shaped the nails					
Softened eponychium					
Cleaned nails					
Dried hands					
Applied cuticle remover					

Performance Assessed	1	2	3	4	Improvement Plan
Loosened and removed cuticles					
Nipped dead skin tags					
Cleaned under free edge					
Removed hand from finger bowl					
Removed debris					
Repeated steps on opposite hand					
Applied bleach (optional)					
Buffed nails with high-shine buffer					
Applied nail oil					
Beveled nails					
Applied lotion and massaged					
Removed traces of oil					
Selected polish color					
Applied base coat					
Applied polish color					
Applied top coat					

BASIC PEDICURE PROCEDURE

Performance Assessed	1	2	3	4	Improvement Plan
Checked water temperature					
Soaked feet					
Dried feet thoroughly					
Removed existing polish					
Clipped nails					
Filed nails					
Rinsed foot					

Essential Rubrics continued

Performance Assessed	1	2	3	4	Improvement Plan
Wrapped foot in towel					
Repeated steps on other foot					
Removed dead tissue on first foot					
Exfoliated foot with scrub					
Used foot file					
Brushed nails					
Rinsed foot and dried thoroughly					
Repeated steps on opposite foot					
Applied cuticle remover					
Removed cuticle tissue and skin tags					
Used curette to push soft tissue away from nail plate walls					
Rinsed, brushed, and dried foot					
Applied lotion, cream, or oil					
Massaged foot					
Repeated steps on other foot					
Removed traces of lotion					
Inserted toe separators					
Applied polish					
Sprayed with rapid polish dryer					
Placed feet on towel to dry					

FOOT AND LEG MASSAGE

Performance Assessed	1	2	3	4	Improvement Plan
Performed relaxation movements to the joints of the foot					
Effleurage on top of foot					
Effleurage on the instep					
Effleurage on heel of the foot					
Fist twist compression (deep rubbing)					
Effleurage movement on toes					
Joint movement for toes					
Repeated all movements on the other leg/foot					
Feathered off					
Effleurage on the front of the leg					
Effleurage on the back of the leg					

Essential Review

Complete the following review of Chapter 25, Manicuring, and Chapter 26, Pedicuring, by circling the correct answer.

1. When you perform nail services, you use permanent tools called ____________.

a) equipment
b) implements
c) materials
d) cosmetics

2. Disposable implements include ____________.

a) nail clippers
b) metal pushers
c) tweezers
d) wooden pushers

3. In a manicure service, to shape the free edge you use a/an ____________.

a) wooden pusher
b) metal pusher
c) abrasive file
d) tweezers

4. During a manicure procedure, if you draw blood, the implement should be ____________.

a) cleaned and disinfected
b) rinsed with water
c) bagged and discarded
d) wiped off with cotton

5. The benefit of using nail clippers to shorten nail length is to ____________.

a) create high shine
b) strengthen weak nails
c) reduce filing time
d) reduce splitting

6. To smooth out wavy ridges and create a high shine use a/an ____________.

a) chamois buffer
b) ridge filler
c) abrasive file
d) nail clipper

7. When you perform nail services, those supplies used during a service that must be replaced for each client are called ____________.

a) equipment
b) implements
c) materials
d) cosmetics

Essential Review continued

8. Lamps attached to a manicure table should have a bulb of ____________ watts.
   a) 25 to 30
   b) 30 to 35
   c) 40 to 60
   d) 60 to 75

9. After you use metal implements and before you place them in disinfectant, they must be ____________.
   a) cleaned with a towel
   b) cleaned in autoclave
   c) rinsed in alcohol
   d) washed with soap and water

10. An oil manicure is a recommended treatment for ____________.
    a) flexible cuticles
    b) brittle nails
    c) short nails
    d) nail fungus

11. The implement used to clean fingernails and remove debris is called a ____________.
    a) nail file
    b) nail brush
    c) wooden pusher
    d) chamois buffer

12. All nondisposable implements must be ____________ in a disinfectant solution.
    a) quickly rinsed
    b) dipped slightly
    c) wiped thoroughly
    d) fully immersed

13. Removing nail cosmetics from their containers is accomplished with a ____________.
    a) wooden pusher
    b) plastic or metal spatula
    c) metal pusher
    d) cotton swab

14. Certain products such as alcohol, nail polish, nail monomers, and nail primers are considered to be ____________.
    a) harmful
    b) sanitizers
    c) self-disinfecting
    d) strengtheners

15. As an added service in a manicure, a hand massage may be given before ____________.
    a) polish
    b) pushing cuticles
    c) soaking fingers
    d) filing

Essential Review continued

16. After an oil manicure, before base coat is applied, you must ____________.

    a) soak fingers in finger bowl
    b) remove all traces of oil
    c) apply cuticle remover
    d) wash hands thoroughly

17. When removing nail polish from nails with wrap resins, a/an ____________ product is recommended.

    a) acetone
    b) oily
    c) non-acetone
    d) potassium

18. The best way to prevent excessive odors and control vapors from nail services in the salon is to use ____________.

    a) plastic trash can
    b) ventilated receptacles with lids
    c) multiple paper bags
    d) metal receptacle with self-closing lid

19. Products designed to hasten the drying of nail polishes may be sprayed on or applied with a ____________.

    a) wooden pusher
    b) cotton swab
    c) metal pusher
    d) dropper

20. One of the functions of a top coat or sealer is to make the nail polish ____________.

    a) dry more quickly
    b) adhere to nail plate
    c) resistant to chipping
    d) appear thick and smooth

21. Nail hardeners include those with reinforcing fibers such as nylon, protein, and ____________.

    a) potassium
    b) formaldehyde
    c) acetone
    d) UV gels

22. The base coat creates a colorless layer on the natural nail that improves ____________.

    a) adhesion of polish
    b) and smoothes ridges
    c) discoloration and stains
    d) strength and rigidity

23. Another name for nail polish is ____________.

    a) lotion
    b) cream
    c) lacquer
    d) oil

24. Yellow surface discoloration or stains on fingernails can be removed with ____________.

a) cuticle removers
b) penetrating oils
c) polish removers
d) nail bleaches

25. Products used to soften dry skin around the nail plate and to increase the flexibility of natural nails are ____________.

a) cuticle removers
b) penetrating oils
c) polish removers
d) nail bleaches

Essential Discoveries and Accomplishments

In the space below, jot some notes about what concepts of this chapter were hardest for you to understand or remember. Imagine finding yourself suddenly in the role of "teacher" and consider what you would tell your "students" about these concepts. Share your Essential Discoveries with some of the other students in your class and ask if they are helpful to them. You may want to revise your discoveries based on good ideas shared by your peers.

Discoveries:

____

____

____

____

____

____

____

____

____

____

____

List at least three things you have accomplished since your last entry that relate to your career goals.

Accomplishments:

____

____

____

____

____

CHAPTER 27–29

Advanced Nail Techniques

This chapter contains information and activities related to Chapters 27, 28, and 29 of *Milady Standard Cosmetology*, 2012 edition.

A Motivating Moment: "There are no evil thoughts except one: the refusal to think."

—Ayn Rand

Essential Objectives

After studying this chapter and completing the Essential Companion components, you will be able to:

1. **Identify the supplies, in addition to your basic manicuring table, that you need for nail tip application.**
2. **Name and describe the types of nail tips available and why it is important to properly fit them for your client.**
3. **List the types of fabrics used in nail wraps and explain the benefits of using each.**
4. **Demonstrate the stop, rock, and hold method of applying nail tips.**
5. **Demonstrate the Nail Tip Application Procedure.**
6. **Demonstrate the Nail Tip Removal Procedure.**
7. **Demonstrate the Nail Wrap Application Procedure.**
8. **Demonstrate the main difference between performing the Two-Week Fabric Wrap Maintenance and the Four-Week Fabric Wrap Maintenance.**
9. **Demonstrate how to remove fabric wraps and what to avoid.**

Essential Objectives continued

10. Explain monomer liquid and polymer powder nail enhancement chemistry and how it works.
11. Describe the apex, stress area, and sidewall, and tell where each is located on the nail enhancement.
12. Demonstrate the proper procedures for applying one-color monomer liquid and polymer powder nail enhancements over tips and on natural nails.
13. Demonstrate the proper procedures for applying two-color monomer liquid and polymer powder nail enhancements using forms over nail tips and on natural nails.
14. Describe how to perform a one-color maintenance service on nail enhancements using monomer liquid and polymer powder.
15. Demonstrate how to perform crack repair procedures.
16. Implement the proper procedure for removing monomer liquid and polymer powder nail enhancements.
17. Describe the chemistry and main ingredients of UV gels.
18. Describe when to use the one-color and two-color methods for applying UV gels.
19. Name and describe the types of UV gels used in current systems.
20. Identify the supplies needed for UV gel application.
21. Determine when to use UV gels.
22. Discuss the differences between UV light units and UV lamps.
23. Describe how to apply one-color UV gel on tips and natural nails.
24. Describe how to apply UV gels over forms.
25. Describe how to maintain UV gel nail enhancements.
26. Explain how to correctly remove hard UV gels.
27. Explain how to correctly remove soft UV gels.

Essential Advanced Nail Techniques

Why do I need to learn about advanced nail techniques to be successful?

The nail industry experienced great expansion when the first acrylic artificial nail extensions were introduced in the early 1970s. The popular singer and actress Cher started a trend of very long nails which were squared off at the ends. By the 1980s, manufacturers had developed products which created very natural-looking artificial nails. It was then that the nail industry became the fastest growing area in the entire field of cosmetology and it continues to grow. Cosmetologists who fine-tune their skills with manicuring, pedicuring, and advanced nail techniques can earn a very good income.

Cosmetologists should study and have a thorough understanding of advanced nail techniques because:

- Offering advanced nail services expands your service offerings and enables clients to have a "one stop shop" experience in your salon.
- Learning the proper technique for applying and removing nail tips will aid in helping your client keep her natural nails in the best possible health and condition.
- Understanding the types and uses of nail wraps will enable you to determine the appropriate wrap for your client's specific needs.
- An understanding of the chemistry of UV gel products will allow you to choose the best system and products to use in your salon.
- An understanding of how UV gel nails are made, applied, and cured will allow you to create a safe and efficient salon service.
- Clients often become loyal and steadfast when they receive excellent advanced nail services, maintenance, and removal.

Essential Concepts

What do I need to know about advanced nail techniques in order to provide a quality service?

You will need to become familiar and experienced with a variety of advanced nail techniques from nail tips and wraps to acrylic nail applications. It has been said that with today's technology, there is no reason for anyone who wants long beautiful nails not to have them. As a professional cosmetologist, you need to be prepared to deliver those services that will meet that need.

Essential Experience 1

Windowpane Monomer Liquid Polymer Powder (MLPP)

Windowpaning is the process of transferring key elements, points, or steps in a lesson into visual images that are hand sketched into the squares or *panes* of a matrix. Let your mind think in pictures and sketch the essential concepts printed in each of the following windowpanes. Don't be concerned with your artistic ability. Use lines and stick figures to depict the concepts requested.

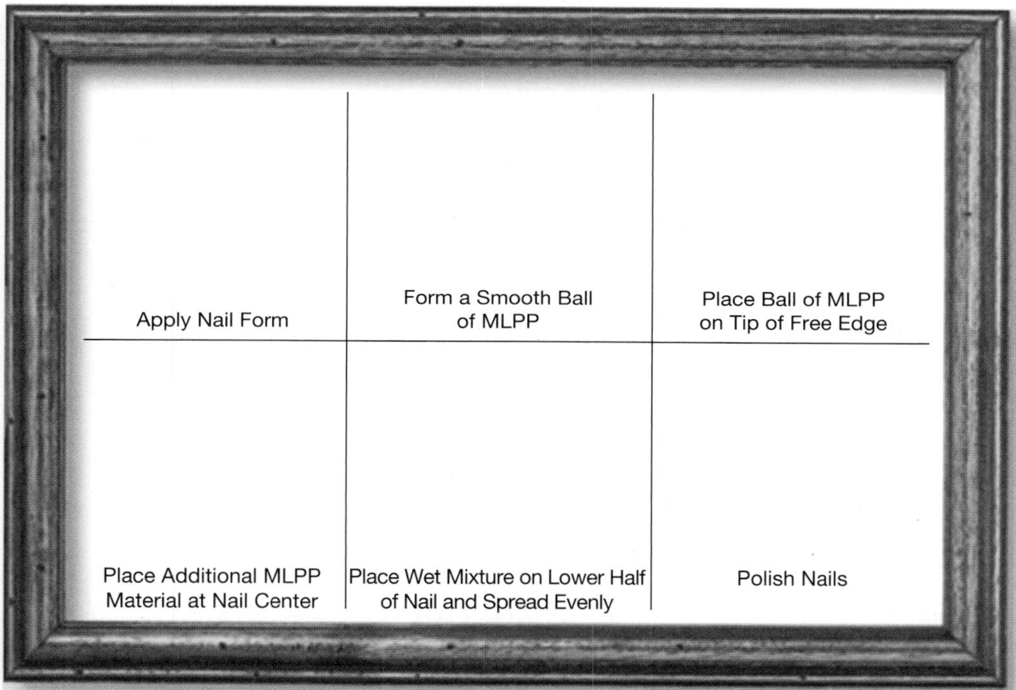

2 Essential Experience

Pre-Service Procedure

Number the following steps in order for an advanced nail technique pre-service procedure.

Cleaning

_______ Rinse implements

_______ Wear gloves

_______ Immerse implements in disinfectant

_______ Clean implements with soap, warm water, and nail brush

_______ Remove gloves and wash hands

_______ Store implements in clean, dry container

_______ Fill disinfectant container and immerse cleaned implements

_______ Place fingerbowl with warm water and nail brush on table

_______ Prepare drawer with extra cleaned materials

_______ Have client wash his/her hands

_______ Greet client

_______ Remove implements, rinse, and dry

_______ Clean manicure table and drawer

_______ Prepare arm cushion

_______ Place abrasives and buffers

_______ Prepare for waste disposal

_______ Place polishes

_______ Perform consultation

_______ Use clean towels

_______ Make client comfortable

Essential Experience 3

Post-Service Procedure

Number the following steps in order for an advanced nail technique post-service procedure.

_______ Record information. Record service information, products used, observations, and retail recommendations on the client consultation card.

_______ Home maintenance. Proper home maintenance will ensure that the nail service looks beautiful until your client returns for another service.

_______ Schedule next appointment. Escort the client to the front desk to schedule the next appointment and to pay for the service. Set up date, time, and services for your client's next appointment. Write the information on your business card and give it to the client.

_______ Retail products. Depending on the service provided, there may be a number of retail products that you should recommend for the client to take home. This is the time to do so. Explain why they are important and how to use them.

_______ Thank client. Before you return to your station and the client leaves the salon, be sure to thank her for her business.

_______ Follow pre-service procedures. Follow steps for disinfecting implements in the pre-service procedure. Reset work area with disinfected tools.

_______ Prepare work area. Remove your products and tools, then clean your work area and properly dispose of all used materials.

4 Essential Experience

Word Scramble

Using the clues provided, unscramble the terms below.

Scramble **Correct Word**

aosylrev _ _ _ _ _ _ _ _

Clue: Any wraps, acrylic, or gel applied over the entire natural nail plate or tip.

remirp _ _ _ _ _ _

Clue: Used to help adhere enhancements to the natural nail.

aetoddyrrh _ _ _ _ _ _ _ _ _ _

Clue: Substance used to remove surface moisture and tiny amounts of oil left on the natural nail plate.

ernmoom _ _ _ _ _ _ _

Clue: Substance made up of many small molecules that are not attached to one another.

irnguc _ _ _ _ _ _

Clue: Hardening process that occurs when powdered and liquid acrylic are combined to form nails.

istp _ _ _ _

Clue: Pre-formed artificial nails applied to the tips of the natural nails.

mryeolp _ _ _ _ _ _ _

Clue: Hard substance formed by combining many small molecules, usually in a long chain-like structure.

nagricnlabe _ _ _ _ _ _ _ _ _ _ _

Clue: Redefining the shape of the acrylic nail during a fill procedure.

pclusdertu _ _ _ _ _ _ _ _ _ _

Clue: Artificial nails created by combining a monomer liquid and polymer powder to form a nail enhancement.

slge _ _ _ _

Clue: Strong, durable artificial nails that are brushed on the nail plate.

Essential Experience continued 4

spwar — — — — —

Clue: Corrective treatments that form a protective coating for damaged or fragile nails.

ytaasltc — — — — — — — — —

Clue: Any substance having the power to increase the velocity of a chemical reaction.

5 Essential Experience

Word Search

After determining the correct word from the clues provided, locate the words in the word search puzzle.

Word	Clue
________________	Refers to an entire family of thousands of different substances that share closely related features
________________	Hardening process for acrylic nails
________________	Gel nail that hardens when exposed to a special light source, either ultraviolet or halogen
________________	Substance made from many small molecules that are not attached to each other
________________	Corrective treatment that forms a protective coating for damaged or fragile nails
________________	Gel nail that hardens when an activator or accelerator is sprayed or brushed on
________________	Any wrap, acrylic, or gel applied over the entire natural nail plate
________________	Hard substance formed by combining many small molecules, usually in a long chain-like structure
________________	Point where the nail plate meets the tip before it is glued to the nail
________________	Substance that improves adhesion and prepares surface for bonding
________________	Redefining the shape of acrylic nails during a fill procedure

Essential Experience continued 5

A	C	R	Y	L	I	C	N	A	I	L	S	R	Q	X	M	Q	Z
D	S	V	B	J	N	P	O	T	S	N	O	I	T	I	S	O	P
I	R	Y	P	G	F	X	L	C	E	L	U	M	B	C	E	H	P
N	E	N	A	Y	T	R	G	H	U	U	M	O	G	I	I	R	M
N	B	O	S	L	A	Z	Y	I	D	P	U	W	A	P	I	O	G
W	A	L	H	U	R	L	A	D	E	F	J	C	V	M	N	L	E
G	L	I	P	Q	B	E	R	Y	B	D	H	A	E	O	E	S	O
N	A	G	E	D	B	J	V	E	T	B	N	R	M	G	P	I	S
I	N	H	T	E	Z	Q	D	O	V	R	E	E	D	P	U	A	F
P	C	T	J	N	R	S	L	I	C	O	R	E	K	M	A	C	E
P	I	G	W	K	I	C	C	O	R	I	R	W	I	T	Q	M	N
A	N	E	M	L	E	U	N	Q	P	U	L	C	L	K	T	Y	A
R	G	L	P	R	H	X	R	O	C	P	Y	Y	U	P	G	O	N
W	N	Q	Z	W	I	H	L	T	W	J	J	K	R	R	E	A	D
L	L	K	U	U	C	Y	H	M	Z	C	Q	T	D	C	I	Q	C
I	H	L	Y	L	M	G	M	X	U	B	G	D	X	A	A	N	N
A	O	T	P	E	I	N	P	H	D	L	Q	W	Y	M	V	Y	G
N	T	O	R	L	Z	Q	Y	X	K	T	Z	S	J	G	S	M	B

6 Essential Experience

Client Consultation

Develop several open-ended questions that you would use in a client consultation prior to an advanced nail technique service and write them in the space provided.

1. ____

____

2. ____

3. ____

____

4. ____

5. ____

6. ____

____

____

____

7. ____

____

____

8. ____

9. ____

____

Essential Experince 7

Steps for Applying Two-Color MLPP Enhancements Using Forms

In your own words list the steps for applying two-color monomer liquid polymer powder nail enhancements using forms in the space provided.

1. ______________________________

2. ______________________________

____

3. ______________________________

____

4. ______________________________

5. ______________________________

____

____

____

____

____

____

____

____

____

6. ______________________________

____

____

____

____

____

____

____

____

7 Essential Experience continued

7.

8.

9.

10.

Essential Experience continued

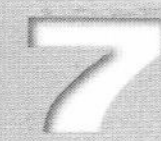

11.

12.

13.

14.

15.

16.

17.

18.

7 Essential Experience continued

19. ____

____

20. ____

____

____

____

21. ____

22. ____

23. ____

____

24. ____

____

25. ____

Essential Rubrics

Rubrics are used in education for organizing and interpreting data gathered from observations of student performance. It is a clearly developed scoring document used to differentiate between levels of development in a specific skill performance or behavior. A rubric is provided in this study guide as a self-assessment tool to aid you in your behavior development.

Rate your performance according to the following scale.

(1) Development Opportunity: There is little or no evidence of competency; assistance is needed; performance includes multiple errors.

(2) Fundamental: There is beginning evidence of competency; task is completed alone; performance includes few errors.

(3) Competent: There is detailed and consistent evidence of competency; task is completed alone; performance includes rare errors.

(4) Strength: There is detailed evidence of highly creative, inventive, mature presence of competency.

Space is provided for comments to assist you in improving your performance and achieving a higher rating.

NAIL TIP APPLICATION PROCEDURE

Performance Assessed	1	2	3	4	Improvement Plan
Removed polish					
Cleaned nails					
Pushed back eponychium					
Removed cuticle tissue					
Buffed nail/removed shine					
Applied dehydrator					
Sized tips					
Applied adhesive					
Slid on tips with stop, rock, and hold procedure					
Trimmed nail tip					
Finished blending using medium- to fine-grit buffing block					
Shaped nail					

TIP REMOVAL PROCEDURE

Performance Assessed	1	2	3	4	Improvement Plan
Soaked tips and nails in acetone					
Gently slid off softened tip using pusher					
Did not pry tip off nail					
Buffed nail with fine block buffer					

NAIL WRAP APPLICATION PROCEDURE

Performance Assessed	1	2	3	4	Improvement Plan
Removed existing polish					
Cleaned nails					
Pushed back the eponychium and removed the cuticle					
Removed the oily shine by buffing lightly with a medium/fine abrasive					
Shaped free edges of natural nails to match shape of nail tip stop point					
Removed dust with clean, dry, disinfected nail brush					
Applied nail dehydrator					
Applied nail tips if desired					
Cut fabric to width and shape of nail plate or tip					
Applied layer of resin wrap to entire surface					
Kept resin off skin					
Removed backing from fabric and gently fit over nail plate					
Placed fabric 1⁄16-inch (1.5 mm) away from sidewall and eponychium					

Essential Rubrics continued

Performance Assessed	1	2	3	4	Improvement Plan
Pressed to smooth it onto the nail plate using plastic					
Trimmed fabric if necessary					
Drew a thin coat of wrap resin down center of nail using extender tip					
Did not touch the skin					
Used plastic to make sure resin was evenly distributed					
Applied wrap resin accelerator according to manufacturer's instructions					
Kept wrap resin accelerator off skin					
Applied second coat of wrap resin					
Sealed free edge with wrap resin by running extender tip on edge of nail					
Applied second coat of wrap resin accelerator					
Shaped and refined nails using medium/fine abrasive					
Applied nail oil					
Buffed wrapped nail to a high shine with fine buffer					
Applied lotion and performed hand and arm massage					
Had client wash hands at sink to remove traces of oil, dust, and contaminants					
Applied polish					

TWO-WEEK FABRIC WRAP MAINTENANCE PROCEDURE

Performance Assessed	1	2	3	4	Improvement Plan
Removed existing polish with non-acetone remover					
Cleaned natural nails					
Pushed back eponychium and carefully removed cuticle from the nail plate					
Lightly buffed the nail plate to remove oily shine					
Removed dust with nail brush					
Applied nail dehydrator					
Applied wrap resin to new nail growth area					
Spread resin with extender tip					
Did not touch skin					
Applied wrap resin accelerator according to manufacturer's instructions					
Applied wrap resin to entire nail plate to strengthen and reseal nail wrap					
Applied second coat of wrap resin accelerator					
Shaped and refined nail wrap with medium/fine abrasive to remove high spots					
Applied nail oil					
Buffed wrapped nails to a high shine with fine buffer					
Applied hand lotion and massaged hand and arm					
Removed traces of oil using a small piece of cotton or plastic-backed cotton pad					
Applied polish					

Essential Rubrics continued

FOUR-WEEK FABRIC WRAP MAINTENANCE PROCEDURE

Performance Assessed	1	2	3	4	Improvement Plan
Removed existing polish					
Cleaned nails with nail brush, liquid soap, and warm running water					
Pushed back the eponychium and gently removed the cuticle					
Buffed nail with medium/ fine abrasive to smooth and remove shine					
Did not file into the natural nail surface					
Removed dust with brush					
Applied nail dehydrator					
Cut fabric large enough to cover new growth area and slightly overlap old wrap					
Applied wrap resin to the fill area					
Spread with extender tip or brush-on adhesive					
Did not touch skin					
Gently fit fabric over new growth area and smoothed					
Applied wrap resin					
Did not touch skin					
Applied wrap resin accelerator according to manufacturer's instructions					
Applied second coat of wrap resin					
Applied second coat of wrap resin accelerator					
Applied wrap resin to entire nail to strengthen and seal wrap					
Apply wrap resin accelerator					

Performance Assessed	1	2	3	4	Improvement Plan
Shaped and refined nails using medium/fine abrasive to remove high spots and imperfections					
Did not cut or damage skin around eponychium and sidewalls					
Applied nail oil					
Buffed nails to a high shine					
Applied hand lotion and massaged hand and arm					
Removed traces of oil using cotton ball or plastic backed pad and non-acetone polish remover					

FABRIC WRAP REMOVAL PROCEDURE

Performance Assessed	1	2	3	4	Improvement Plan
Soaked nails in acetone					
Used pusher to slide softened wraps away from nail plate					
Did not pry off wrap					
Gently buffed natural nail with fine abrasive to remove wrap resin					
Conditioned skin around nail plate with nail oils or lotions					

Essential Review

Complete the following review of Advanced Nail Techniques, Chapters 27 through 29, by circling the correct answer.

1. UV gel enhancements rely on ingredients from the ____________ family.
   a) resin wrap activator
   b) monomer liquid polymer powder
   c) acrylonitrile butadiene styrene
   d) fiberglass wrap material

2. UV gels contain ____________, which are liquids.
   a) monomers
   b) polymers
   c) oligomers
   d) primers

3. Acrylates and methacrylates are used in making ____________.
   a) fiberglass wraps
   b) sculptured nails
   c) UV gels
   d) nail tips

4. The step that makes UV gel nail enhancements different from all other nail enhancements is ____________.
   a) soaking
   b) filing
   c) clipping
   d) curing

5. UV lamp intensity or concentration is more important than rating a UV light unit based on ____________.
   a) voltage
   b) ohms
   c) amperes
   d) wattage

6. UV gel product is held and spread with ____________.
   a) synthetic brushes
   b) wooden pushers
   c) natural brushes
   d) metal pushers

7. The product used to improve adhesion of UV gels to the natural nail plate is called ____________.
   a) UV gel glue
   b) UV gel paste
   c) UV gel primer
   d) UV gel buffer

8. A medium-abrasive (180) grit is used for ____________.
   a) priming the tip
   b) natural nail preparation
   c) dehydrating the eponychium
   d) conditioning the nail

Essential Review continued

9. UV gel #1 is called ____________.
   a) base coat gel
   b) builder gel
   c) primer coat gel
   d) sealer gel

10. When cured, UV gels have a tacky surface called a/an ____________.
   a) integumentary layer
   b) aggressive layer
   c) contour layer
   d) inhibition layer

11. What is used to enhance the adhesion of acrylic nails?
   a) dehydrator
   b) primer
   c) initiator
   d) catalyst

12. A process that joins together monomers to create very long polymer chains is called ____________.
   a) rebalancing
   b) molecular reaction
   c) chain reaction
   d) positive reaction

13. Catalysts are added to the ____________ and used to control the set or curing time.
   a) powder
   b) liquid
   c) adhesive
   d) dehydrator

14. Benzoyl peroxide is a/an ____________ that is added to the powder to start a chain reaction which leads to the creation of long polymer chains.
   a) initiator
   b) dehydrator
   c) catalyst
   d) primer

15. Using the wrong powder with your chosen liquid could result in nails that are ____________.
   a) too thick and cloudy
   b) too thin and cloudy
   c) not properly cured
   d) not ready for polish

16. The amount of monomer and polymer used to create a bead is called the ____________.
   a) product density
   b) product consistency
   c) mixture formula
   d) mix ratio

Essential Review continued

17. If equal amounts of liquid and powder are used to create a bead, it is called a/an ____________.

a) wet bead
b) medium bead
c) dry bead
d) oily bead

18. If twice as much liquid is used as powder, the bead is called a ____________.

a) wet bead
b) medium bead
c) dry bead
d) oily bead

19. Using the proper mixture of powder and liquid ensures proper set and maximum ____________ of the nail enhancement.

a) flexibility
b) durability
c) adaptability
d) resilience

20. If too little powder is used, the nail enhancement can become ____________.

a) stronger
b) brittle
c) discolored
d) weaker

21. ____________ primer is corrosive to the skin and potentially dangerous to the eyes.

a) Alkaline-based
b) Monomer-based
c) Acid-based
d) Alcohol-based

22. The use of dappen dishes to hold acrylic products helps to ____________.

a) minimize evaporation
b) maximize evaporation
c) minimize condensation
d) maximize condensation

23. For use with acrylic products, the best brushes are composed of ____________.

a) sable hair
b) mink hair
c) synthetic fiber
d) bristle fiber

24. For nail service applications, gloves made of ____________ work best.

a) nitrile polyester
b) nitrile polymer
c) benzoyl polymer
d) benzoyl monomer

Essential Review continued

25. Nail enhancements are hard enough to ____________ if they make a clicking sound when lightly tapped with a brush handle.

a) nip and trim
b) clip and trim
d) polish and finish
d) file and shape

26. Nail enhancement that are not properly maintained have a greater tendency to ____________.

a) lift and break
b) split and chip
c) grow and strengthen
d) grow slower

27. The method for maintaining the beauty, durability, and longevity of the artificial nail enhancement is known as ____________.

a) servicing
b) rebalancing
c) reconstructing
d) restructuring

28. Nipping an acrylic nail may perpetuate a lifting problem and can damage the ____________.

a) nail bed
b) eponychium
c) hyponychium
d) nail plate

29. Odorless products harden more slowly which creates the tacky layer called the ____________.

a) exhibition layer
b) assertion layer
c) inhibition layer
d) sticky layer

30. ____________ in the powder with the brush may be needed with low-odor products in order to create the proper mix of powder and liquid.

a) Multiple circular motions
b) Minimal circular motions
c) A single stroke
d) Multiple vertical dipping

31. When handling nail adhesive, nail technicians should ____________.

a) avoid touching skin
b) apply to free edge only
c) apply to eponychium
d) apply to sidewalls

32. The product that acts as the dryer that speeds up the hardening process of the wrap overlay is called ____________.

a) resin activator
b) resin dehydrator
c) cyanoacrylate accelerator
d) wrap accelerator

Essential Review continued

33. Natural oil and shine are removed from the nail plate with a/an ____________.

a) antibacterial soap
b) abrasive
c) adhesive
d) nail wrap

34. Nail tips are attached to the nail plates by using a ____________.

a) cotton-tipped wooden pusher
b) small nail brush
c) stop, rock, and hold procedure
d) stop, rock, and slide procedure

35. Softened nail tips are removed by ____________.

a) rubbing them off
b) nipping them off
c) pulling them off
d) sliding them off

36. A thin, elongated board with a rough surface is called ____________.

a) an abrasive
b) an adhesive
c) a buffer
d) a file

37. Nail-size pieces of cloth or paper that are bonded to the top of the nail plate with nail adhesive are called ____________.

a) repair patches
b) nail wraps
c) no-light gels
d) buffer wraps

38. A piece of fabric cut to completely cover a crack or break in the nail is called ____________.

a) a repair patch
b) a nail wrap
c) a no-light gel
d) a fiberglass resin

39. A thin, natural material with a tight weave that becomes transparent when adhesive is applied is ____________.

a) linen
b) fiberglass
c) silk
d) paper

40. An implement designed especially for use on nail tips is called a ____________.

a) nail clipper
b) nail nipper
c) nail cutter
d) tip cutter

Essential Discoveries and Accomplishments

In the space below, jot some notes about what concepts of this chapter were hardest for you to understand or remember. Imagine finding yourself suddenly in the role of "teacher" and consider what you would tell your "students" about these concepts. Share your Essential Discoveries with some of the other students in your class and ask if they are helpful to them. You may want to revise your discoveries based on good ideas shared by your peers.

Discoveries:

____

____

____

____

____

____

____

____

____

____

____

List at least three things you have accomplished since your last entry that relate to your career goals.

Accomplishments:

____

____

____

____

____

CHAPTER 30

Seeking Employment

A Motivating Moment: "Success is not measured by what you accomplish but by the opposition you have encountered, and the courage with which you have maintained the struggle against overwhelming odds."
—Orison Swett Marden

Essential Objectives

After studying this chapter and completing the Essential Companion components, you will be able to:

1. **Understand what is involved in securing the required credentials for cosmetology in your state and know the process for taking and passing your state licensing examination.**
2. **Start networking and preparing to find a job by using the Inventory of Personal Characteristics and Technical Skills.**
3. **Describe the different salon business categories.**
4. **Write a cover letter and resume and prepare an employment portfolio.**
5. **Know how to explore the job market, research potential employers, and operate within the legal aspects of employment.**

Essential Employment Seeking

Why do I need to learn about seeking employment while I am still in training?

Learning about seeking employment is all part of planning your career, which is an essential part of planning your life. If you set a goal on the first day of school to become a successful salon owner or a well-known international platform artist, you must begin your journey toward that goal by obtaining your first career-related position. It's important for you to recognize that when you complete your course of study, your training has really just begun. You have become a student in lifelong learning. Therefore, that first job needs to be suited to your interests, talents, and goals. In addition, it should provide opportunities for your continued growth and professional development. It is not realistic to believe you can obtain your license and find exactly what you are looking for on your first job inquiry. By beginning your search while you are in school, it is far more likely that you will secure an appropriate position upon graduation.

Cosmetologists should study and have a thorough understanding of how to prepare for and seek employment because:

- You must pass your State Board Exam to be licensed and you must be licensed to be hired; therefore, preparing for licensure and passing your exam is your first step to employment success.
- A successful employment search is a job in itself, and there are many tools that can give you the edge—as well as mistakes that can cost you an interview or a job.
- The ability to pinpoint the right salon for you and target it as a potential employer is vital for your career success.
- Proactively preparing the right materials, such as a great resume, and practicing interviewing will give you the confidence that's needed to secure a job in a salon you love.

Essential Concepts

What do I need to know about seeking employment in order to achieve success in my career?

In addition to developing important personal characteristics such as a positive attitude, desire, and commitment, you will need to identify your talents, skills, and interests to determine the type of salon for which you are best suited. You will learn how to target these salons and observe them in action to confirm whether you want to pursue an employment interview. You must learn to develop an action-oriented resume that will catch the potential employer's eye in a few seconds. You will need to properly prepare for the ever-important job interview. In our society, first impressions matter a great deal. You may have already learned in life that the best qualified applicant does not always get the best job. In fact, the job often goes to the applicant who projects the best image and comes across best during the interview. Thus, learning how to prepare for the interview and how to present yourself during the interview are critical to obtaining the most appropriate position upon graduation.

1 Essential Experience

Personal Data Page

In preparation for accurate and prompt completion of an employment application, it is beneficial to prepare a personal data page that contains generally the same information. Gather all the necessary information ahead of time and list it on the form provided. It will then be easy to transfer the applicable information to the application form used by your potential employer.

Name ____________________ Over age 18: _____ Yes _____ No

Address ____

Telephone ________________ E-mail ________________

Position Desired ________________ Date Available ____________

Education

High School ________________ Graduate: _____ Yes _____ No

Post-secondary ________________ Diploma: _____ Yes _____ No

Post-secondary ________________ Diploma: _____ Yes _____ No

Post-secondary ________________ Diploma: _____ Yes _____ No

Employment History

Where ____________________ When ________________

Position ________________ Reason Left ________________

Where ____________________ When ________________

Position ________________ Reason Left ________________

Where ____________________ When ________________

Position ________________ Reason Left ________________

Significant Skills ________________________________

____

Awards and Recognitions ____________________________

Essential Experience 2

Mind Map Steps in Seeking Employment

Mind mapping creates a free-flowing outline of material or information. Using the central or key point of seeking employment, diagram the different procedural steps you will need to complete in order to obtain the best possible position. Use terms, pictures, and symbols as desired. Using color will increase your retention of the material. Keep your mind open. Don't worry about where a line or word should go as the organization of the map will usually take care of itself.

3 Essential Experience

Windowpane Clinic Achievements

Windowpaning is the process of transferring key elements, points, or steps in a lesson into visual images that are hand sketched into the squares or *panes* of a matrix. Let your mind think in pictures and sketch the essential concepts printed in each of the following windowpanes. Don't be concerned with your artistic ability. Use lines and stick figures to depict the concepts requested for creating an achievement-oriented resume.

Total Regular Clients
Clients Served Weekly
% Clinic in Texture Services
Client Ticket Average
Client Retention Rate
% Clinic in Retail
% Clinic in Haircolor
Attendance Record
Other Accomplishments

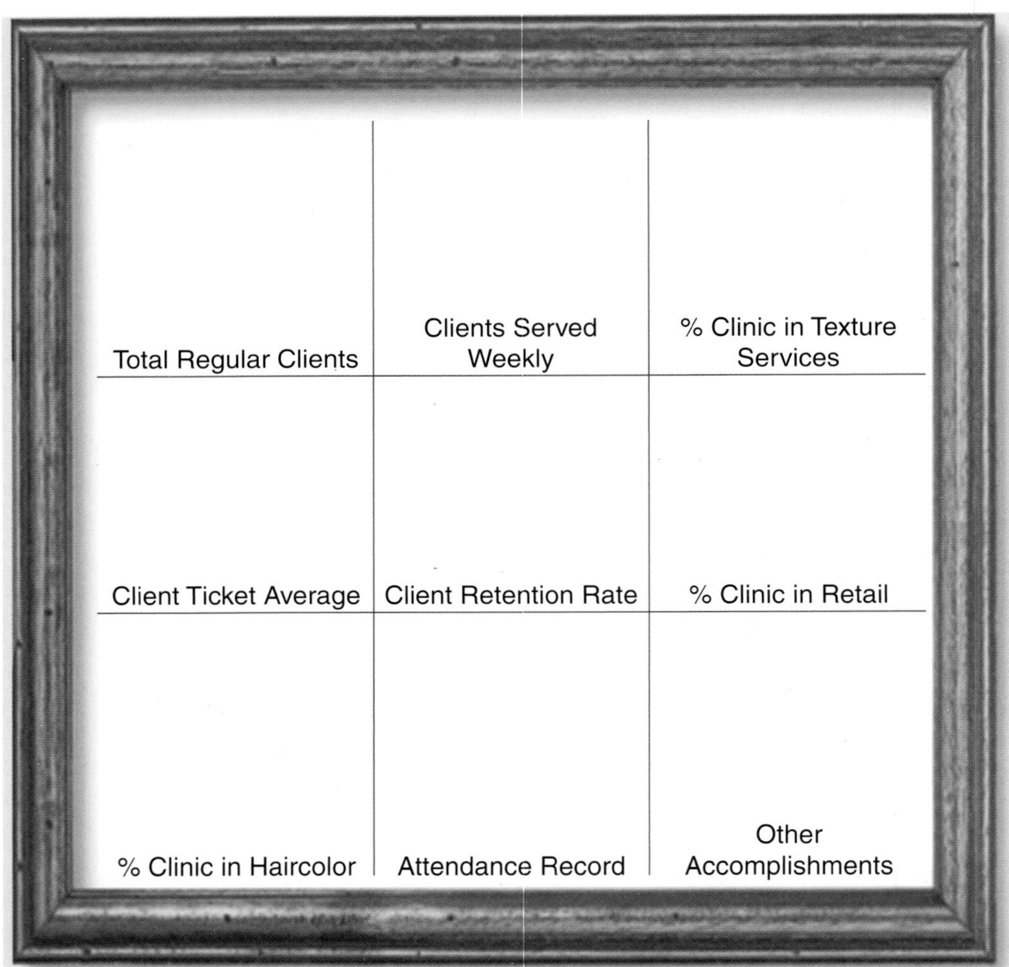

Essential Experience

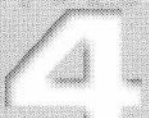

Cover Letter

Using the format described in Chapter 30, Seeking Employment, page 976, *Milady Standard Cosmetology*, 2012 edition, write a cover letter to accompany your resume when applying for a job.

Date ______________________________

Your Name ______________________________

Your Address ______________________________

City/State ______________________________

Salon Name ______________________________

Salon Address ______________________________

City/State ______________________________

Dear ______________________________,

____

____

____

____

____

____

____

Very cordially yours,

(Signature here)

Your Name

Enclosure

5 Essential Experience

Interview Preparation

Listed below are several potential questions that may be asked during your interview. Using the space provided, answer the questions to the best of your ability. This exercise will help you be more thoroughly prepared for that important interview.

What did you like best about your training? ______________________________

____

Are you punctual and regular in attendance? ______________________________

What skills do you feel are your strongest? ______________________________

____

What skills do you feel are your weakest? ______________________________

____

Are you a team player? __________ Please explain: ______________________

____

Are you flexible? __________ Please explain: ______________________________

____

What are your career goals? ______________________________________

____

What days/hours are you available to work? ______________________________

Do you have your own transportation? ______________________________

What obstacles, if any, would prevent you from keeping your commitment to full-time employment? ______________________________

____

What assets will you bring to the salon and this position? ______________

____

Essential Experience continued 5

Who is the most important person you have met in your work/education experience and why? ______________________________

____

Explain some strategies you would use in handling a difficult client. ________

____

How do you feel about retailing? ______________________________

____

What is your philosophy about attending continuing education programs, seminars, and shows? ______________________________

____

Are you willing to personally invest in your professional development?

____

____

Describe ways in which you feel you provide excellent customer service.

____

____

Please share some examples of consultation questions you might ask a client. ______________________________

____

List steps you would take to build a solid client base and ensure that clients return. ______________________________

____

6 Essential Experience

Word Scramble

Using the clues provided, unscramble the terms below.

Scramble **Correct Word**

ticedduve gninsaoer _ _ _ _ _ _ _ _ _   _ _ _ _ _ _ _ _ _

Clue: Used to reach logical conclusions.

loftropoi _ _ _ _ _ _ _ _ _

Clue: Collection of documents that reflect your skills.

usemer _ _ _ _ _ _

Clue: Summary of education and experience.

krow chiet _ _ _ _   _ _ _ _ _

Clue: Commitment to delivering worthy service for value received.

yolpemmten _ _ _ _ _ _ _ _ _ _

Clue: Something you pursue upon graduation.

nucomcamiinot _ _ _ _ _ _ _ _ _ _ _ _ _

Clue: Something needed to interact effectively with clients.

trigeytin _ _ _ _ _ _ _ _ _

Clue: Commitment to a strong code of moral and artistic values.

frenchais _ _ _ _ _ _ _ _ _

Clue: Having a national name and image consistent with the organization.

shemtnilbatse _ _ _ _ _ _ _ _ _ _ _ _ _

Clue: A place where you may obtain employment.

weevtiinr _ _ _ _ _ _ _ _ _

Clue: A meeting where your qualifications are considered.

Essential Experience 7

Why I Chose Cosmetology

One of the most important tasks you can complete in preparing your professional portfolio and in preparing for an effective interview is writing a brief statement about why you have chosen a career in cosmetology. In the space provided, write such a statement. Remember to include such points as an explanation of what you love about your new career; a description of your philosophy about the importance of teamwork and how you see yourself as a contributing team player; and a description of methods you would employ to increase clinic and retail revenue.

Essential Review

Using the following words, fill in the blanks below to form a thorough review of Chapter 30, Seeking Employment. Words or terms may be used more than once or not at all.

10 seconds	**contacts**	**portfolio**
2 minutes	**course content**	**practice**
20 seconds	**crib notes**	**qualifying**
20	**documents**	**responsibilities**
30	**down-time**	**resume**
50	**drawings**	**self-confident**
60	**easiest**	**self-motivation**
70	**English**	**smiling**
80	**family member**	**solidified**
90	**half million**	**speed**
370,000	**hardest**	**studying**
appropriate	**ideals**	**test-wise**
assumptions	**illegal**	**timing**
attention	**integrity**	**transferable**
autobiography	**legal**	**true/false**
broad	**motivation**	**two million**
bullheadedness	**multiple choice**	**willpower**
career goals	**negative**	**work ethic**
cheating	**network**	
conclusions	**neutral**	

1. Top professionals in the field of cosmetology were not born successful; they achieved success with their ________________, energy, and persistence.
2. Of all the factors that will affect your test performance on the licensing examination, the most important is your mastery of ________________.
3. A test-wise student begins to prepare for test-taking by practicing the daily habits and time management that are an important part of effective ________________.

Essential Review continued

4. On test day, it is a good idea to arrive early with a _______________ attitude; be alert, calm, and ready for the challenge.
5. When taking a test, answer the _______________ questions first.
6. Deductive reasoning is the process of reaching logical _______________ by employing logical reasoning.
7. When applying deductive reasoning in test-taking, watch for "key" words or terms and look for _______________ conditions or statements.
8. When taking a _______________ test, read the entire question carefully, including all the choices.
9. An effective tip when preparing for the practical examination is to participate in "mock" licensing examinations, including the _______________ of applicable examination criteria.
10. Completion of the Inventory of Personal Characteristics and Technical Skills helps you identify any areas needing further _______________ and determine where to focus the remainder of your training.
11. One key characteristic that will not only help you get the position you want but will help you keep it is _______________.
12. You have a strong _______________ when you believe that work is good and you are committed to delivering worthy service for the value received from your employer.
13. In the United States alone, the professional salon business numbers over _______________ establishments that employ more than 1,682,600 million active cosmetologists.
14. A basic value-priced salon may be a good starting place for a recent graduate because it provides for practice on many types of haircuts, which increases self-confidence and _______________.
15. A _______________ is a written summary of your education and work experience.
16. The average time a potential employer will spend scanning your resume to determine if you should be granted an interview is about _______________.
17. When writing a resume, it is more important to focus on your achievements rather than your _______________.
18. Skills which you have already mastered at other jobs that can be put to use in the new position are known as _______________.

Essential Review continued

19. An employment portfolio is a collection, usually bound, of photos and _______________ that reflect your skills, accomplishments, and abilities in your chosen career field.
20. One way to determine if your portfolio portrays you and your career skills in the most positive light is to run it by a _______________ party for feedback and suggestions about how to make it more interesting and accurate.
21. When visiting salons prior to requesting an employment interview remember that it is important to never burn your bridges, but rather to build a _______________ of contacts who have a favorable opinion of you.
22. _______________ is the universal language.
23. On an employment application questions regarding race, religion, or national origin are considered to be _______________.
24. Make sure your resume focuses on information that is relevant to your _______________ goals.
25. Having a complete and thorough knowledge of the subject matter and understanding the strategies for taking tests successfully means that you are _______________.

Essential Discoveries and Accomplishments

In the space below, jot some notes about what concepts of this chapter were hardest for you to understand or remember. Imagine finding yourself suddenly in the role of "teacher" and consider what you would tell your "students" about these concepts. Share your Essential Discoveries with some of the other students in your class and ask if they are helpful to them. You may want to revise your discoveries based on good ideas shared by your peers.

Discoveries:

List at least three things you have accomplished since your last entry that relate to your career goals.

Accomplishments:

CHAPTER 31

On the Job

A Motivating Moment: "The place to begin building any relationship is inside ourselves, inside our circle of influence, our own character."

—Stephen R. Covey

Essential Objectives

After studying this chapter and completing the Essential Companion components, you will be able to:

1. **Describe what is expected of a new employee and what this means in terms of your everyday behavior.**
2. **List the habits of a good salon team player.**
3. **Describe three different ways in which salon professionals are compensated.**
4. **Explain the principles of selling products and services in the salon.**
5. **List the most effective ways to build a client base.**

Essential On the Job

Why do I need to learn about making the transition from school to work?

It has been said that as much as 80 percent of your career success will result from personal attributes such as your people skills, your ability to communicate, your visual integrity, and your goal orientations. If only 20 percent of your career success has to do with your technical skills, it stands to reason that there are many more qualities you need to work on to achieve that desired level of success. The cosmetologists who achieve that goal, who stay with the profession longer than the rest, who own or work in successful salons and enjoy all the rewards of success, all started out with stars in their eyes. However, they knew it took more than just a dream. They knew it would take commitment and hard work, and they made sure they were prepared for every opportunity that knocked.

As professionals-in-training they came to school early and stayed late as needed. They accepted those late clients without whining; they wrapped and rewrapped those design texture services on mannequin after mannequin to ensure quality and competitive speed. They read industry journals and stayed abreast of the daily changes happening within the field of cosmetology. The important thing to remember here is that as a professional-in-training, you are about to become a full-fledged, licensed professional.

If you consider yourself among this elite class, you know that you were not born but made yourself who you are today by your own desires and energies and persistence. You recognize that being a stylist is not a nine-to-five job four days a week. It's being there whenever your clients need you. You know that it is going the extra mile, taking the extra client, biting back those angry words that spring up when a client is rude or a coworker is unfair. It is paying your dues, mastering your craft, building self-confidence, and developing strong personal pride in your accomplishments.

Cosmetologists should study and have a thorough understanding of what it is like on the job because:

- Working in a salon requires each staff member to belong to and work as a team member of the salon. Learning to do so is an important aspect of being successful in the salon environment.
- There are a variety of ways that a salon may compensate employees. Being familiar with each way and knowing how they work will help you to determine if the compensation system at a particular salon can work for you and what to expect from it.

Essential On the Job continued

- Once you are working as a salon professional, you will have of financial obligations and responsibilities, so learning the basics of financial management while you are building your clientele and business is invaluable.
- As you build your clientele and settle into your professional life, there will be opportunities for you to use a variety of techniques for increasing your income, such as retailing and upselling services. Knowing and using these techniques will help you to promote yourself, build a loyal client base, and create a sound financial future for yourself.

Essential Concepts

What do I need to know about making the transition from school to work in order to maintain satisfaction and success on the job?

While you are probably highly excited about having your first paying job in your new career, there are a number of responsibilities that go along with that paycheck. Your school environment has been a relatively safe and comfortable one. Here, you have had the opportunity to practice service after service to get to the desired results. On the job, your clients will expect the desired results the first time around. In school you have had to deal with the institution's tardy policy, which is probably quite lenient compared to that of a salon. Clients are not very forgiving when you are not at work at the appointed time to provide their service.

While in school you probably had more flexibility in dealing with your personal schedule as it related to your class schedule. On the job you will be expected to be at work every day as scheduled, promptly, and ready to work when you arrive. At school you may have had the opportunity to do your hair or your makeup after you clocked in—not so in the workplace. If you just did not feel like going to school on any given day, perhaps you just did not go. A job with a paycheck brings with it an expectation of more maturity than that.

You need to realize that, on the job, you are responsible for many more decisions and for performing in a professional manner at all times, even when you do not feel like it. On the job you will need to be focused on constantly building a business rather than watching the clock to see how long it is until your required hours have been clocked. In addition, you will need to concentrate on furthering your knowledge and skills to remain abreast of all the new trends, tools, and techniques your new job presents. All in all, it's an exciting new opportunity—one that has many rewards accompanied by many responsibilities.

1 Essential Experience

Evaluate Your Skills—Are You Job Ready?

Take a few minutes to think back over your training and your clinical experience and reflect on all you have learned that you did not know when you started. Give yourself a hearty pat on the back for your accomplishments. Then evaluate your skills and check off those in which you feel confident. If you need more practice, indicate by checking the improvement column. Then make a personal commitment to improve in those areas.

Subject Area	Competent	Need Improvement
Infection control	_____	_____
Product knowledge	_____	_____
Hair chemistry	_____	_____
Shampooing	_____	_____
Haircutting		
Blunt shapes	_____	_____
Graduated shapes	_____	_____
Layered shapes	_____	_____
Clipper cutting	_____	_____
Other cutting techniques	_____	_____
Hair texturizing		
Texture services	_____	_____
Relaxer services	_____	_____
Mixing solutions	_____	_____
Wrapping	_____	_____
Processing	_____	_____
Haircoloring		
Color wheel	_____	_____
Levels of color	_____	_____
Brush application	_____	_____
One process	_____	_____
Two process	_____	_____

Essential Experience continued 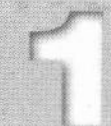

Subject Area	Competent	Need Improvement
Retouch	_____	_____
Foil highlights	_____	_____
Mixing color (tube and liquid)	_____	_____
Style finishing		
Blowdry	_____	_____
Round brush	_____	_____
Curling iron	_____	_____
Wet sets	_____	_____
Styling aids	_____	_____
Client communications		
Eye contact	_____	_____
Handshake	_____	_____
Open-ended questions	_____	_____
Active listening	_____	_____
Developing rapport	_____	_____
Client consultation		
Greeting	_____	_____
Analysis	_____	_____
Recommendations	_____	_____
Client record keeping	_____	_____
Client development	_____	_____
Client retention	_____	_____
Client referrals	_____	_____
Client rebooking	_____	_____
Retail product sales	_____	_____
Ticket upgrading	_____	_____
Salon/clinic teamwork	_____	_____
Work ethic	_____	_____
Productivity	_____	_____
Receptionist duties	_____	_____
Industry knowledge	_____	_____

1 Essential Experience continued

Subject Area	Competent	Need Improvement
Time management	_____	_____
Goal setting	_____	_____
Personal finances	_____	_____
Job hunting skills	_____	_____
Career planning	_____	_____

Essential Experience 2

Technical Skills Improvement

Based on the analysis you completed in Essential Experience 1, create a plan of action for every area you checked as needing improvement. Record your plan in the space provided.

3 Essential Experience

Career Management

In today's market there are more jobs available than there are stylists to fill them. Thus, you owe it to yourself and your potential new employer to find the best fit possible. Once you have made that decision, stick with it and give it your absolute best as long as you can. Job-hopping early in your career is not good for your professional development or your reputation. Following are several pointers that will help you right from the start. In the column Plan of Action, explain how you intend to make the most of each suggestion.

Pointer	Plan of Action
Master the techniques you learned in Chapter 30, Seeking Employment, to ensure you find the right job for your strengths and preferences.	
Understand that your income grows when you work harder, build a sound client base, volunteer for extra clients, sell retail, and show initiative and ambition.	
Arrive for work at least fifteen minutes prior to your first client, dressed and groomed, ready to work.	
Have your station set up and ready for each scheduled service before the client arrives.	
Know that your clients and the salon are relying on you to be there. Only call in sick if you are absolutely sick.	
Have realistic expectations of how much money you will earn your first year. It takes time to build a loyal client base.	
Build a realistic personal budget and stick to it. Don't spend more than you make!	
Continue to study, train, and expand your personal and technical skills.	
Join your local cosmetology association and attend meetings faithfully.	

Essential Experience 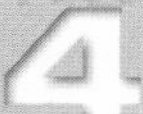

Teamwork

As a contributing team member in the salon, you will be called upon to deal with a variety of problems or situations on a regular basis. In order to build your teamwork skills while you are in school, work with a couple of other classmates. Consider the following situations and how you would handle them in the workplace. Record your results in the space provided.

1. You each arrive for work with a fully booked schedule for the day. The manager and two other stylists have been stricken with the flu and will not make it into work today. You and your teammates have to decide how to handle the clients of the other three stylists. What do you do?

___

___

___

2. Your salon owner is remodeling the facility, which includes reorganizing the space and assigning new work stations to everyone. With a partner discuss and develop some criteria the owner could use in assigning new stations because some spaces are more desirable than others.

___

___

___

3. The salon's manager states the plan of implementing a retail bonus plan for all stylists and asks for your help in developing the policy. With a partner create a retail bonus plan that you would recommend for adoption.

___

___

___

5 Essential Experience

The Job Description

Assume the role of owner of a highly successful salon. Write a job description for a junior stylist, listing all the factors you deem appropriate to the position.

Essential Review

Using the following words, fill in the blanks below to form a thorough review of Chapter 31, On the Job. Words may be used more than once or not at all.

client	**doubt**	**immature**	**salon**
client consultations	**feelings or desires**	**increasing**	**serving**
commissions	**financial**	**job description**	**temptation**
compensation	**grateful**	**mathematical**	**ticket upgrading**
conflict	**hourly**	**respectful**	**transition**
		retailing	

1. When you become the employee of a salon, you will be expected to put the needs of the ____________ and ____________ ahead of your own.
2. Making the ____________ from school to work can be difficult.
3. The number one thing to remember when you are in a service business is that your work revolves around ____________ your clients.
4. In the salon you will have to quickly get used to putting your own __________________ aside and putting the needs of the salon and the client first.
5. Getting to work on time is ____________ not only to your clients but also to your coworkers who will have to handle your clients if you are late.
6. Remember that it is an honor to have a job that will provide you and your family with financial stability, so be very ____________.
7. Although you may not like or agree with the salon manager or her rules, you must give her the benefit of the ____________.
8. Thinking that you will never need to learn anything more once you are out of school is ____________ and limiting.
9. Given the stress of a typical salon, there will be lots of opportunities for you to become negative or to have conflicts with your teammates. Resist the ____________ to give in to maliciousness and gossip.
10. The most difficult part of being in a relationship, whether it is a personal or professional relationship, is when ____________ arises.

Essential Review continued

11. When assuming a new position, you are agreeing to do everything as it is written down in a ______________, so if you are unclear about something or need more information, it is your responsibility to ask.
12. Being paid an ____________ rate is usually the best way for new salon professionals to start out.
13. _____________ are paid on percentages of your total service dollars and can range anywhere from 25 percent to 60 percent, depending on your length of time at the salon and your performance levels.
14. When deciding whether a certain _____________ method is right for you, it is important to be aware of what your monthly expenses are and to have a personal financial budget and plan in place.
15. Ask a senior stylist to sit in on one of your ____________________ and to make note of areas where you can improve.
16. Although a career in the beauty industry is very artistic and creative, it is also a career that requires _____________ understanding and planning.
17. Many people are afraid of the word budget because they think it will be too restrictive on their spending, or because they think they need to be _____________ geniuses in order to work with a budget.
18. You will want to think about other ways to increase your income, including spending less money and _____________ service prices.
19. ___________________ or upselling services is the practice of recommending and selling additional services to your clients, which may be performed by you or by other practitioners in the salon.
20. _____________ is the act of recommending and selling products to your clients for at-home hair, skin, and nail care.

Essential Discoveries and Accomplishments

In the space below, jot some notes about what concepts of this chapter were hardest for you to understand or remember. Imagine finding yourself suddenly in the role of "teacher" and consider what you would tell your "students" about these concepts. Share your Essential Discoveries with some of the other students in your class and ask if they are helpful to them. You may want to revise your discoveries based on good ideas shared by your peers.

Discoveries:

List at least three things you have accomplished since your last entry that relate to your career goals.

Accomplishments:

CHAPTER 32

The Salon Business

A Motivating Moment: "If you will call your troubles experiences, and remember that every experience develops some latent force within you, you will grow vigorous and happy, however adverse your circumstances may seem to be."

—John Homer Miller

Essential Objectives

After studying this chapter and completing the Essential Companion components, you will be able to:

1. **Identify two options for going into business for yourself.**
2. **Understand the responsibilities of a booth renter.**
3. **List the basic factors to be considered when opening a salon.**
4. **Distinguish the types of salon ownership.**
5. **Identify the information that should be included in a business plan.**
6. **Understand the importance of record keeping.**
7. **Recognize the elements of successful salon operations.**
8. **Explain why selling services and products is a vital aspect of a salon's success.**

Essential Salon Business

Is the knowledge of business really so important to someone who just wants to be a hair designer?

Absolutely! Even if you never own your own salon, you need to understand the key principles of building and operating a business to ensure your own success. Most individuals entering this exciting field dream of owning their own salon one day. The fact is that more than just a few cosmetology graduates actually turn that dream into reality. The more you know about managing and operating an efficient business, the more valuable you become to your future employers.

Cosmetologists should study and have a thorough understanding of the salon business because:

- As you become more proficient in your craft and your ability to manage yourself and others, you may decide to become an independent booth renter or even a salon owner. In fact, most owners are former stylists.
- Even if you spend your entire career as an employee of someone else's salon, you should have a familiarity of the rules of business that affect the salon.
- To become a successful entrepreneur, you will need to attract employees and clients to your business and maintain their loyalty over long periods of time.
- Even if you think you will be involved in the artistic aspect of salons forever, business knowledge will serve you well in managing your career and professional finances, as well as your business practices.

Essential Concepts

What do I need to know about the salon business in order to be successful?

There are many factors to consider before taking the step into ownership or even management. Knowledge of business principles, bookkeeping, business laws, insurance, salesmanship, and psychology is crucial for the successful salon owner or manager. Serving people is one thing; managing people is quite another. Just knowing about business is not enough. You need to develop leadership, self-control, and sensitivity. This whole area of business calls for planning, supervision, control, evaluation, and, above all, teamwork.

Essential Experience 1

Salon Research

Research at least five salons in the area where you may want to work. Your mission is to determine which salon is most suited to your needs. Rate each category on a scale of 1 to 10, with 10 being considered the best. Explain your rating. Use the chart below to track your findings.

Category	Salon 1	Salon 2	Salon 3	Salon 4	Salon 5
Location/Active Business Nearby					
Demographics/ Income Area					
Adequate Parking					
Direct Competition Nearby					
Exterior Appearance and Design (attractive)					
Interior Appearance and Design (attractiveand efficient)					
Retail Sales Awareness					

2 Essential Experience

Matching Exercise

Match each of the following essential terms with its definition.

______	**Salon Policies**	**1.**	Summarizes your plan and states your objectives
______	**Executive Summary**	**2.**	Long-term picture of what business is to become
______	**Marketing Plan**	**3.**	Description of key strategic influences of the business
______	**Vision Statement**	**4.**	Outlines employees and management levels and describes how business will run
______	**Mission Statement**	**5.**	Outlines research obtained regarding the clients the business will target
______	**Supporting Documents**	**6.**	Includes projected financial statements
______	**Organizational Plan**	**7.**	Includes owner's resume, personal information, and legal contracts
______	**Financial Documents**	**8.**	Ensure all clients and employees are treated fairly and consistently

Essential Experience 3

Income and Expenses

Assume the following facts:

- Your monthly revenue goal is $10,000.
- The ticket average in your salon is $20 per client.
- Your salon is open 5 days per week or an average of 22 days per month.

Based on the above information, determine how many clients you will have to serve per day and how many stylists you will have to employ to reach your revenue goal.

____

____

____

Once you have obtained the above information, apply the percentages taken from Chapter 32, The Salon Business, Table 32–1, page 1018, of your text to the $10,000 gross revenue to determine what your salon net profit will be for the month.

Salaries:	$10,000 × 53.5%	=	$ ________
Rent:	$10,000 × 13%	=	$ ________
Supplies:	$10,000 × 5%	=	$ ________
Advertising:	$10,000 × 3%	=	$ ________
Depreciation:	$10,000 × 3%	=	$ ________
Laundry:	$10,000 × 1%	=	$ ________
Cleaning:	$10,000 × 1%	=	$ ________
Light and Power:	$10,000 × 1%	=	$ ________
Repairs:	$10,000 × 1.5%	=	$ ________
Insurance:	$10,000 × .75%	=	$ ________
Telephone:	$10,000 × .75%	=	$ ________
Miscellaneous:	$10,000 × 1.5%	=	$ ________
	Total Expenses:		$ ________
	Net Profit:		$ ________

3 Essential Experience continued

Now, consider what would happen if you were unable stay within the recommended guidelines of your budget. Perhaps your rent is more than the above amount. Maybe you are having to pay more for a cleaning crew or you have several telephone lines and your telephone bill runs around $300 per month. It's important to consider all these factors when setting up a business because the only way to make more money is to increase revenue or reduce expenses or a combination of both.

Essential Experience 4

Salon Computer Systems

Research at least three different salon computer systems used for Point of Sale and client tracking. List the features and benefits of each and report to the rest of the class your recommendations for purchase.

System 1:

____

____

____

____

____

____

System 2:

____

____

____

____

____

____

System 3:

____

____

____

____

____

____

5 Essential Experience

Job Descriptions

Write a position description for a stylist and a receptionist in your salon. Be thorough and specific. Outline their general responsibilities as well as their specific duties. Use additional paper as needed.

Stylist: ____

____

____

____

____

____

____

____

____

____

____

Receptionist:

____

____

____

____

____

____

____

____

____

____

Essential Experience 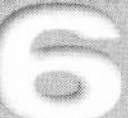

Advertising

In the space provided, design a 3″× 5″ newspaper ad for your salon.

In the space provided, write a thirty-second radio ad promoting your salon and its services.

7 Essential Experience

Crossword Puzzle

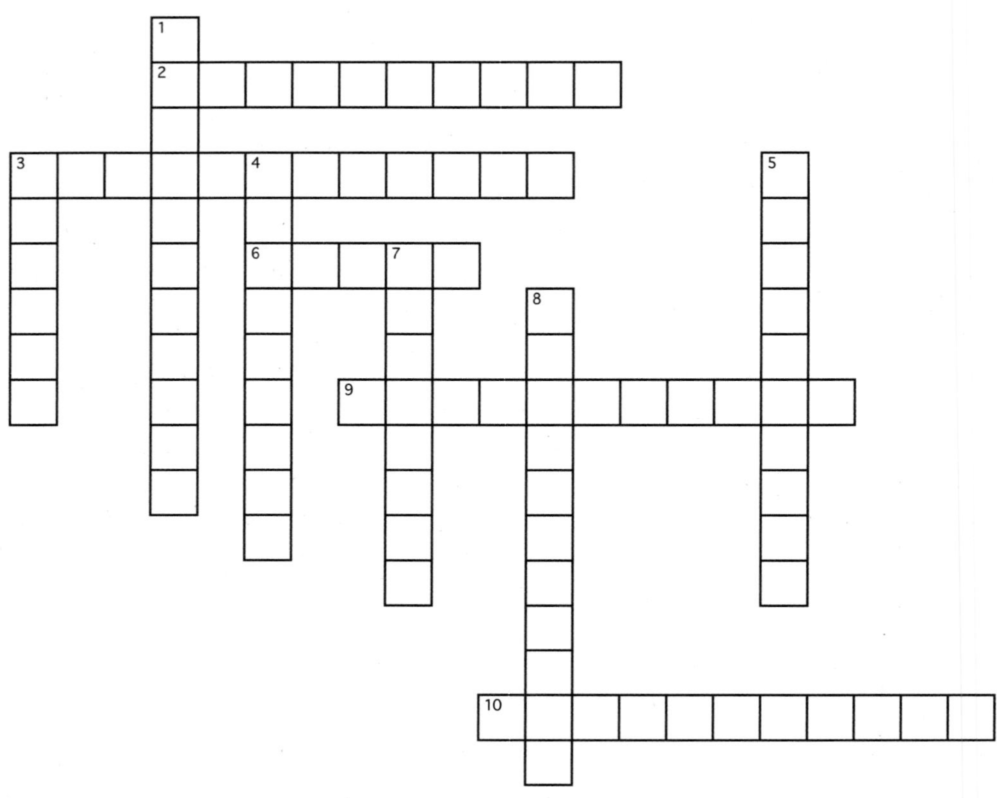

Across

Word	Clue
________________	**2.** Advertising that allows for close contact with the potential client
________________	**3.** The quarterback of the salon
________________	**6.** Must state all provisions that pertain to the landlord and tenant
________________	**9.** Ownership is shared by two or more people
________________	**10.** Ownership is shared by stockholders

Down

Word	Clue
______________	**1.** Should be 3 percent of your gross income
______________	**3.** Supplies sold to the client
______________	**4.** Complaints are often handled on this
______________	**5.** Proprietor is owner and manager
______________	**7.** Largest expense in the salon
______________	**8.** Supplies used in the daily business operations

8 Essential Experience

Interviewing Personnel

Select a partner and role-play interviewing that person for employment in your salon. Prepare in advance a list of questions you wish to ask him or her. List the questions and his or her responses below.

Essential Review

Using the following words, fill in the blanks below to form a thorough review of Chapter 32, The Salon Business. Words or terms may be used more than once or not at all.

advertising
booth rental
business plan
capital
consumption supplies
correct grammar
equal
excellent customer service
health
incoming phone calls
indispensable
investment capital
location
mortgage
nerve center
noncompete agreement
overall attitude
quality inventory
quarterback
retail
sole proprietorship
tact

1. Supplies used in daily business operations are called ________________________.
2. An important aspect of the salon's financial success revolves around __________ sales.
3. A satisfied client is the very best form of ____________.
4. The lifeline of the salon is ______________________.
5. When handling complaints by phone, respond with self-control, _________, and courtesy.
6. When using the telephone, you should have a pleasant voice, speak clearly, and use __________________.
7. A well-trained receptionist has been referred to as the ____________ of the salon.
8. The reception area of the salon has been referred to as the _______________ of the salon.
9. When interviewing potential employees, consider their level of skill, personal grooming, communication skills, and _______________.
10. Money needed to start a new business is known as _________.
11. In a successful business, a good accountant and an accounting system are _______________.

Essential Review continued

12. Smooth business management depends on many factors, including sufficient ________________.

13. Another factor that is critical in a successful business is the delivery of ________________________.

14. If purchasing an existing salon from another individual, it is imperative for the agreement to include a ______________________.

15. In a partnership, ownership is not necessarily _________.

16. When the salon is owned by a single individual, who is most often the manager, it is known as a __________________.

17. A written description of your business as you see it today or foresee it in the next five years is known as a ______________.

18. One of the most important factors to consider when planning the success of your salon is __________.

19. ____________ is a desirable situation for practitioners who have many steady clients and do not have to rely on the salon to stay busy.

20. Included among the many obligations of a booth renter are keeping records, paying taxes, maintaining inventory, advertising, and carrying adequate malpractice and _________ insurance.

Essential Discoveries and Accomplishments

In the space below, jot some notes about what concepts of this chapter were hardest for you to understand or remember. Imagine finding yourself suddenly in the role of "teacher" and consider what you would tell your "students" about these concepts. Share your Essential Discoveries with some of the other students in your class and ask if they are helpful to them. You may want to revise your discoveries based on good ideas shared by your peers.

Discoveries:

List at least three things you have accomplished since your last entry that relate to your career goals.

Accomplishments: